Generalism in Clinical Practice and Education

Generalism in Clinical Practice and Education

Edited by
Sophie Park and Kay Leedham-Green

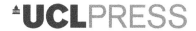

First published in 2024 by
UCL Press
University College London
Gower Street
London WC1E 6BT

Available to download free: www.uclpress.co.uk

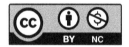
ISBN: 978-1-80008-544-2 (Hbk.)
ISBN: 978-1-80008-543-5 (Pbk.)
ISBN: 978-1-80008-542-8 (PDF)
ISBN: 978-1-80008-545-9 (epub)
DOI: https://doi.org/10.14324/111.9781800085428

We dedicate this book to three wonderful people: Derek Frankland, Sophie's father, who was committed to social equity and education throughout his life, Elisabeth Leedham-Green, Kay's aunt 'Baj', historian, archivist and expert on 'the sharing of knowledge', and to Alistair Park for his patient support on the production of this book.

Contents

List of figures

List of tables

List of contributors

Henry Aughterson is a health researcher, final-year medical student at UCL and aspiring GP. He is now completing medical school, after having just taken three years out to complete a PhD at UCL exploring the mental health benefits of 'social prescribing', using ethnographic and other qualitative methods.

Alice Clack is a consultant obstetrician and gynaecologist currently working as a fellow with the Centre for Sustainable Healthcare in their sustainability in quality improvement education team. She has a background working in clinical education and quality improvement in West Africa, and works voluntarily with Health for Extinction Rebellion.

Nicola Clarke is a GP in South London and a Fellow for the Enhancing Generalist Skills London Trailblazer. She has an interest in flourishing and wellbeing and is studying for a Master's in Medical Education with UCL.

Tanya Cohen is part of the primary care Experts by Experience Patient Group at UCL. She is a former member of the UCL Public and Patient Involvement (PPI) Advisory Group and has been an active member of the Medical Education PPI team since its inception in 2019, including PPI representation at Health Education England (HEE) meetings. Tanya has a wealth of experience as a patient and carer. She also has 25 years of professional experience as a television producer, specialising in medical and character-led observational documentaries.

Charles Coombs is completing his undergraduate medical degree at UCL. His research has focused on structural reform of general practice within the UK and internationally. He completed a summer internship with the National Institute for Health Research (NIHR) School for Primary Care Research (SPCR) in 2021 to further develop his research on micro teams. He is an Army medical bursar and will join the Royal Army Medical Corps on completing his degree.

Anya de Iongh is an occupational therapist working in Scotland, having retrained after almost a decade of working as a patient leader in the fields of self-management support, medical education and patient involvement in research and medical publishing, both locally and nationally. This included work as a self-management coach directly supporting patients, working as Patient Editor at the BMJ and in regional strategic and service development roles. She began this work following a significant illness in 2009, which had a long-standing impact throughout her twenties.

Claire Duddy is an information specialist and health researcher based at the Nuffield Department of Primary Care at the University of Oxford. Her research to date has focused on the implementation of diagnostic and screening tests in primary care settings. She has a keen interest in realist research approaches and has supported numerous realist review and evaluation projects. She is an Associate Fellow of the Higher Education Academy and co-tutor on the University of Oxford's Realist Reviews and Realist Evaluation postgraduate taught course.

Graham Easton is a GP and Professor of Clinical Communication Skills at Queen Mary University of London. His career, combining general practice, medical education and medical journalism, has inspired his special interest in how narratives influence communication. He was a senior producer and presenter in the BBC Radio Science Unit, spent several years as an editor at the BMJ, and his research at the Institute of Education explored how lecturers use narratives in medical teaching. He has written several books, including *The Appointment* – the story of a morning surgery told from inside the mind of a GP.

Jens Foell trained in Germany in rehabilitation medicine with special focus on musculoskeletal disability. He moved to the UK where he retrained as a GP. He worked in the deindustrialised areas of North West and North East England, in an inner-city practice and as an academic GP in London; he currently lives in North Wales. His research interests are the management of pain, mental health problems and social issues in community settings with a special focus on pain communication. He is active in under- and postgraduate medical education.

Nina Fudge is a Lecturer in Social Science at Queen Mary University of London. She is a THIS Institute-funded Research Fellow and a Fellow of the Higher Education Academy. With a background in social anthropology, Nina has an interest in the use of ethnographic methods for understanding health, and the systems and practices of healthcare and research. Her research interests include long-term conditions, polypharmacy, and concepts and practices of knowledge production in biomedical research.

Dame Hazel Genn is Professor of Socio-Legal Studies and Director of the UCL Centre for Access to Justice, which she founded in 2013. She is a leading empirical legal researcher and expert on access to civil justice. Her work has influenced policymakers in relation to the provision of legal aid and the social and health effects of unmet legal need. In 2016–18 she developed the activities of the Centre for Access to Justice to include a health justice partnership with a GP practice in

East London, delivering free social welfare legal services to low-income and vulnerable patients within the practice. She is currently directing a National Strategy for Health Justice Partnership, funded by The Legal Education Foundation.

John Gillies OBE is currently an Honorary Professor of General Practice in the Usher Institute and Co-director of the Global Compassion Initiative, both in the University of Edinburgh. He worked in rural Malawi in the 1980s and was a GP in rural Scotland for many years. He served as Chair of RCGP Scotland from 2010 to 2014 and was deputy director of the Scottish School of Primary Care from 2015 to 2019. He has published on rural general practice, generalism, philosophy of medicine and medical humanities.

Nigel Hart is the Associate Director for General Practice and Primary Care in the Centre for Medical Education at Queen's University Belfast. He is responsible for General Practice teaching in the Queen's University medical curriculum and also leads the General Practice Academic Research Training Scheme. His research interests include health inequalities, addressing unmet clinical need, and medical education. He practises as a general practitioner in west Belfast, Northern Ireland.

Jane Hopkins was initially employed as a Home Office Research Associate before training as a psychiatric (forensic) social worker. She maintained her interest in research throughout her 40 years as a practitioner and, on retirement in 2006, was recruited as a lay adviser to the Health and Social Care Workforce Research Unit (HSCWRU) at King's College London and has contributed to many NHS England 'task and finish' groups, working parties and committees. Since 2014, she has been the lead public contributor on a long-term, three-site study based within the Primary Care and Population Health Unit at UCL. As a registered severely sight-impaired person, Jane also acts as a freelance adviser on accessibility issues to major corporations and as a trainer for their public-facing staff.

Eleanor Hothersall is Head of MBChB at the University of Dundee, and an Honorary Consultant in Public Health in NHS Tayside, Scotland. Her interests are in widening participation in medicine, inequalities in health and education, and assessment, with a particular focus on contextual topics which are traditionally hard to assess. She has a national role in the development of the new Medical Licensing Assessment, and is Co-Chair of the Public Health Educators in Medical Schools group, which is a Special Interest Group of the Faculty of Public Health.

Emma Hyde is a diagnostic radiographer currently working as an Associate Professor at the University of Derby. Her PhD research defined informed measures of patient-centred care in diagnostic radiography. Her aim is to support both students and qualified practitioners to be as person-centred as possible. In addition to her university role, Emma is also Clinical Director of the Personalised Care Institute, which provides training that supports health and care staff to deliver personalised care. She is also a member of the International Community of Practice for Person-Centred Practice, and is President of the UK Imaging & Oncology (UKIO) Congress 2024–5. Emma is a Fellow of the Higher Education Academy and was awarded a National Teaching Fellowship by Advance HE in 2020.

Ben Jackson is Director of Primary Care Education at Sheffield Medical School. His teaching and research focus on clinical supervision, integrated learning, and health inequities. During the COVID-19 pandemic, he co-led the national general practice undergraduate virtual learning group which developed Virtual Primary Care. His current research includes a realist evaluation of clinical supervision in general practice and the FAIRSTEPS study on actions that address inequities through primary care. He practises general practice in Conisbrough, Doncaster, UK.

Martina Kelly is a family physician and Professor of Family Medicine in Cumming School of Medicine, University of Calgary. Martina oversees family medicine teaching in the undergraduate medical program, fostering conversations on generalism across faculty, as the school launches a new curriculum centring on generalism. Martina is also co-chair of the Undergraduate Education Committee of the Canadian College of Family Physicians, which is working to promote generalism in undergraduate curricula in Canada.

John Launer is a GP, family therapist, educator and writer. He has written or edited 10 books on primary care and related topics, including *Narrative-Based Practice in Health and Social Care: Conversations Inviting Change* and *How Not To Be A Doctor, and Other Essays*. He has given presentations and run workshops around Europe, in the United States, Canada, Australia and Japan. John is president of the Association of Narrative Practice in Healthcare, an honorary associate clinical professor at UCL and a regular columnist in the BMJ.

Sadie Lawes-Wickwar is a health psychologist registered with the Health and Care Professions Council (HCPC), an Associate Fellow of the British Psychological Society (AFBPS) and a Fellow of the Higher Education Academy (FHEA). Sadie is Lecturer in Medical Education at UCL and Lead for UCL's Primary Care Medical Education Experts by Experience Group. She is a member of the national Doubleday Medical Schools Patient Partnership Collaborative. Her teaching and research focus on patient-centred community health services, health communication, the psychosocial impact of long-term conditions, patient and public involvement in medical education and behavioural medicine.

Kathleen (Kay) Leedham-Green is a senior research fellow at the Medical Education Research Unit of Imperial College London, and previously led the early years primary care curriculum at King's College London. She provides faculty development to clinical educators and has published extensively on education for sustainable healthcare, health service innovation and quality, patient and learner engagement, and preparedness for practice. She is a member of the ASPIRE Board at the Association for Medical Education Europe, on the editorial board at BMC Medical Education, and on the education and quality improvement committees at the Centre for Sustainable Healthcare, Oxford.

Rebecca Mackenzie is an academic GP trainee at King's College London, and qualified from UCL in 2020. Motivated by the positive impact of providing high-quality healthcare, she has completed numerous quality improvement (QI) qualifications, including the Institute of Healthcare Improvement's Improvement Capability Course, and NHS England's Quality, Service Improvement and Redesign College Programme. With this knowledge, she has led an award-winning student QI initiative, designed a QI training course and curriculum at UCL, received multiple QI prizes, and been a member of the Quality and Safety Committee at UCL Hospital.

Clare MacRae is a general practitioner and was awarded a Medical Research Council Clinical Research Training Fellowship in 2021. Her PhD, at the University of Edinburgh, involves using data science to better understand the interplay between health geography and multimorbidity, and exploring methodologies for measuring long-term conditions and multimorbidity using electronic health records. She works clinically as a GP (NHS Lothian) and is a Member of the Royal College of Paediatrics and Child Health and the Royal College of General Practitioners.

Kamal Mahtani is a Professor of Evidence-Based Healthcare at the Nuffield Department of Primary Care Health Sciences, University of Oxford. With a focus on translational science, Kamal specialises in the generation, synthesis and implementation of evidence into practice and policy. For over 10 years, he has been an influential teacher of evidence-based healthcare, nurturing the development of students at both undergraduate and postgraduate levels. In his role as Director of the MSc in Global Healthcare Leadership at the University of Oxford, Kamal is also shaping the next generation of healthcare leaders. Kamal remains connected to real-world healthcare delivery as a practising NHS general practitioner. This dual role enables him to bridge the gap between research and clinical practice.

Fiona McKenzie specialises in helping healthcare focus on what matters to patients, carers and the public. Living with three long-term conditions, she has a unique understanding of health promotion, healthcare delivery and transformation. With almost four decades of personal experience and over a decade working in the field, she founded the consultancy Human-Centred Health to help organisations improve the quality of care and research by collaborating with patients, carers and the public. She has been on the Editorial Board of the *Health Expectations* journal since 2018 and helped develop the ICHOM Set of Patient-Centred Outcome Measures for Overall Adult Health.

Stewart Mercer is a general practitioner and Professor of Primary Care and Multimorbidity at the University of Edinburgh, where he is also Deputy Director of the Advanced Care Research Centre, and Acting Director of the Centre for Homelessness and Inclusion Health. He was Director of the Scottish School of Primary Care from 2014 to 2020, and is a former Director of Quality at RCGP Scotland. Stewart helped to establish the GPs at the Deep End group, and remains an active member of the Scottish Deep End Steering Group. He has extensively researched multimorbidity, deprivation and general practice.

Frances Mortimer is Medical Director of the Centre for Sustainable Healthcare (CSH) in Oxford, UK, where her focus is on embedding sustainability into clinical culture and patient care. Frances has led CSH's work with clinical specialties and medical education; she first identified CSH's four principles of Sustainable Clinical Practice and developed the 'SusQI' framework for incorporating sustainability into quality improvement in healthcare. Frances studied medicine at Oxford University and at the Royal Free & UCL Medical School, graduating in 2003 before working and training for five years in the UK National Health Service.

Jane Myat has been a GP partner at the Caversham Group Practice in north central London for the last 26 years. She is the co-founder of The Listening Space, a therapeutic garden in the middle of her practice that supports a range of gardening, arts, craft, cooking and walking opportunities for patients. Jane is a council member for the College of Medicine, an ambassador for the Fathom Trust and the Patient Revolution, and a quiet leading voice in community-based healing, sometimes referred to as social prescribing.

Nitisha Nahata is a portfolio GP in London and medical educator, having completed her PGCert in Medical Education from the Royal College of Physicians/UCL and associate Fellowship from the Higher Education Academy. She has held various roles in the NHS, education and private sectors and has experience in clinical audits, presentations and quality improvement projects in these different settings. As lead for the GP Assistantship module for final-year UCL MBBS students, she introduced quality improvement in the module redesign. This further fuelled her interest in the topic and its uses in generalism.

Danielle Nimmons is a GP and Alzheimer's Society Clinical Training Fellow based at UCL. She is currently conducting a PhD exploring mental health identification and support in people living with dementia. Her interests include multimorbidity and undergraduate medical education, and she developed and continues to be a module lead for Multimorbidity, which is a module of UCL's intercalated BSc programme. She is a Fellow of the Higher Education Academy (FHEA) and was awarded UCL's prestigious Excellence in Medical Education Award 2020–21.

Emily Owen is a Research Fellow in the Department of Primary Care and Population Health at UCL. Her research focuses on disadvantaged populations, health inequalities, primary healthcare organisation and design, and realist approaches to evaluation and evidence synthesis. Her PhD comprised a series of realist evaluations of multi-component interventions with disengaged students and young people who were outside of education and employment. Since completing her PhD, Emily has been involved in several realist reviews with colleagues in the UK and Sweden.

Sophie Park is a GP in Hertfordshire and Professor of Primary Care and Clinical Education at the University of Oxford. She is honorary Professor of Primary Care and Medical Education at UCL, where she was previously Director of Undergraduate Medical Education (Community and Primary Care) and Head of Teaching for the Research Department of Primary Care and Population Health. Sophie is Chair of the International Society of Academic Primary Care (SAPC) Education Research Special Interest Group, an Executive member of the NIHR Clinical Education Research Incubator Group, and Director of the London Best Evidence in Medical Education (BEME) International Collaboration Centre (BICC). Her research uses qualitative and evidence synthesis approaches to examine delivery and organisation of generalist clinical care and learning systems. She is committed to patient partnership in her clinical and academic work, founding a primary care clinical education PPI advisory group at UCL, and focusing on patient perspectives and inclusion in methodologies within her research.

Lindsey Pope is a GP and a Professor of Medical Education at the University of Glasgow where she is the Director of Community-Based Medical Education at the Undergraduate Medical School. She is currently Co-Director of the Scottish School of Primary Care and the Specialty Adviser for General Practice to the CMO for Scotland. She is also a GMC Education Associate and an Examiner for the Royal College of GPs. She has published on educating in general practice, medical careers, doctors' wellbeing, equality, diversity and inclusion (EDI) and assessment.

Eliot Rees is a National Institute for Health and Social Care Research (NIHR) Academic Clinical Fellow in General Practice at UCL and a Lecturer in Medical Education at Keele University. He was previously a Clinical Teaching Fellow in Assessment at UCL Medical School. He currently serves on the item writing group for the Applied Knowledge Test (AKT) component of the UK Medical Licensing Assessment (MLA). He co-edited *Starting Research in Clinical Education* for Wiley-Blackwell.

Helen Reid is a GP and Clinical Senior Lecturer (Education) in Queen's University Belfast's School of Medicine, Dentistry and Biomedical Sciences, where she leads the Year 4 Medical programme, centred around primary care. She holds a medical education MPhil and PhD with expertise in critically oriented qualitative research. Current research ranges from affordances of clinical workplace learning to mental health detention processes and domestic abuse. Helen is currently an Associate Editor at *Perspectives on Medical Education* and Fellow of the Academy of Medical Educators.

Jane Riddiford co-founded *Global Generation,* a London-based environmental education charity in 2004. Her doctoral study focused on Leadership for Community Development. She is the author of *Learning to Lead Together: An Ecological and Community Approach*, published by Routledge in 2022. In 2018 Jane was first diagnosed with breast cancer which was the catalyst for co-leading a range of green social prescribing initiatives with her GP, Dr Jane Myat. In 2022 Jane returned to live in Aotearoa New Zealand and is currently leading Ruamahanga Mauri oho, a wetland and riparian forest restoration project with community involvement on family land in the South Wairarapa.

Rupal Shah is a GP trainer and Associate Dean within the Multiprofessional Faculty Development Unit (London and South East) on behalf of Health Education England, with a particular interest in generalism. She has been a partner in the same general practice in Battersea for 18 years. With Jens Foell, she is co-author of *Fighting for the Soul of General Practice: The Algorithm Will See You Now*. She has published widely in the field of medical education.

Deborah Swinglehurst is a GP in Suffolk and Professor of Primary Care at Queen Mary University of London, with an international profile as a qualitative researcher. She adopts innovative methodologies at the interfaces between medicine, social science and linguistics and publishes widely on the complexities of medical generalism. Her research is grounded in clinical practice and builds robust theoretically informed 'practice-based' evidence for clinicians and policymakers. She won the 2019 RCGP/SAPC John Fry Award for her contribution to the discipline of general practice through research and scholarship.

Sara Thompson is a GP, academic and yoga teacher with an interest in lifestyle and preventive medicine. She practises in a large urban general practice where she teaches yoga for staff, and has helped set up a craft group for patients and staff to improve wellbeing. In her academic role, Sara has designed and delivered a well-received and popular Lifestyle Medicine in Primary Care module, as well as sessions on wellbeing and preventing burnout within the medical school 'essential study skills toolkit'.

Jessica Ying-Yi Xie is an academic Foundation Doctor and UCL Medical School graduate. She has led projects in medical education and nutrition, presented her award-winning research at international level and is first author for multiple publications. Through an internship with the National Institute of Health Research, she collaborated with the UCL Primary Care team to design and implement the first Culinary Medicine course to be integrated into the core curriculum at a European medical school. She continues to advocate for nutrition education for healthcare professionals through quality improvement projects.

Foreword

John Launer

Some years ago, a GP colleague of mine arranged an admission to hospital for one of his patients and then visited her there a few days later, to see how she was getting on. He happened to arrive during a ward round and found the consultant and a group of junior doctors standing by her bed. As soon as the patient recognised him approaching, she turned to the other doctors, beamed at them and proudly announced, 'And here's my own doctor, my real doctor!'

What she said spoke volumes. It reflected the distinction that people often make between hospital specialists who deal in diseases and parts of people, and GPs who look after illnesses and whole persons. But my colleague believed – and I'm sure he was right – that it implied a far more important difference than the one between primary and secondary care. He thought it testified to a deep-seated and commonly held idea that a real doctor offers certain dimensions of care that others do not. Among other things, these include continuity of care, an understanding of biography as well as biology, an interest in people's stories and an awareness of their social context.

If he was right, his patient was paying tribute to some of the key features of what is now widely termed 'generalism'. Other features of generalism are set out in this groundbreaking and comprehensive book on the subject. They include respect, the ability to use multiple forms of knowledge, collaborative working, pragmatism and flexibility. As Sophie Park, Kay Leedham-Green and Tanya Cohen point out in their opening chapter, not every GP is a generalist but you do not have to be a GP to become a generalist either. Generalism is a stance or an attitude of mind to which every doctor should aspire.

For all sorts of reasons, the encounter that took place on the hospital ward would be far less likely to happen nowadays. We are, by common agreement, living through a crisis in medicine. The crisis is multidimensional. In many countries, it includes under-resourcing of health services, or a gross imbalance between the financing of cost-effective services in the community and hyper-specialised technological ones. It encompasses a prioritisation of the market and commodification of medical treatment over population health and workforce planning. Along with this – and with related pressures like the influence of pharmaceutical companies – there are ever-widening health inequalities between different social and ethnic groups, as well as over-exploitation of the natural resources around us. Many of us who work within medicine and health, not only in the United Kingdom but worldwide, share a general feeling that 'we cannot go on like this'.

If there is a silver lining to this cloud, it is our belief that there are remedies for this situation. Among these, the promotion of generalism as a key ingredient of any future enterprise is crucial. The different chapters of this book describe in detail and with vivid examples what needs to be done at every point in the system to infuse it with generalist values, whether these are about interactions with individual patients, cooperation in multiprofessional teams, or interventions at the organisational or political level. Different authors in this book, whether clinicians, patients or academics, cover clinical practice, education and assessment, research and quality improvement. They write too about social accountability, health justice, sustainability, wellbeing, personalised care and many other topics that now preoccupy doctors, other health professionals and the public.

Generalism will not solve all our problems, but as the different contributions to this volume all illustrate, no project to turn around the juggernaut of the medical-industrial complex is likely to succeed without it. Any doctor of the future, this book suggests, may still want to remain a specialist in their chosen field, whether this is family medicine or a subspecialty of neurosurgery. But no doctor should practise without also being capable of generalism. To be a generalist is to be a thinking and feeling human being, a citizen of one's community and a resident of this planet, before being just a doctor. Or to put it another way, it is to claim the right to call oneself a real doctor. *Generalism in Clinical Practice and Education* points the way.

Acknowledgements

Epistemic justice is at the heart of this book and the process through which it was co-produced: valuing, sharing and applying a range of different expertise and knowledge. We are profoundly grateful to patients, carers and colleagues who engaged in this journey with us: to explore, examine and extend our collective knowledge about doing generalism and being a generalist. This has involved deep critical reflexivity about how we make meaning of our professional and personal worlds and lives: exploring the collisions, overlaps and interfaces between different forms of knowledge, ways of working and being, and the systems, structures and relationships which enable these to connect and grow. Honesty, trust, vulnerability and a generous spoonful of good humour have enabled us to value and explore the troublesome and joyous spaces which exist in between the accepted certainties of our time and disciplines. This process has made visible the interconnections and humanity in what we do. Together we have interwoven collective efforts to celebrate how things are and can be done: to flourish in how we live our lives and support the lives of others. Wherever and whenever you encounter this book, we hope it provides an opportunity for you to consider your own situation and practice, helping to navigate the fragile, complex and dynamic nature of clinical care and education.

Thank you for taking time to read these pages. Gratitude to all those who have contributed to this book, providing iterative feedback and encouragement to each other throughout. Enormous thanks to Pat for her straightforward, honest and supportive editorial guidance and feedback. To John Launer and Esther de Groot for comments on earlier drafts. Thanks to our colleagues, family, friends and each other for support, kindness, patience and nourishment during the writing process. Particular thanks to Alistair for his tenacious capacity to keep us and the writing process going through to dissemination.

About this book

This book is for a broad readership: you might be a practising clinician, an educator, a clinical academic, a patient, a leader or a learner. It will support you in practical and conceptual approaches to generalist clinical encounters, education, and organisation of care. It has been co-produced by over 40 expert clinicians, patients, educators and academics from the UK, Europe, Australia and Canada. Generalism within these contexts has a rich history and an established academic knowledge base. We therefore hope that exploring generalism within these contexts will be of interest in the widest sense.

When done well, generalism has the potential to transform patient and population outcomes in ways that are equitable, sustainable and responsive to evolving patient and population health needs. Although generalism is rooted in primary care and family medicine, it can be and is enacted both individually and collaboratively within specialties and allied health professions: the knee surgeon who also attends to dietary risks; the ward nurse who coordinates a personalised discharge plan; the occupational therapist who focuses on what matters to individuals; the geriatrician who works collaboratively across multiple sectors; and the dentist who improves access for people with special care needs. We use examples from multiple contexts throughout this book; however, we are unapologetic that the majority are from a primary care perspective. Primary care clinicians see all types of patients holistically from cradle to grave and have developed ways of working, organising and learning that appear in many other professional contexts, but have been honed within this context. When we use the term 'generalist', however, this is not synonymous with general practitioner. Generalists can be people within any clinical setting or group who instinctively adjust their remit in response to patient and population needs.

This book not only contextualises the factors past and present that have shaped what generalism is today; it is future-facing, proposing possibilities for expansion and enhancement. Generalism is inherently practical and widely applicable and we hope that everyone who reads this book will be able to implement some aspects. The clinical examples throughout this book are either fictitious or shared with permission.

Part I: Core concepts

Part I contains five chapters. These aim to provide the reader with a conceptual understanding of what generalism is and why it is important. Chapter 1 introduces an overarching philosophy of practice. Chapter 2 explores how generalism can manifest as a team process across multi-professional contexts. Chapter 3 presents a critical patient perspective. Chapters 4 and 5 describe how generalist knowledge is constructed and used within clinical practice and research.

1
What is generalism and why is it important?

Sophie Park, Kay Leedham-Green and Tanya Cohen

Introduction

Generalism is an inclusive and holistic form of clinical practice that, due to its innate breadth, remains poorly defined or understood. The concept of generalism, however, is increasing in prominence as healthcare systems worldwide respond to the rising complexity of population health needs and other challenges, such as ensuring sustainable and equitable access.

One of the core strengths of generalism is its adaptability: the ability to move flexibly to accommodate particular contexts or individual patient needs. Although we provide examples of generalism in practice throughout the book, these are not intended to describe one 'right' way to do generalism. Rather, by providing you with a rich description of how a problem *might* be negotiated, we hope you will think critically about how you could use a similar approach (or not) in your own practice. Throughout the book, we emphasise the importance of critical reflexivity: the ability to question and be curious about yourself and others, and to use this to inform how and when you choose to act in particular ways. When we describe a clinical example, there is almost always more than one possible way to approach it. We invite you to consider explicitly (for example, 'thinking aloud') what influences or shapes *your* intention and preference for a particular option. How does this align or differ from the preferences of a colleague, peer or patient, and why? This process includes thinking about ways of knowing, doing, learning and organising clinical practice. Also, the value systems that inform what 'good' looks like in relation to each of these. We celebrate a multiplicity of approaches, and throughout the book share ways of moving with agility between forms of knowledge and ways of doing. This critical curiosity enables us to value not only biomedical excellence but also a wide range of other important and valuable ways of knowing; to examine their relevance to the current situation or challenge; and to select this knowledge to inform practice and ways of doing.

The Health Foundation in 2011 highlighted generalism as a way of thinking, a distinct paradigm of clinical practice (1) which is:

> at root, a way of thinking and acting as a health professional and, more than that, a way of looking at the world. It is possible to be a generalist in any specialty or profession and, equally, it is possible to work as a General Practitioner without being a true generalist. The essential quality is that the generalist sees health and ill-health in the context of people's wider lives, recognising and accepting wide variation in the way those lives are lived, and in the context of the whole person.

The work of a generalist is dynamic, scoping their focus and attention, accruing knowledge about a patient and their community over time, and using this to inform decisions about how, when and why to implement (or not) an element of healthcare at a particular moment in time. What is clear is that, when done well, generalism is beneficial for patients, clinicians and broader healthcare ecosystems. The situated, conditional and dynamic nature of generalist work, however, means that it is inherently politically and ethically challenging, creating both rewards and frustrations for patients and clinicians alike.

A reductive definition of generalism risks oversimplifying something that is innately complex; therefore, we begin by proposing an integrative philosophy of practice and then discuss how generalism might be enacted clinically through a set of guiding principles. This philosophy was co-produced with our co-authors: patients, academics and practitioners with international perspectives. It has arisen from our meetings with them and their writing. We hope it will give you a framework on which to hang your reading as you continue through the book.

A philosophy of generalism

We have constructed this philosophy as ways of being, knowing, judging and doing (Figure 1.1). These categories reflect the philosophical domains

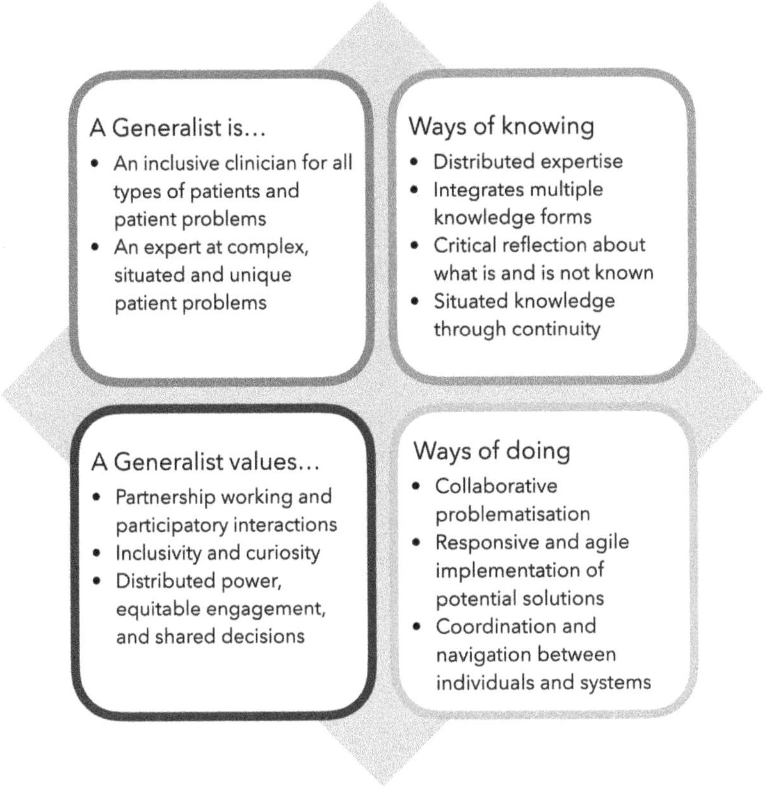

A Generalist is...
- An inclusive clinician for all types of patients and patient problems
- An expert at complex, situated and unique patient problems

Ways of knowing
- Distributed expertise
- Integrates multiple knowledge forms
- Critical reflection about what is and is not known
- Situated knowledge through continuity

A Generalist values...
- Partnership working and participatory interactions
- Inclusivity and curiosity
- Distributed power, equitable engagement, and shared decisions

Ways of doing
- Collaborative problematisation
- Responsive and agile implementation of potential solutions
- Coordination and navigation between individuals and systems

Figure 1.1 A philosophy of generalism for clinical practice. © Sophie Park and Kay Leedham-Green

of ontology, epistemology, axiology and praxis which are also discussed in relation to research practices in Chapter 4. We have created an illustrative example for each section. If you prefer starting with a tangible example rather than theory, you might wish to read the examples first.

Rather than jump straight into this philosophy of generalism, we invite you first to reflect for a moment on your own philosophy of practice. Do you identify with a particular professional group? How do you perceive that profession in relation to others, and yourself in relation to patients? What types of patients and patient problems fit within your professional remit? From what perspective and by what means do you judge the quality of the care that you provide? What do you look for when updating and researching your practice, or teaching others? How do you identify, prioritise and address patient and population health needs, including future needs? What do you do if your patient or their problem is beyond your remit? How and when do you collaborate? How does the organisation of health and social care in your context enhance or inhibit your profession, and how will your profession respond to future challenges or be shaped by future contexts?

Ways of being

Generalists are inclusive and holistic practitioners who are able to work with all types of patients and problems. They can support people at all stages of life who may have undifferentiated symptoms, minor or major illnesses, chronic conditions, and complex, situated and contextual issues. They are sustainable clinicians attending to patient health as well as disease and they work to address population health inequalities.

A generalist focuses on the person – 'What does this person need now?' – rather than on their own area of expertise or preferred approach. This may seem an obvious place to start a clinical interaction, but an expansive clinical remit has implications. Seeing health needs from the perspective of people rather than a clinician's own specialised skill set means that generalists work comfortably with symptoms and illnesses that may pass without ever coalescing into a named disease. A generalist might be the first person to diagnose a major illness, but they also treat people with everyday health needs that may not have an associated specialty, but nonetheless matter to people. Generalists see symptoms, illnesses and diseases as dynamically enmeshed with people's life circumstances: the poorly nourished baby, the teenager with a sexually transmitted disease, the arthritic carer. This is where generalists lean in and engage rather than disengage. And, because a generalist sees a person within their life context and life narrative, they attend to potential future concerns and wellbeing rather than focusing solely on today's 'presenting complaint'. This invites secondary questions within a consultation: 'Why have they come today?' 'Why has this person become unwell, and what can be done about that?' and, perhaps, 'Why might this person become unwell in the future and how can this be navigated?' or even 'What does "well" look like from this person's perspective?'

Example 1.1: Jay the trainee (identifying as a generalist)

Jay spent much of his undergraduate and early postgraduate training in urban hospitals, seeing a constantly revolving set of patients, either acutely unwell in the emergency room, admitted to the wards, or in clinics being assessed for complex procedures and treatments. Jay was always curious about the people he met and often frustrated that they had not accessed help at an earlier stage, or had underlying or additional issues addressed. Jay still remembers a young homeless person on his cardiology rotation, admitted for infective endocarditis after using an unclean needle, discharged back on to the streets after a heart valve replacement without further support. The operation itself was a success, but the impact on the person less so. This is when Jay decided to become a generalist.

Ways of knowing

If a clinician is going to work with all types of patients and all types of patient problems this requires a very special approach to knowledge. Although most generalists would call themselves 'lifelong learners' with a 'can do' attitude, they cannot know everything. Generalism therefore requires clinicians to have an awareness of, and a humble and open attitude to, not knowing. But how does a generalist know what to do, when they do *not* know? Observing a generalist in action will quickly reveal that they rely on what we term 'distributed expertise'. This means they acknowledge, construct and implement a wide range of knowledge forms as needed and work with the knowledge and expertise of others. For example, if a menopausal patient attends because their hormone replacement therapy is not working as they had hoped, a generalist might further explore the patient's expectations and experiences; consult local prescribing guidelines and spend some time looking up the benefits and side effects of alternative combinations with the patient at their side; if they feel unsure, ask a colleague with a special interest for their opinion or make a referral; or, if they are unable to meet their patient's need today, share a reliable information resource and invite them back. This approach to knowledge means that generalists are not only able to consider all types of problems, but they can accommodate a particular person's situation *and* adapt to continuously evolving therapeutic guidelines and population health needs.

Generalists adopt personalised approaches to complex problems. This requires generalists to integrate and implement 'situated knowledge' (knowledge that is unique to a person or place) with other forms of knowledge. Examples of situated knowledge include what someone's home life is like, how their situation has changed over time, or what opportunities exist for teenage parents in a local area. Situated knowledge is not written down in any textbook, and therefore takes time to build and connect. Biomedical and other forms of clinical knowledge need to be connected with situated knowledge for each to be effectively implemented. Generalists, therefore, benefit from continuity with people and with places, so that they can construct and use situated knowledge.

Ways of knowing are dependent upon how we use language or attribute meaning to particular terminology. For example, the word 'complexity' might be used by a specialist to mean an atypical or technically complicated condition or 'patient case'. In contrast, 'complexity' might be used by a generalist to mean interconnected or situational factors, making a patient situation unique or challenging to manage using monolithic or linear guidelines.

Finally, because generalists work with complex problems such as multimorbidity in addition to diseases with established guidelines, they embrace multiple knowledge forms and different types of evidence. For example, a flare-up of chronic pain might require different lenses (medical, anatomical, psychological, behavioural and/or sociological), with the final approach negotiated through curiosity, listening and relevance.

In summary, generalists reflect on what is *not* known as well as what is; they embrace distributed expertise (acknowledging and implementing the expertise and knowledge of others); they construct situated knowledge through continuity with people and places; and they integrate multiple knowledge forms, applying different lenses to complex problems.

Example 1.2: Fiona the health visitor (using distributed expertise)

Fiona originally trained as a midwife but decided to move across to health visiting as she felt she could make more of a difference to a child's start in life by seeing families longitudinally at home. She said that one of the things she learned is that you can never know the answer to every question a new parent asks, from 'Which is the best type of nappy?' to 'How can I leave my abusive partner safely?' For simple questions, she tries to help people find information and supports them in reflecting on its relevance and quality. Where she identifies a potentially serious problem, she discusses it with her team and/or refers onwards. Where there is no simple answer, she explores the problem and its context with curiosity, sharing information and resources as needed, and helps the person construct an informed plan that fits their specific situation. With these strategies for finding and using knowledge and expertise, Fiona feels able to operate safely and effectively whatever the question.

Values

The ways of being and knowing outlined above are not separate from generalist values; rather, they arise *from* their values. Focusing first and foremost on what matters to people, rather than a clinician's own field of expertise, arises through a generalist value system. This does not mean that other value systems are wrong; they are complementary. A generalist's value system not only defines their clinical approach, it also defines how they judge what 'good practice' looks like, and how they position themselves in relation to others. For example, can the quality of generalist care be adequately measured through biomedical markers of disease control? Is there a place for more complex patient-defined and patient-reported measures? Is the disease-based knowledge of a clinician more important than the knowledge that a person brings about their own body, experience and context?

Exploring what someone values, how they judge what good is, and how they position themselves in relation to others, gives clues as to their value system. We argue that generalists value things like inclusivity, curiosity, continuity, collaboration, adaptability and participation; they invite multiple perspectives when judging what 'good' is, including the perspectives of patients and communities alongside the perspectives of clinicians and academics. They position themselves *with* colleagues and patients: sharing knowledge, sharing decisions, asking for and integrating the perspectives of others.

Example 1.3: Participatory and person-centred approaches

Marta is a social worker and trainer. She is currently working with her local library service which is being converted into a flexible community space for people with complex needs. It will have a social space, a garden and a creative space in addition to the current quiet reading and lending space. Marta has been asked to support the mixed team of librarians, administrators, social workers and mental health professionals who will deliver the new service. Her goal is to ensure that it is constructed around the needs of the people who will use it. Her main challenge, she says, is working with professionals who are often entrenched advice-givers. Marta includes service users in her workshops to help the group develop curiosity and respect for others and a shared sense of purpose. Today Marta has invited representatives from a local community group for people with learning disabilities. They will work with her team to co-create a design brief and evaluation strategy for the social space together with a team leader from a neighbouring area where a similar service has already been set up.

Ways of doing

Generalism is enacted in ways that are rarely straightforward or procedural. Of course, generalists need to be familiar with national consensus guidelines and procedures, but they often need to adapt or select approaches so that they are relevant to a particular situation. Generalism is a mindful and skilled navigation of multiple points of possibility: exploring broadly, connecting diverse types and sources of knowledge, involving people in clinical reasoning and decisions, and implementing those decisions in ways that are dynamic and responsive.

We have distilled the ways of doing generalism into four overarching principles: expansive exploration, connecting knowledge, participatory processes, and adaptive implementation (Figure 1.2). These principles underpin the practices described throughout this book. Each principle can be used equally within clinical encounters, educational and academic activities, and within policy, innovation and improvement. In this chapter, we present a brief overview of how these principles might be applied within clinical practice (explored further in Part IV, Chapters 15–18) and some wider implications.

Expansive exploration

Within generalist clinical practice there is a broad spectrum of legitimate clinical attention within an encounter. Attention can be directed to, for instance: a single disease; multiple diseases; symptoms of ill

Expansive Exploration	Connecting Knowledge
• Attention to root causes, current and future needs • Attention to social and environmental determinants • Holistic needs assessments • Proactive case finding • Inductive and deductive approaches • Embracing complexity • Narrative approaches	• Integrating different types and sources of knowledge • Embracing distributed expertise • Bringing multiple lenses to complex problems • Creating spaces for dialogue • Sharing information and ideas • Valuing continuity
Participatory Processes	**Agile, Adaptive Implementation**
• Partnership approaches • Collaborative problematisation • Sharing power, knowledge and decisions • Mutually active engagement • Collaborative integrated working • Patient and public involvement • Attention to justice, dignity and equity	• Responding to changing context and needs • Personalised approaches • Practical wisdom and critical reflexivity • Continuous improvement and innovation • Working safely with unknowns • Regular review and response • Intersectoral approaches

Figure 1.2   Principles of generalism. © Sophie Park and Kay Leedham-Green

health with an absence of disease; prevention of ill health and well-being support; management of long-term conditions; the interface between health and social care; or historical and economic challenges shaping a patient's social determinants of health. Stott and Davies in 1979 examined over one hundred UK general practice consultations (2) and identified four key categories of focus: management of presenting problems, modification of help-seeking behaviours, management of continuing problems, and opportunistic health promotion. Iona Heath defines further subtle gradations of clinical focus: stress, illness, disease (possible to manage locally), and disease requiring referral to other services or teams (3). Clinicians have tended to focus their clinical attention on confirming or excluding the presence of disease. It is, she argues, legitimate to give attention to any or all of stress, illness and disease within a generalist clinical encounter, engaging at the boundaries and intersections between each. This can be explicit ('I am stressed, please help'), or implicit: a patient bringing something to a consultation as a potential disease, which becomes re-problematised within the clinical interaction as an illness, or stress, while remaining a relevant and legitimate concern for both to recognise and attend to. Part of the role of the generalist is to act as a gatekeeper, and indeed gate-opener, to specialist and community services. The efficiencies and effectiveness of a healthcare system are further amplified if generalist interactions also involve discussing the boundaries and intersections between stress, illness and disease. What needs to be classified as a disease at this point in time, and what requires a different lens? Explicitly involving people in these decisions avoids over-medicalising or over-investigating them; instead, treating them with respect and thereby minimising harms and maximising benefits. This process is fluid and dynamic and clinicians must think critically and explicitly about the value and consequences of constraining the focus of a consultation or broadening and collaboratively refocusing its scope. This broader scope of practice and the fluid and real-time negotiation of issues enable a more balanced sharing of power (both clinician and patient bring relevant elements of knowledge).

Scoping the potential focus or 'spotlight' of clinical attention is complex and value-laden and has significant implications for resource allocation. Sometimes investment in expansive exploration rather than narrowing the focus of attention can mean longer-term efficiencies: for example, signposting to community services for people experiencing social isolation, or considering trauma and/or distress rather than dismissing or overtreating idiopathic pain. Depending on the circumstances, available time and patient expectations, some wider considerations might be explicitly discussed, while others might be implicit but inform how a clinician focuses their questions or examination.

We are not suggesting that it is possible or necessary to broaden the scope at every encounter. The generalist is, however, constantly selecting *with* the patient what to focus on within an interaction: collaboratively and creatively exploring, agreeing and formulating the problem or focus *together* before seeking possible solutions or next steps. Instead of positioning the patient as bringing problems or 'presenting complaints', or even as 'being a problem' if their complaint does not feel relevant to a clinician's field of expertise, generalists collaboratively negotiate where to focus clinical attention with their patient.

Example 1.4: Kamal and Dr Jay (a generalist consultation)

Kamal has COPD and chronic knee pain following an operation a few years ago. Kamal has come to see Dr Jay about a flare-up in chronic knee pain which is keeping him up at night. Dr Jay asks Kamal about himself while he examines the joint. Kamal explains that he has retired early to care for his father who has dementia. Dr Jay asks Kamal why he thinks his pain has flared up, and what he thinks might help. Perhaps a medicines review is needed, or a behavioural approach such as walking every day and keeping a pain diary, or understanding today's pain in the context of carer fatigue and applying for respite care, or a combination of all three. Kamal explains that he hasn't been taking his painkillers as he distrusts them. He agrees that the pain isn't helped by being cooped up all day with his father. He thinks walking might help and this was suggested by his surgeon, but he can't leave his father alone. He doesn't want respite care as his dad would be too stressed, and in any case, he can't afford to go anywhere. Dr Jay explores Kamal's concerns about analgesia and deprescribes the strong painkillers his surgeon had given him. Kamal agrees to try simple analgesia before bed every day for a week to see whether that helps and to come back if it doesn't. Dr Jay describes a new service at the library which includes a dementia-friendly social space and advice service for carers. Kamal agrees to take his dad along and try it out. Dr Jay reflects and writes a note to check up on Kamal's mood the next time he visits. Dr Jay sees Kamal next at his father's care-planning appointment. Kamal's mood appears brighter. He has joined a network of carers via the library and both he and his father have had their financial and social support reviewed. His knee is still sore, but no longer wakes him at night.

Attending to what is *not* said, as well as what is, can help shape a clinician's understanding of where people locate their distress and broaden the range of acceptable solutions considered. In the example above, Kamal did not directly express distress about his role as a carer but this was held by Dr Jay as potentially relevant and he 'opened a gate' to a community service. Generalists not only attend to what people might explicitly expect from an encounter but also explore what is missing or unmet. Thus, a generalist might just as readily suggest referral or access to a resource for a patient in need (despite their not previously having articulated or acknowledged this as a problem) as discuss with a patient why an investigation might not be clinically informative.

Expansive exploration might feel like opening a Pandora's box of unsolvable problems, and proactive care might feel like more work despite longer-term efficiencies. Broadening the scope of clinical attention does not mean that the generalist must deal with or action all problems at all times. Naming something as 'a problem' can in itself provide therapeutic value or become a catalyst for change beyond the consulting room. An example might be asking a patient what they could do about a housing or relationship problem. There is extraordinary skill inherent in this process, and when done well, it can open up a range of contrasting, vivid opportunities to those actively involved. The focus shifts from 'What can I identify that I can solve?' towards a more collaborative and inclusive approach to problem identification and acknowledgement: 'What will help this patient, and can I support them with this?' This requires both clinician and patient to accept that not all identified problems might have an immediately available solution, and not all problems are solvable by the clinician or patient, but they can still discuss issues that are beyond their own scope of direct action, and use their interaction to establish what they can do together and what each can work on independently or with others (for example, multidisciplinary team, community resources, lawyer) supplementing what can be achieved within the consultation.

Participatory processes

Navigating generalism's broad clinical remit is challenging and requires the participatory engagement of patients, carers and others. Generalists work in a potentially infinite problem space and people often come with undifferentiated or diffuse symptoms. There are various hypothetic-deductive diagnostic strategies that aim to help generalists work safely within this space. John Murtagh (4) proposes systematically considering the most probable, dangerous and easily missed diagnoses, and whether the patient is trying to communicate a psychosocial problem. Norbert Donner-Banzhoff argues that including or excluding every possibility through direct questioning and hypothesis testing is unfeasible and actually unhelpful in generalist contexts: the range of potential problems is too high and the frequency of positive findings too low. He examined hundreds of consultations in the general practice setting in Germany (5) and found that there is a practical reason why generalists work more collaboratively with their patients. It is only by giving patients and carers the opportunity and encouragement to describe everything they find worrisome, changed, or both, that the generalist can hope to narrow this infinite problem space to the point where hypothesis testing becomes productive. He describes a process of inductive foraging (extended active listening) and triggered routines (for example, to characterise a symptom or check for 'red flags') which occur before a diagnosis is even considered. If hypothesis testing or triggered routines start too early in the interaction, they become counterproductive as the clinician is forced into deductive mode before the problem space is sufficiently narrowed. In generalist contexts, more participatory and patient-centred approaches result in better clinical reasoning.

This collaborative process of identification, appreciation and integration of why a patient has come can also strengthen a patient's agreement and use of the management plan and contribute to a stronger and more trusting relationship, enhancing future continuity of care. In using an explicit 'think aloud' approach to reasoning, the clinician is sharing the boundaries of their decision-making rationale, enabling the patient to be more confident about re-attending if something unexpected arises and making visible areas of dissonance which might need further attention. If there is unaddressed dissonance, this can disrupt opportunities for future care. For example, if a patient feels that a clinician offered inappropriate advice, 'missed' or 'dismissed' symptoms, it can reduce trust and confidence and a patient's willingness to seek help if symptoms persist or to agree to suggested actions in the future. Understanding which lens(es) the patient is using to make sense of their experiences, alongside critical awareness by the clinician of their own preferred or familiar lenses, can help map out a far wider range of potential sense-making opportunities and approaches (Figure 1.3).

Participatory processes are not without challenges. There are potential pitfalls in distributing power and decision-making responsibilities between clinicians, patients, carers and others. For example, if the balance is tipped heavily towards the patient's experience, the clinician may find it hard to move the conversation beyond emotional suffering. Or, if decisions are transferred completely to the patient, they may feel overwhelmed or burdened with the responsibility to make a 'good decision'. Instead, the frame and focus of clinical interactions need to remain agile, with the clinician holding a space in which both patient and clinician can explore and develop. This requires mutual

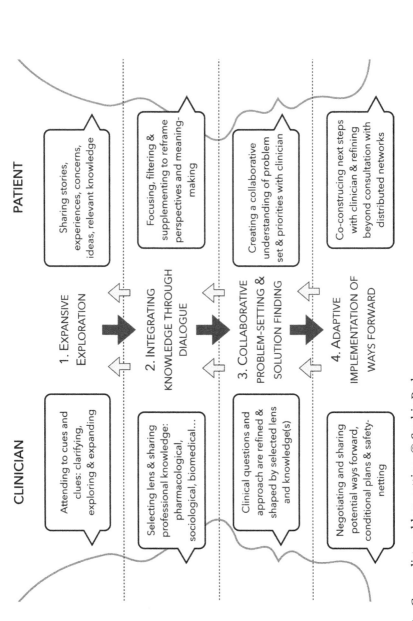

PATIENT

Sharing stories, experiences, concerns, ideas, relevant knowledge

Focusing, filtering & supplementing to reframe perspectives and meaning-making

Creating a collaborative understanding of problem set & priorities with clinician

Co-constructing next steps with clinician & refining beyond consultation with distributed networks

1. EXPANSIVE EXPLORATION

2. INTEGRATING KNOWLEDGE THROUGH DIALOGUE

3. COLLABORATIVE PROBLEM-SETTING & SOLUTION FINDING

4. ADAPTIVE IMPLEMENTATION OF WAYS FORWARD

CLINICIAN

Attending to cues and clues: clarifying, exploring & expanding

Selecting lens & sharing professional knowledge: pharmacological, sociological, biomedical...

Clinical questions and approach are refined & shaped by selected lens and knowledge(s)

Negotiating and sharing potential ways forward, conditional plans & safety-netting

Figure 1.3 Generalist problem-setting. © Sophie Park

engagement, trust and curiosity in decision-making. A generalist may need to help a patient balance short-term gains with longer-term complications. For example, a patient might benefit from a referral for insomnia therapy but want sleeping tablets. This is commonly described as the difference between needs and wants: the latter being an easy or transactional short-term 'win', but unhelpful in the context of a relationship which values continuity, trust and long-term care. When done well, sharing knowledge and responsibility can be refreshing to both patient and clinician, as both become actively engaged in the decision-making process. Tim Rapley describes how the process of sharing power, knowledge and decisions is not confined to a one-off consultation event, but a distributed continuum over time beyond the consultation (6). A patient might welcome the opportunity to pause a decision so that they can read selected information and discuss sensemaking and options with others. Similarly, a clinician might benefit from discussing a patient's unmet needs with colleagues or engaging in further reading themselves before suggesting a course of action.

Connecting knowledge

Patients and clinicians are human beings; however, both can lose sight of one or other element of the 'human' and their 'being'. Treating clinicians and patients as human beings involves an integration of lenses. The 'human' lens focuses attention on the physical body, the disease object, or the biomedical science relating to the disease pattern. The additional focus on 'being' explores the situated nature of being human: their experiences, their circumstances, their context, and their relationships with others. In Chapter 15, Graham Easton writes about the importance of storytelling within clinical interactions. In the example above, Dr Jay invites Kamal's story by simply asking him about himself. Listening to, engaging with and navigating another's story is key to human empathy. Rebecca Solnit in her book *The Faraway Nearby* describes how stories enable us to put ourselves into another's place: to put ourselves in another's story, or to tell ourselves their story (7). Enabling a space within a consultation to listen and exchange knowledge as two human beings invites a broader range of ideas and issues as relevant and/or interrelated.

Connecting disparate forms and sources of knowledge presents generalists with a problem: they are no longer focusing on a single type or set of knowledge (for example, biomedical), but balancing a range of interrelated knowledge forms. Knowledge is no longer fixed and boundaried but dynamically constructed and ever-expanding. They must connect and navigate this wider knowledge space during a clinician–patient interaction, with each participant shaping the nature of the dialogue and the potential outcomes. Part of the expertise of the generalist is in recognising which knowledge sets are relevant and where that knowledge is incomplete. Acknowledging such gaps, knowing when to pause, or how to connect with other resources and people to enhance a person's care requires humility and explicit vulnerability.

Adaptive implementation

Working with ongoing uncertainty requires adaptive approaches to the implementation of potential ways forward, including revisiting decisions if symptoms persist or change. Many people's problems never cross clear diagnostic or interventional thresholds but remain in a zone of uncertainty. Generalists apply practical wisdom, balancing when to act with when to wait and see. The threshold or 'cut-off' shaping whether or when something is medicalised, held for future review, or explored in other ways will vary, depending on how well the clinician and patient know and trust each other, and their respective experiences, concerns and preferred approaches (8). The relationship between patient and clinician becomes more important, requiring mutual trust and openness to enable an effective exchange and co-production of how to proceed.

Adaptive implementation presents challenges, particularly for relatively inert clinical systems and educational curricula. Clinical education has typically been about producing clinicians who implement evidence-informed solutions to predetermined problems. Similarly, systems and processes are often set up to constrain options to fixed guidelines. This may be entirely appropriate for a simple infection or isolated problem. Complex, real-world problems, however, seldom have a single best solution and choices may need to be revisited. Generalism is often implemented in ways that are contextual and adapted to individual situations, framed within a distributed web of knowledge production. There is creative potential arising within and from clinical encounters for combining disease-based and procedural knowledge with more complex knowledge forms about the person and their situation. The clinician no longer positions themself as all-knowing, although they are of course introducing, connecting and filtering expert knowledge; rather, they are co-producing relevant knowledge during an encounter, including inviting the expertise of others. Generalists become positioned as part of a collective community of professional and personal ways of knowing. The patient also shifts from being a passive recipient of care at a single point in time to someone participating in multiple exchanges of information, knowledge and personal experience over time.

So, through interaction and negotiation, clinicians and patients explore an expansive range of possibilities, collaboratively problem-set and prioritise, then use their collective knowledge and expertise to formulate a plan most fitting for that person at that moment in time, which may be revisited or adapted according to need.

Wider implications

Generalism has profound implications for clinical education, explored in Part II (Chapters 6 and 7). It has an exceptionally broad and dynamic knowledge base and requires learners to integrate multiple knowledge paradigms: biomedical sciences, clinical guidelines, psychological, behavioural and social sciences, communicative and procedural knowledge, and situated knowledge. The pedagogies associated with the acquisition of clearly defined 'codified' knowledge, such as anatomy and physiology, therefore need to be supplemented with approaches that stimulate criticality, curiosity, reflexivity and practical wisdom – learning from and with patients and peers. The development of situated knowledge and practical wisdom requires longitudinal connections between learners, patients, practitioners and places. Generalist knowledge requires curricula to be dynamically connected with evolving practice and research, and responsive to local patient and population health needs, rather than fixed. Assessments need to examine how learners explore expansively, work collaboratively, integrate knowledge and manage uncertainties.

Similarly, there are important implications for how services are designed and organised, explored in Part III (Chapters 8–14). Generalism as a way of working does not happen in a vacuum. A healthcare system includes many interconnected elements, such as hospital-based services, specialist services that operate in community settings, social care services, pharmacists, dentists and general practitioners. Each element relies on and contributes to the efficiency and effectiveness of the others. Generalism as a way of working requires enabling systems, processes and resources if it is to flourish within this wider health and social care ecosystem. Generalists often find themselves addressing gaps in other services – 'holding work' for people who cannot get a hip replacement, 'listening work' for people who cannot get a mental health referral, emergency antibiotics for people who cannot get a dental appointment. Generalists require a responsive functioning specialist healthcare system, just as much as specialists need generalists. Generalism needs the various sectors within a healthcare system to be coordinated so that one cost centre is not incentivised to push people as problems into a neighbouring cost centre, but instead to work collaboratively across sectors.

Generalists sometimes act as a pivot between specialist and intersectoral services, signposting and helping people navigate between them. As discussed above, generalists, particularly within primary care and emergency services, are sometimes thought of as gatekeepers to the wider healthcare system, triaging which diseases can be managed now and which require referral (9,10). We also described how gatekeeping is not merely limiting access to resources: there is also a simultaneous responsibility to act as 'gate-opener'. This is particularly important in areas of social deprivation where the generalist attends to how healthcare is accessed and distributed. Generalists balance the needs and wants of different individuals, assessing how these can be met equitably in relation to the resources and possibilities of a particular health or social care system. Generalism therefore benefits from systems that prioritise people who are vulnerable and/or frail or who have complex or enduring needs. Examples include scheduling a weekly clinic in a hostel for homeless people or a visiting system for people living with frailty, or inviting people with multimorbidity or complex conditions for regular review.

Focusing holistically on patient and population health outcomes has structural implications for how health and healthcare are organised and resourced. Ill health is driven by social and environmental factors, such as poverty, education, nutrition and housing. Sociopolitical inattention to these factors adds compound pressures to generalist services as they provide comprehensive, universal healthcare to people with undifferentiated problems. Generalism therefore requires healthcare resources to flow towards rather than away from areas of population need (to build capacity) and for population health to be prioritised, including the social, economic and environmental determinants of health (to reduce demand). Investment in ever more technical solutions to disease without addressing the determinants of health is neither efficient nor sustainable. We argue that the values that a generalist brings to their practice should be mirrored when making resource allocation decisions and designing services. Patients and communities should be involved as partners with academics and clinicians to co-produce service innovation and improvement ideas. Doing generalism well therefore requires investment in spaces (time and headspace as well as physical and online spaces) so that patients, carers, communities, learners, specialists, generalists, academics and practitioners can connect and learn from each other in ways that are responsive and dynamic.

Healthcare data and monitoring systems also need to be optimised for generalism. If monitoring is too loose, there is a risk of rogue or unprofessional practices; however, if systems are too tight they risk stifling the creative and adaptive approaches that generalists bring. Most health service data are collected for single-hypothesis observational research (is pathway A better than pathway B?). This mode of data use is often hard to translate into generalist practice as decisions are negotiated and contextualised rather than prescribed. We argue that generalism is supported by more complex data-driven tools (such as AI, inductive approaches and semantic technologies). Shared data can then be used to identify emerging areas of excellence; to encourage the diffusion of successful service innovations and improvement ideas; to make visible areas of care that are not working well; and to identify unmet population needs.

Example 1.5: Organising end-of-life care around people's needs

End-of-life care was not working well locally. Care homes were understaffed at weekends and there was a tendency to call an ambulance for people who were approaching end of life, rather than employ extra staff to support them. The most vulnerable people, those without families or friends to advocate for them, were most likely to be admitted. Once in hospital, people were often overtreated, hospitalised for weeks, or even admitted to intensive care. Step-down care was also difficult as the care homes sometimes refused to take people back if they were unstable. After reading a particularly painful account of end-of-life care that had been flagged on Care Opinion (an open data feedback platform), the local clinical commissioning group decided to set up an integrated system that was centred around the needs of people rather than service needs. Patients and families were consulted about their preferences and needs, the care homes had training and support to provide high-quality end-of-life care, and community advocates were employed for the most vulnerable. The service was resourced through the cost savings associated with fewer hospitalisations. The service was positively evaluated by patients and families and was less resource-intensive overall. After sharing the evaluation at a regional meeting, it was adopted or adapted by neighbouring areas.

Conclusion

Knowledge changes all the time and people and contexts are constantly evolving and developing. Personalised approaches to care require a shift in the organisations and systems which govern, prioritise and support particular approaches to knowledge creation and use. We have made significant steps over the last century towards a more balanced and inclusive acceptance of approaches to science and practice; however, many of our established clinical and education systems and institutions remain focused exclusively on biomedical and disease-based knowledge.

Generalist practice is an exciting space, constantly operating at the interface between different sets of knowledge, and boundaries between what is and is not known. This might be the intersection between a biomedical and experiential lens to make sense of an interaction, or acknowledging the interfaces between stress, illness and disease in formulating a problem-set and plan, or acknowledging the limits of one form of knowledge or indeed 'not knowing'. Through critical reflexivity clinicians can safely create an inclusive and expansive approach to clinical practice: one that embraces a range of knowledge forms and ways of knowing; recognises the value of relational expertise in supporting knowledge deduction and induction; is able to interconnect forms of knowledge; and is able to apply and implement this in a meaningful way in the individual context and situation of a particular patient at one moment in time. As you continue through this book, we hope this philosophy will help you to recognise and articulate generalist approaches, to engage in new ways of reasoning and thinking, and even when a suitable option appears unavailable, to feel confident to negotiate an adaptive and responsive way forward.

References

1. Finlay I, Cayton H, Dixon A, Freeman G, Haslam D, Hollins S, et al. Guiding Patients Through Complexity: Modern medical generalism. Report of an independent commission for the Royal College of General Practitioners and the Health Foundation. 2011. Available from: www.health.org.uk/publications/guiding-patients-through-complexity-modern-medical-generalism (accessed 2 May 2023).
2. Stott N, Davis R. The exceptional potential in each primary care consultation. *J R Coll Gen Pract*. 1979;29(201):201–5.
3. Heath I. Divided we fail. *Clin Med*. 2011;11(6):576.
4. Murtagh J. Common problems: a safe diagnostic strategy. *Aust Fam Physician*. 1990;19(5):733–4.
5. Donner-Banzhoff N. Solving the diagnostic challenge: a patient-centered approach. *Ann Fam Med*. 2018;16(4):353–8.
6. Rapley T. Distributed decision making: the anatomy of decisions-in-action. *Sociol Health Illn*. 2008;30(3):429–44.

7. Solnit R. *The Faraway Nearby*. Granta Publications; 2013. Available from: https://books. google.co.uk/books?id=UnRgkYpxFiMC (accessed 18 February 2024).

8. Michiels-Corsten M, Bösner S, Donner-Banzhoff N. Individual utilisation thresholds and exploring how GPs' knowledge of their patients affects diagnosis: A qualitative study in primary care. *Br J Gen Pract*. 2017;67(658):e361–9.

9. Starfield B, Shi L, Macinko J. Contribution of primary care to health systems and health. *Milbank Q*. 2005;83(3):457–502.

10. Park S, Abrams R. Alma-Ata 40th birthday celebrations and the Astana Declaration on Primary Health Care 2018. *Br J Gen Pract*. 2019;69(682):220.

2
Generalism across disciplines
Martina Kelly, Rupal Shah, Nicola Clarke and Jens Foell

Introduction

Conflicting conceptions of truth are not new, nor are the benefits of mutual respect and collaboration. The parable of the blind men and the elephant is shared across many cultures. A group of blind men meet an elephant – an animal they have not encountered before. To describe the elephant to other members of the group, each man reaches out and feels a different part of the elephant – the fan-like ear, the spear-like tusk, the tree-trunk-like leg and so on. Each then describes the elephant based on their experience. Each account is different. They cannot agree on a unified account of the elephant, each making 'truth-claims' as absolute, ignoring other people's limited accounts. In some accounts, conflicts arise as the blind men discredit each other's contributions. In others, they start listening to each other, to appreciate the full elephant.

While interpretations of this story are manifold, in this chapter, we use the parable to explore the notion of 'generalism across disciplines' – work that can be collaborative but is often contested and rooted in disciplinary identity – ways of knowing, doing and being. In a way, the idea of 'generalism across disciplines' is an oxymoron – how can disciplines defined by their specialty knowledge 'think and act' in generalist ways? Thus a challenge is posed. How do we collaborate across disciplines to realise generalism while respecting disciplinary ways of knowing and being, to avoid conflict, territorial tussles and 'turf' wars?

In this chapter, building on ideas from Chapter 1, we invite readers to critically reflect on if, how and what generalism happens in their specific discipline, to consider how aspects of generalism are enabled or inhibited by cross-disciplinary factors within their context, and to articulate strategies for how generalism could be reinforced and enhanced to benefit patient care. You may be reading this chapter as a manager of a ward or a team, or as a doctor, specialist nurse, physiotherapist or physician assistant. Questions to consider include:

- What does 'thinking and acting' as a generalist look like in your discipline? Can you think of examples from your practice?
- What facilitates 'doing generalism' in your discipline?
- Are there barriers to generalism in your discipline?
- How might disciplines work together to realise generalism in your context (a morning huddle, for example) or across different contexts (a hospital-based palliative care team providing community support)?

To facilitate reflection, we provide examples from clinical and educational literature. Many of the examples come from clinical medicine, reflecting the authors' discipline. To critically appraise these examples, we integrate ideas from social science on the structure of professional knowledge, and how these influence interactions between disciplines. However, we hope the examples used are relevant to all disciplines as often the tensions, challenges and opportunities for inter- and intra-professional work are mirrored across disciplines.

The chapter opens by exploring the nature of disciplines and the commonly used terms interprofessional and intraprofessional, often used to describe work 'across disciplines'. To elucidate the 'work' of generalism across disciplines, the concept of 'boundary work' is introduced. Boundaries provide a useful metaphor to play with possibilities of generalism across disciplines; on the one hand, boundaries can be defining, rigid or official, but boundaries are also porous, existing as liminal spaces, and can be expanded to reconceptualise taken-for-granted positions. The idea of boundaries is increasingly used in social science research to understand how professions work (or do not work) together (1,2). Before applying the concept of 'boundary work' to professional practice, we first pause to acknowledge some other 'elephants in the room', other boundaries – epistemic, jurisdictional and institutional boundaries – that need to be conceded for collaborative boundary work to flourish. To progress generalism across disciplines, some hard sociohistorical truths need to be identified and mapped. With this groundwork laid, we share examples of boundary work, and work with these ideas to consider how generalism can be enacted across disciplines in clinical practice. Finally, we conclude by thinking about how ways of doing generalism across disciplines can be advanced using 'boundary working tools' – exploring boundaries by 'knowledge brokering', and 'trading zones' – skills inherent to generalism. These approaches, we propose, could progress imaginative conversations to facilitate a thriving generalism that spans the workplace and workforce.

Section 1: Definitions and delineations – what is a 'discipline'?

Disciplines are defined by the possession of a specific domain of knowledge. Professional disciplines are characterised by the possession of a designated set of knowledge and skills, institutionalised in curriculum, ethics and a community of practice. Membership is regulated by competencies, certification and peer review. Sociological literature is rich with descriptions of how different healthcare disciplines define, regulate and defend their expertise (3–6). In general, negotiating expertise is fraught, imbued with power differentials, such that challengers often need to appeal to the discursive norms of the dominant profession (2). Professional territorial tussles are informed by differences in professional identities and core beliefs – what constitutes knowledge, safe practice, and quality in patient care. Disciplines, however, are neither 'static nor monolithic' (7) – relationships in and across disciplines evolve and flux, in response to changing knowledge, healthcare policies, public expectations and needs.

Cross-disciplinary practice: terminology

Interprofessional boundaries: refer to how professions work *across* professions – for example, medical–nursing boundary, the boundary between ophthalmologists and opticians (8), blurry boundaries in 'mental health work'.

Intraprofessional boundaries: refer to boundaries *within* occupations. Differentiation between medical specialties has a long history – for example, disparities between general practitioners and specialists. Increasingly, delineation between specialties is also contested – for example, is performing gastroscopy the remit of the gastroenterologist or the surgeon (9)? What distinguishes the work of specialist and ward nurses? Within professions, power differentials also exist between different levels of seniority which impact who gets heard, and when.

Interdisciplinary boundaries: demarcate between healthcare professionals (doctors, nurses, physiotherapists, social workers and so on) based on the discipline in which they specialise – for example, cardiology or neurology. Interdisciplinary boundaries can be either intraprofessional or interprofessional.

Section 2: 'Boundary work'

Boundary work is a term used to describe purposeful, individual and collective efforts to influence boundaries, demarcations and distinctions affecting groups (Table 2.1) (2). While initially coined to distinguish between science and 'non-science' (10), the term has since been used to explore boundaries in a range of disciplines (2). Hinrichs, for example, advocates the concept of boundaries as fundamental to researching interdisciplinarity (11). Langley, in a recent review, outlined approaches to boundary work (2). Competitive boundary work focuses on how people defend and contest boundaries, while collaborative boundary work focuses on practices to develop and sustain patterns of collaboration. The significance of the idea of boundary work arises from its role in studying the dynamics of collaboration, inclusion and exclusion that influence work practices and learning (12). Thinking about boundaries places an analytical focus on hierarchies, social structures, knowledge and knowledge production (13). Working across disciplines is not merely about acquiring new areas of responsibility but also about recognising and finding ways to negotiate dynamics of resistance. Boundaries 'can be crossed, confused, consolidated and collapsed – they can also be reconceived, redesigned or replaced' (14). Strategies of boundary work – crossing, reasserting, replacing, reframing and expanding – have relevance to help us consider how to progress generalism in cross-disciplinary contexts such as healthcare. The notion is also of relevance to generalism, as inherently generalism is boundary work; it works at the interface of illness and health, person and population (15).

A small caveat before progressing: first, to recognise that not all boundaries are negative – they can be necessary to accomplish collaborative work. Also, interdisciplinarity is not always better than disciplinarity, nor are all disciplines 'silos' – in fact, Albert and colleagues show that cross-disciplinary communication is well-established in some communities (16).

Elephants in the room: epistemic and jurisdictional boundaries

The challenge of conceptualising 'generalism across disciplines' is further reinforced by pervasive dyadic models of specialism and generalism, often reported as competitive, defined by knowledge expertise (training) or locale of work (primary, secondary, tertiary care). Take, for example, some titles from the literature: 'A comparison of outcomes resulting from generalist versus specialist care for a single discrete medical condition', 'A comparison of the management of venous leg ulceration by specialist and generalist community nurses: a judgment analysis', or 'Centralized or decentralized perinatal surgical care for rural women: a realist review

Table 2.1 Types of boundary work, with examples from health literature (based on Langley, 2019)

Type of boundary work	Purpose	Practices	Examples from health literature
Competitive	Boundaries used to protect territory and exclude others	Defending Contesting Creating Blurring	(17): examined how nurse managers influenced boundaries between doctors, nurses and assistant roles in England, as a response to government policy promoting role flexibility. (18): studied how nurses and healthcare assistants advance their occupational status. Low-status groups focused on similarities and high-status group on distinctions (see p.30).
Collaborative	Boundaries realigned to enable collaboration	Negotiating Downplaying Blurring	(5): compared how doctors and nurses in different hospital wards negotiated everyday work, identifying 3 approaches – separating, replacing and intersecting. This study shows the complex interplay between disciplines and context (see p.37). (19): ethnographic study of various health professionals implementing a new clinical pathway, by downplaying boundaries, as 'we', when patients are the focus. This study shows how boundary work can be facilitated by identifying a 'boundary object', in this example, patients, as the focus for work.

of the evidence on safety'. While the conclusions of these studies often advocate for collaborative boundary work, the unintentional messaging of this research perpetuates dualistic thinking to legitimise power differentials between disciplinary groups. Let's consider what we can learn from social science to help us understand this some more.

Epistemic boundaries and hierarchies of knowing

Epistemic boundaries are boundaries based on knowledge claims. Let's take an example from medicine. The term 'professional dominance', for example, harks back to the 1970s (3). The medical profession was dominant in the division of labour, in which other professions were obliged to work under 'medical orders' or 'supervision', gatekeeping access to care, testing and treatment (interprofessional boundaries). While much has changed since the 1970s, 'knowledge-gatekeeping' hierarchies continue to permeate interdisciplinary boundary work, often embedded in biomedical expertise and technological competencies held as 'gold standards' of evidence-based medicine. Expertise is also hierarchical, for example, expressed in vertical rank ordering – for example, junior doctor, senior nurse, terms such as 'sub-specialist' and 'allied health professional'. Within professions 'knowledge elites', such as those involved in academic research or devising clinical standards, maintain professional control to establish, advance and communicate knowledge of a given profession (intraprofessional boundaries) (4,17).

In contrast, generalism has struggled to find its place as a foundational element of knowing. Generalism has often been described in clinical literature as an absence – for example, lack of further training. Generalists from across disciplines have often been 'lumped together' in US studies, with little acknowledgement of differing disciplinary training – for example, internal medicine, general paediatrics or family medicine. In other contexts, 'generalists' refers to, for example, community workers or ward nurses, contrasting with specialist nurse practitioners or professionals with focused areas of practice in physiotherapy or pharmacy. Language also plays an important role, where 'generalist' knowledge is claimed as 'specialist' (18). Furthermore, as outlined in Chapter 1, generalist epistemology is often more distributed and participatory, to reflect horizontal decision-making, where different forms of 'knowing' are variably considered in relation to the presenting problem. Key to the craft of generalism is the ability to: (1) recognise salient information, sometimes described as 'inductive foraging' (19); (2) prioritise, sort, rank what is most important; and (3) personalise care, moving statistical generalities of evidence-based medicine to the nitty-gritty of this person or family, in this context, at this time and moment (15).

Collaborative boundary work values both vertical and horizontal ways of knowing. Well-characterised disease-centred models of care advance scientific discovery, new technologies and treatments. Horizontal 'ways of knowing' are well-suited to multifactorial, complex and unexplained problems. Recognising, prioritising and personalising care values variability, rather than trying to remove it as a confounder or source of bias.

Jurisdictional boundaries

Historically, 'the physician and surgeon retained the hospital, but the general practitioner retained the patient' (20). Inter- and intraprofessional work was clearly demarcated by context. Contemporary health policy and support for the development of multidisciplinary teams eschew that dichotomy – and even propose new disciplines and new roles. For example, the USA, Canada and Japan increasingly train 'hospitalists' as physicians, often trained in family medicine, but who work primarily in hospitals. General Practitioners with an Extended Role (GPwER) comprise a variable workforce in diverse settings in the UK. Nurse practitioners and physician assistants are increasingly common in hospital and community settings. In the UK, policy statements such as 'HR in the NHS Plan: More Staff Working Differently' (21) or the recent NHS Long Term Workforce Plan (22) support and envision new models of working, 'improving productivity by working and training in different ways, building broader teams with flexible skills' and more 'flexible deployment'. In Canada, the 'Patient Medical Home Model' (Example 2.1) proposes a one-stop shop, available to patients at the community level, with accessibility to team-based models of care that seamlessly cross interdisciplinary boundaries (50). This simplistic, almost evangelical aspiration to promote knowledge sharing and mitigate boundaries fails to acknowledge a wide evidence base in clinical, sociological and organisational literature that highlights the boundary work required to facilitate this work (6,23–26). This literature has evolved since Friedson's work in the 1980s, moving away from an over-deterministic model of medical dominance, to recognise the 'delicate ordering of healthcare work' (27). Jurisdictions may not be self-evident in the swampy lowlands of clinical practice but are actively negotiated and claimed in day-to-day interactions. This move is acknowledged through terms such as 'negotiated order', or 'negotiated context' (5). This approach acknowledges that boundary work is harder for 'newer' disciplines, whose influence is constrained by the subordinate role in healthcare organisational hierarchies (28). Perhaps most striking, is that despite decades of advocacy for 'teamwork', most professions continue to learn in disciplinary silos at undergraduate and postgraduate levels (see Chapter 9 for further discussion).

Example 2.1: Reshaping generalism in Canada through the Patient's Medical Home

Many of the concepts above are embedded in the Canadian model of the 'Patient's Medical Home'. This team-based model of care embeds core principles of generalism, modelled across different healthcare professionals (such as nursing, social work, pharmacy, nutritionists, mental health). Teams work together to provide patient care that is accessible and local. Team compositions vary, in accordance with local needs; for example, in areas with high populations of ethnic diversity, this may include having services available in different languages that are culturally sensitive, in other areas this may involve tailoring services such as home outreach teams for elderly patients or parenting classes in newer communities.

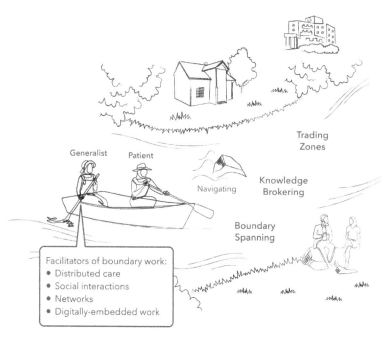

Figure 2.1   Generalist boundary work. © Sophie Park, 2024

One last elephant

One final acknowledgement when considering generalism across disciplines is that often the 'work on the ground' is not determined by or at the discretion of disciplines but imposed by institutional priorities, funding structures, policymakers and politics. Healthcare is predominantly organised around well-characterised disease categories, with outcome measures that are easy to measure and document (15). Consequently, messy, multifactorial, poorly defined problems are either unacknowledged, ignored or 'passed around' between disciplines, in an endless cycle. Most of us are well aware of these structural barriers and work to circumnavigate them, so for this chapter, while we recognise the moral distress caused and the administrative burden of these systems, we focus on what is/may be possible to individual readers within the scope of their discipline.

Section 3: Generalism across disciplines, examples of 'knowing and doing'

So, having dug into some foundational concepts, let's apply 'boundary work' across disciplines to exemplify and progress generalism in healthcare (Figure 2.1). To do this, we draw on some core ideas of generalism – generalism as 'holistic thinking' and generalism as 'adaptive expertise'.

Generalism as a way of knowing – 'connecting' knowledge across disciplines

Holistic thinking is the bedrock of generalist practice. It requires more than 'joining up all the dots' but also the ability to step back and see 'the big picture'. It also imbues a sense of 'being with' when responding to a patient presentation, where the clinician and patient work together to 'figure things out'. Holistic thinking as valuable to patient care is recognised across medicine (29), nursing (30,31), physiotherapy (32,33) and other health professions to counter reductionism and an increasingly fragmented experience of healthcare. While many models of 'holistic thinking' exist, perhaps one of the most well-known is the 'bio-psycho-social' (BPS) approach – with many 'add-ons' developed over the decades (29). This approach emphasises the integration of biological, psychological and social dimensions of care and is commonly taught in many medical schools across the world. While predominantly associated with family medicine, it is widely used in disciplines such as obstetrics and gynaecology, paediatrics, psychiatry and other professions such as dentistry and social work (29,34–38). Since its original publication in 1977, the BPS approach has evolved and is recognised as a central tenet of person-centred medicine and relationship-centred care. BPS can be used as a tool for collaborative boundary work, and as a problem-solving approach to articulate and promote holistic thinking, thereby promoting generalism as a way of thinking and acting, in and across disciplines. A word of caution, however, as terms are not always interpreted similarly across disciplines – for example, when studying how nurses and healthcare assistants manage their occupational status (Example 2.3), the author demonstrated how claims of 'ownership' vis-à-vis 'holistic thinking' were used to defend disciplinary boundaries. Nurses denied the contribution of healthcare assistants to holistic care, designating their role as 'helpers'. In contrast, healthcare assistants emphasised 'teamwork', to blur boundaries between the two groups.

Pause and reflect

- How might a BPS approach promote collaborative boundary work in your discipline? Or across disciplines?
- How can the BPS model facilitate holistic thinking that
  a) crosses generalist and specialist physician disciplines?
  b) crosses health profession disciplines?
- If running an educational session (intra- or interprofessional) how could the BPS model be used to support generalism across disciplines?

In clinical practice and education, the BPS approach is often given lip-service, used to neatly 'divide' the patient up (39), where different disciplines (inter- or intraprofessional) 'chop up' care, and therapies are selected and applied accordingly. Each discipline 'owns' a particular dimension of care – the social worker, nurse, dietician and physician 'collaborate' but in a synchronous and distributed fashion. While some could argue that this is 'multidisciplinary' teamwork – does it achieve the integration of disciplinary ways of knowing that treat the whole person? For teamwork to be effective, work in and across disciplines is required. This is often illustrated through the use of participatory processes such as partnered care, collaborative problematisation and shared decision-making, representing more horizontal approaches to care. Ironically, these approaches are often embedded through the relational continuity of team members – something rarely planned for, or accredited, but which often supports generalism as key to success in praxis.

Pause and reflect

- Based on your experience of teamwork, what barriers and facilitators exist within your workplace to hinder or support collaborative boundary work on generalism?
- How can you, as an individual, support collaborative boundary work on generalism?
- What structural changes are required to develop collaborative boundary work on generalism?

Generalism as doing – generalism adapts to context

One of the biggest challenges and strengths when discussing generalism is its variability. There is no neat definition, nor one-size-fits-all model. Its secret superpower is its adaptability. Generalism is shaped by and responds to context, which is also where generalism across disciplines is considered and interrogated. All too often, context, or healthcare settings, become contested competitive spaces of ownership, as disciplines define and defend 'who knows best' or which discipline 'owns' expertise. This is particularly prevalent in literature following a) the introduction of new technology or b) the implementation of new policies (2). In the clinical literature, this tension is also prevalent where generalists adapt skills and services to resource deficits – for example, when working with structurally vulnerable populations with limited access to care, such as cultural minorities or rural and remote communities (40,41).

However, in the spirit of thinking forward, we present two examples of collaborative boundary work which demonstrate generalism across disciplines:

1. Macro-level generalism: participatory approaches to integrate mental healthcare into an HIV programme of care in Ethiopia (Example 2.2).
2. Meso-level generalism (or not): examining doctor–nurse interaction in Italian hospital wards (Example 2.3).

Example 2.2: Collaboratively reframing mental health for integration of HIV care in Ethiopia

In this example (42,43), a group of psychiatrists from the USA and Ethiopia collaboratively worked with generalist healthcare providers to introduce mental health services for patients with HIV. Generalist clinicians in Ethiopia spanned physicians, nurses and mental health workers and worked in a range of settings, from community hospitals to outreach community work [diverse professional knowledge and contexts]. The study outlines how different disciplines, including expert patients, collaborated to introduce training and programme development tailored to the cultural context, that worked across a range of disciplines [adapting to local needs]. Specialists recognised the need to adapt mainstream diagnostic criteria, which tended to focus on single disorders, to make mental health issues more accessible to generalist clinicians [adapting to context; moving from single-disease models to working with multimorbidity], and worked [facilitated focus groups] with several stakeholders including doctors, nurses, administrators and expert patients [participatory practices, inclusion of patients as part of the team].

While programme administrators preferred standardised questionnaires to help justify funding decisions, the stigmatised nature of mental health issues made them unsuitable for community use. The team, using a participatory approach, therefore devised questions to open up discussion of mental health-related topics [from disease models to symptom clusters]. To offset single-disease models, the team devised 'clinical clusters' (in contrast to the use of DSM criteria), each mapped to some brief interventions. Idealised treatments were modified [adapting to local resources], following best evidence, to support patients – for example, offering 'pulsed' treatments over having to commit to prolonged treatment in the absence of trained staff [integrating evidence-based knowing with local knowing of what will work, for whom]. Working with stakeholder disciplines new forms were developed, using patient-based language [collaboratively creating new knowledge]. With patient input, barriers to care which included financial access to medications led to collaboration between funded HIV programmes and mental health services so patients could access services and treatments [flexible approaches to care; sharing knowledge across disciplines; mutual learning]. Knowledge exchange between services led to mental health workers learning about the diagnosis of HIV, facilitating greater access to government-funded services. Community-based approaches such as empathic interaction and cognitive reframing were acknowledged and integrated into the programme [adapting to local team strengths and approaches].

The study highlights the thoughtfulness and time it takes to work across disciplines, including a recognition of how specialist and generalist knowledge can be integrated and adapted to resource availability. The study also showcases how commitment from different stakeholders – from government, administration, clinicians and patients – supported engagement with the project for patient benefit.

Example 2.3: Separating, replacing, intersecting: the influence of context on the construction of the medical–nursing boundary

In this ethnographic study (5), interactions between nurses and physicians in a hospital were examined in three wards: a neurology ward, a surgical ward and an intensive care unit (ICU). While the focus was not on 'generalism' per se, the data shown exemplify how the principles of generalism can be leveraged across disciplinary boundaries. The author uses three 'ways of doing' to show how different levels of negotiation of work were impacted by the context. In the neurology ward, doctors and nurses worked separately; each had their own jurisdiction of knowledge and labour, and no attempts were made to cross disciplinary boundaries. In the surgical ward, as surgeons were predominantly in the operating theatre, nursing staff 'replaced' doctors on the ward, managing many day-to-day issues. Knowledge was shared, however, during ward rounds, when doctors asked for nursing input and expertise; this was reflected through the use of open-ended questions, or nurses put forward ideas and concerns, where both disciplines negotiated decision-making – for example, about the need for a referral. Generalist 'knowing' in the discipline of surgical care was acknowledged and exchanged [working together across 'ways of knowing', 'specialist' and 'holistic']. In intensive care, nurses and physicians 'intersected' to collaborate on patient care, whereas a physician quote showed 'reciprocal feedback is crucial, we need to listen carefully' [integrated care, respectful listening]. The author concludes that one of the reasons for different ways of 'doing' was related to differences between holistic and specialised ways of thinking. In the neurology ward, clinical medicine was 'specialised' and nurses' 'holistic thinking' was separated out; the doctors focused on specific symptoms ('a narrow clinical approach'), while nurses cared for the patient in their broader social context. In contrast, in ICU, the sharing of a holistic approach between doctors and nurses obscured their disciplinary boundaries, noted by the author to become an 'identity marker' that distinguished intensivists from other doctors.

Section 4: Next steps – boundaries as continually becoming

In this section, we consider 'next steps' for integrating generalism across disciplines, proposing 'thinking and doing generalism' to 'thinking and doing boundary work' as complementary and synergistic approaches to cross-disciplinary work. We draw on two ideas that originated in anthropology – 'knowledge brokering' and 'trading zones', as a set of boundary-spanning tools.

Generalism as knowledge brokering

Generalism is inherently a form of knowledge brokering – it involves crossing, interpreting and negotiating different forms of knowledge. The term 'knowledge brokering' has become prevalent in scientific literature, an activity that connects and disseminates knowledge and influences policy (44,45). The term originates in anthropology, describing someone who promoted interactions of different cultures. Later the term 'boundary spanner' was used to describe someone who spanned two social groups – it is notable that generalism itself has been described as 'boundary-spanning' (15). Knowledge brokers connect knowledge to stakeholders by building networks and fostering opportunities between knowledge users, forming and sustaining partnerships, facilitating knowledge application and creating new knowledge. Changing epistemic culture does not happen overnight. These approaches require a 'team science' to create convergence across disciplines – for example, different disciplines may use different words for the same thing, or use the same word to mean different things (46). There may also be differences in the way each discipline measures, evaluates or values different concepts and outcomes. Across different disciplines there are opportunities for all healthcare professionals to pause, take stock and reflect on commonly used ideas or terms, to listen to each other mindfully, broker knowledge and promote trust-building. Mutual engagement, building around the patients' best interests, sharing joint enterprise and building common resources are features of communities of practice (47).

Pause and reflect

- Who, if anyone, plays or could play the role of 'knowledge broker' in your context? In some teams, working across several disciplinary 'territories', there can be a role for a specific facilitator, to act as knowledge broker. Alternatively, seeking to 'flatten' hierarchy and embrace horizontal models of care, it may be possible for multiple and conflicting logics to co-exist with creative outcomes.
- Are any core concepts assumed and are there any that could be explored or 'brokered' more thoughtfully? For example, what does 'teamwork' mean in your discipline?
- How might 'broad' ways of thinking, or participatory approaches, be integrated into team discussions or individual interactions across disciplines? For example, might different members of the team outline their disciplinary approach to patient care, each listening and responding, before planning?
- How might boundary work (blurring, negotiating, downplaying) be justified to promote sustainable practices in your team?
- What structural barriers facilitate or mitigate knowledge brokering in your context? How might these be fostered or overcome?

Generalism and 'trading zones'

Boundaries may be considered limiting and enclosing, or expansive – places to meet, connect and exchange ideas. Trading zones is a term originally used to describe how different cultures establish common ground. Trading zones afford opportunities to understand values, 'what counts' and why. Examples in clinical education could, for example, span curriculum development, assessment practices and teaching – consider, for example, inter- or intraprofessional co-teaching as opportunities to unbundle and disperse disciplinary stereotypes. Interdisciplinary work on entrustable professional activities (EPAs) – that is, EPAs that may be useful in different specialties – offers some exciting possibilities in this regard to counter fragmentation and create a collaborative health professions education (48).

Attention to 'how' trading occurs can shift the focus from structures and products to examine social relations, networks and movement across them; turning boundary work into 'do-ing' – negotiating, trading, coalescing, blurring – a lexicon of action to support cross-disciplinary engagement. Treating interdisciplinary work as a verb rather than a noun moves us beyond 'land ownership' to see the river that flows across boundaries complete with eddies, tributaries and confluences (49), generating new ideas and 'ways of seeing'. This is at the heart of generalism – seeing not just the 'map' but seeing it in its sociohistorical economic and political history, four-dimensional thinking that integrates the long view, to foreground how relational continuity across and between disciplines can create fertile ground for new ventures and adventures. Many opportunities currently exist – opportunities to move beyond physical boundaries with the advent of distributed care, increasing use of technology and digitally embedded work.

Pause and reflect

- Can you identify a generalism competency that spans disciplines?
- How might trading zones in 'virtual care' support the integration of generalism across disciplines?
- How might new technologies create novel trading zones for generalism in hospital or community contexts?

Conclusion: when elephants fight, it is the grass that suffers

From our opening parable, we know that insisting on one's interpretation of 'what is true' can lead to conflict and suffering. In the case of healthcare, it is the patient who ultimately loses out. Similarly, it is the patient who inspires and makes all of us in healthcare want to do better. Ideas such as boundary work, knowledge brokering and trading zones offer theoretical and linguistic tools to collaboratively negotiate historical structures across disciplines, inter- and intraprofessionally, while welcoming newer disciplines and building (or rebuilding) a whole-person medicine, by integrating the parts. Perhaps it is an aspirational elephant dream to envision a workplace where different disciplines can integrate generalist approaches across seemingly insurmountable boundaries, but it surely seems worth the effort.

References

1. Klein JT. Typologies of interdisciplinarity: the boundary work of definition. In: Frodeman R, editor. *The Oxford Handbook of Interdisciplinarity*. Oxford University Press; 2017.
2. Langley A, Lindberg K, Mørk BE, Nicolini D, Raviola E, Walter L. Boundary work among groups, occupations, and organizations: from cartography to process. *Academy of Management Annals*. 2019;13(2):704–36.
3. Freidson E. *Professional Dominance: The social structure of medical care*. Transaction Publishers; 1970.
4. Friedson E. The reorganization of the medical profession. *Med Care Rev*. 1985 Spring;42(1):11–35.
5. Liberati EG. Separating, replacing, intersecting: the influence of context on the construction of the medical-nursing boundary. *Social Science & Medicine*. 2017;172:135–43.
6. Martin GP, Currie G, Finn R. Reconfiguring or reproducing intra-professional boundaries? Specialist expertise, generalist knowledge and the 'modernization' of the medical workforce. *Soc Sci Med*. 2009;68(7):1191–8.
7. Klein JT. *Beyond Interdisciplinarity: Boundary work, communication, and collaboration*. Oxford University Press; 2021.
8. Stevens FCJ, Diederiks JPM, Grit F, Van Der Horst F. Exclusive, idiosyncratic and collective expertise in the interprofessional arena: the case of optometry and eye care in The Netherlands. *Sociology of Health & Illness*. 2007;29(4):481–96.
9. Zetka JR Jr. Occupational divisions of labor and their technology politics: the case of surgical scopes and gastrointestinal medicine. *Social Forces*. 2001;79(4):1495–520.
10. Gieryn TF. Boundary-work and the demarcation of science from non-science: strains and interests in professional ideologies of scientists. *American Sociological Review*. 1983;48(6):781–95.
11. Hinrichs CC. Interdisciplinarity and boundary work: challenges and opportunities for agrifood studies. *Agric Hum Values*. 2008;25(2):209–13.
12. Lindberg K, Walter L, Raviola E. Performing boundary work: the emergence of a new practice in a hybrid operating room. *Soc Sci Med*. 2017;182:81–8.
13. Heite C. Setting and crossing boundaries: professionalization of social work and social work professionalism. *Social Work and Society*. 2012;10(2).
14. Greenblatt S, Gunn G. *Redrawing the Boundaries: The transformation of English and American literary studies*. Modern Language Association of America; 1992.
15. Stange KC, Miller WL, Etz RS. The role of primary care in improving population health. *Milbank Quarterly*. 2023;101(S1):795–840.
16. Albert M, Vuolanto P, Laberge S. Re-appraising disciplines: a commentary. *Studies in Higher Education*. 2023;48(3):413–23.
17. Jones L, Fulop N. The role of professional elites in healthcare governance: exploring the work of the medical director. *Soc Sci Med*. 2021;277:113882.
18. Fins JJ. The expert-generalist: a contradiction whose time has come. *Acad Med*. 2015;90(8):1010–4.
19. Donner-Banzhoff N, Hertwig R. Inductive foraging: improving the diagnostic yield of primary care consultations. *European Journal of General Practice*. 2014;20(1):69–73.
20. Stevens R. *Medical Practice in Modern England: The impact of specialization and state medicine*. Yale University Press; 1966.
21. Great Britain. Department of Health. HR in the NHS Plan: More staff working differently, July 2002. Department of Health; 2002. Available from: https://books.google.co.uk/books?id=cWsYzQEACAAJ (accessed 21 February 2024).
22. NHS Long Term Workforce Plan. NHS England; 2023 June. Available from: https://www.england.nhs.uk/wp-content/uploads/2023/06/nhs-long-term-workforce-plan-v1.2.pdf (accessed 31 October 2023).
23. Powell AE, Davies HTO. The struggle to improve patient care in the face of professional boundaries. *Social Science & Medicine*. 2012;75(5):807–14.
24. Bucher SV, Chreim S, Langley A, Reay T. Contestation about collaboration: discursive boundary work among professions. *Organization Studies*. 2016;37(4):497–522.
25. King O, Nancarrow S, Grace S, Borthwick A. Interprofessional role boundaries in diabetes education in Australia. *Health Sociology Review*. 2019;28(2):162–76.

26. Comeau-Vallée M, Langley A. The interplay of inter- and intraprofessional boundary work in multidisciplinary teams. *Organization Studies*. 2020;41(12):1649–72.
27. Hindmarsh J, Pilnick A. The tacit order of teamwork: collaboration and embodied conduct in anesthesia. *Sociological Quarterly*. 2002;43(2):139–64.
28. Currie G, Finn R, Martin G. Accounting for the 'dark side' of new organizational forms: the case of healthcare professionals. *Human Relations*. 2008;61(4):539–64.
29. Ventres WB, Frankel RM. Personalizing the biopsychosocial approach: 'add-ons' and 'add-ins' in generalist practice. *Frontiers in Psychiatry*. 2021;12. Available from: www.frontiersin.org/articles/10.3389/fpsyt.2021.716486 (accessed 21 February 2024).
30. McEvoy L, Duffy A. Holistic practice – a concept analysis. *Nurse Education in Practice*. 2008;8(6):412–9.
31. Watson J. Holistic nursing and caring: a value-based approach. *Journal of Japan Academy of Nursing Science*. 2002;22(1):69–74.
32. Jones MA, Jensen G, Edwards I. Clinical reasoning in physiotherapy. In: Higgs J, Jones MA, Loftus S, Christensen N, editors. *Clinical Reasoning in the Health Professions*. Elsevier; 2008;245–56.
33. Morris JH. Body, person and environment: why promoting physical activity (PA) with stroke survivors requires holistic thinking. *Brain Impairment*. 2016;17(1):3–15.
34. Bedos C, Apelian N, Vergnes JN. Towards a biopsychosocial approach in dentistry: the Montreal-Toulouse Model. *Br Dent J*. 2020;228(6):465–8.
35. Edozien LC. Beyond biology: the biopsychosocial model and its application in obstetrics and gynaecology. *BJOG*. 2015;122(7):900–3.
36. Garland EL, Howard MO. Neuroplasticity, psychosocial genomics, and the biopsychosocial paradigm in the 21st century. *Health Soc Work*. 2009;34(3):191–9.
37. Novy DM, Aigner CJ. The biopsychosocial model in cancer pain. *Current Opinion in Supportive and Palliative Care*. 2014;8(2). Available from: https://journals.lww.com/co-supportiveanddpalliativecare/fulltext/2014/06000/the_biopsychosocial_model_in_cancer_pain.6.aspx (accessed 21 February 2024).
38. Tripathi A, Das A, Kar SK. Biopsychosocial model in contemporary psychiatry: current validity and future prospects. *Indian J Psychol Med*. 2019;41(6):582–5.
39. Rowe H. Biopsychosocial obstetrics and gynaecology – a perspective from Australia. *Journal of Psychosomatic Obstetrics & Gynecology*. 2016;37(1):1–5.
40. Chu C, Umanski G, Blank A, Grossberg R, Selwyn PA. HIV-infected patients and treatment outcomes: an equivalence study of community-located, primary care-based HIV treatment vs. hospital-based specialty care in the Bronx, New York. *AIDS Care*. 2010;22(12):1522–9.
41. Kornelsen J, Iglesias S, Humber N, Caron N, Grzybowski S. GP Surgeons' experiences of training in British Columbia and Alberta: a case study of enhanced skills for rural primary care providers. *Can Med Educ J*. 2012;3(1):e33–41.
42. Wissow LS, Tegegn T, Asheber K, McNabb M, Weldegebreal T, Jerene D, et al. Collaboratively reframing mental health for integration of HIV care in Ethiopia. *Health Policy and Planning*. 2015;30(6):791–803.
43. Jerene D, Biru M, Teklu A, Rehman T, Ruff A, Wissow L. Factors promoting and inhibiting sustained impact of a mental health task-shifting program for HIV providers in Ethiopia. *Glob Ment Health (Camb)*. 2017;4:e24.
44. Thompson MR, Schwartz Barcott D. The role of the nurse scientist as a knowledge broker. *Journal of Nursing Scholarship*. 2019;51(1):26–39.
45. Glegg SM, Hoens A. Role domains of knowledge brokering: a model for the health care setting. *J Neurol Phys Ther*. 2016;40(2):115–23.
46. Bach S, Kessler I, Heron P. Nursing a grievance? The role of healthcare assistants in a modernized National Health Service. *Gender, Work & Organization*. 2012;19(2):205–24.
47. Wenger E. Communities of practice: learning as a social system. *Systems thinker*. 1998;9(5):2–3.
48. Pool I, Hofstra S, van der Horst M, ten Cate O. Transdisciplinary entrustable professional activities. *Medical Teacher*. 2023;45(9):1019–24.
49. Lyon A. Interdisciplinarity: giving up territory. *College English*. 1992;54(6):681–93.
50. College of Family Physicians of Canada. A new vision of Canada: family practice – the patient's medical home. 2019. Available from: https://patientsmedicalhome.ca/vision/ (accessed 2 June 2024).

3
Patient priorities and perspectives

Anya de Iongh and Fiona McKenzie

Introduction

This chapter explores some of the perspectives and priorities of people, patients and public who receive clinical care and engage in clinical learning. Efforts to understand 'patient perspectives' often start with a patient story. To truly understand patient perspectives, we need to hear what the person is saying in the context of who they are, and what matters to them. Our chapter begins with a story of sharing our patient stories.

> ### The story of a patient's story (synthesised from personal and peer network experiences)
>
> I feel the weight of expectation as I prepare. I am expected to make people feel something, to help them connect the personal and factual. Why does it feel like my experience is valued more in this storytelling than it is in the day-to-day clinical interactions?
>
> As I enter the space, I can feel the [students] trying to guess my diagnosis. I feel a moment of guilt – these are busy people with precious space in their crammed curriculum. What can I add within the next few minutes that will stay with them through their career? Is my story enough to change behaviour, and if it isn't, is that because this stuff is hard to change, or because my story isn't 'good enough'?
>
> The trainer who invited me into their lecture covers science and theory. I can't help but feel stupid ... not clever enough to talk about the 'proper' stuff, and left with the 'soft fluffy' story stuff. At the end, a few people say it was 'inspiring' or I was 'brave'. I resist the

gut instinct to cry. It feels like, in artificially separating the storytelling from the science, they have missed the point. Others say it was thought-provoking, and I wonder what happens to those thoughts ...

I might have been able to sow a seed in the minds of those listening, but I'm also exhausted, physically and emotionally, by the process of reliving the details of the hardest days. To have been vulnerable in a room of strangers, to have hope at the insightful questions but also despair at the narrow medically minded thinking in others' questions. I may spend the next day in bed, recovering. The irony of discussing the 'future of healthcare' only to spend the following day battling through current services increases the rhetoric versus reality chasm.

Stories can introduce patient perspectives and priorities but they cannot, on their own, transform clinical education and care. They root the conversation in the real world and can concentrate the audience's mind on a key point, tapping into emotionally driven motivation. These are *potential* advantages; they are not guaranteed every time a story is told. Sometimes listening to a story can be seen as implicit permission to make decisions and refer to them as 'person-centred'.

In this way, stories are a currency, adding legitimacy, and could be considered both tokenism and virtue signalling. David Gilbert describes how the emotional labour of personal narratives can be heavy for patients, weighed down with no further meaningful opportunities to influence behaviour and the frustration of no tangible actions (1). Often a person and a life are distilled down to a single story, selected by professionals, who set the agenda and give the patient permission to talk. In distilling a life into the limited minutes of an appointment, we miss the chance to see the whole person and end up talking more about illness than health.

Defining a patient

In this chapter, the term 'patients' refers to people who have accessed health or care services. Other terms are used in different settings and countries. While highlighting the common humanity of all with a stake in healthcare, we bring particular attention to the perspectives of people who access services. We also use the first person plural, actively labelling where we speak as patients ourselves. We both, however, have other roles within healthcare.

Healthcare systems are centred around patients, but we are not a homogenous group. While patients may have use of services in common, we also have other identities, related and unrelated to our health. These lives beyond healthcare mean our perspectives, priorities and decisions will be different, shaped by different beliefs, backgrounds and communities, among other variables. It is fundamentally important that those working in health and care see patients as fully realised humans who can have the potential and capacity to make decisions. Those providing care need to see us holistically, with whole lives, not just illness, with families and communities, with communication and behavioural needs that affect individual interactions.

We are, or have been, people with the unenviable task of managing the 'work' of being a patient. The invisible work this entails has been impactfully illustrated by Tran and colleagues (2) who researched the burden of treatment. The concept of a patient is inherently individualist, yet 'no man is an island'. The journey that patients, and those close to them, tread means they interact with many different people – with a spectrum of priorities and approaches, including generalists and specialists. This ecosystem that exists around each patient might include staff, families, carers, friends and others. There is no one-size-fits-all composition of those ecosystems which grow and shrink at different stages along our journey, but we as the patient remain present. There is emerging work from Ageing Well Without Children to address how we value all these different roles equally, avoiding stigmatising those without children or non-blood next of kin (3,4). Systems often assume that there are family members who can take on the burden of care in our bubble, but with rising levels of isolation in society, we must normalise other types of ecosystems. The importance of this ecosystem is evident in those heartbreaking stories of isolation and loneliness when it is missing.

Isolation on the ward (Fiona's story)

I don't remember her arrival but her presence is one of the lingering memories of that inpatient stay. She was older, much more frail, and in urgent need of surgery. The surgeons wanted her to be a little more well before they operated. There might have been an infection, and there was a general need for nourishment and hydration. The ward staff were stretched thin and there seemed to be no one to give her the care she so clearly needed. She would ring the call bell to be helped on to the commode but help rarely came in time. Her water glass was left unfilled, her meals largely uneaten. Over my week opposite her, she was declared not well enough for surgery. Her only visitor was a social worker, who came in once, maybe twice, that week for what felt like a few minutes.

Patients in the context of the professionals around them

As described in Chapter 2, an African proverb says that, when elephants fight, it is the grass that gets trampled (5). Commonly, within systems of care, there is a clinical triad at play: patient, specialist and generalist. When what lies within the remit of a generalist or a specialist is debated and tension emerges, it is often patients who can feel trampled. Perhaps this is most evident in the significance given to clinical consultations, as either the pressured pinnacle of a year-long wait or another 20-minute slot in a busy day (6).

We also need to recognise how these relationships are impacted, particularly for generalists, when people have multiple conditions (or comorbidities). The generalist–specialist dyad implies a one-to-one ratio, whereas, in reality, a patient may have several specialists and only one generalist who needs to integrate disparate treatment plans and resolve any contradictions. The generalist needs to see the medical 'whole' of these different conditions, and also the person as a whole.

Moreover, the role of generalists is not solely fulfilled by healthcare professionals. Indeed, patients often fulfil the role of a generalist and specialist themselves in the way they self-care, self-manage and navigate symptoms, services and support. Some tasks of self-care might be seen as the patient acting as a generalist, while self-management of a specific long-term condition might reflect the patient as a specialist. Given the inevitable juggling act for patients between tasks that span generalist and specialist roles, the emerging concept of 'versatilist' becomes helpful, because it breaks down this binary distinction and introduces blended roles that reflect our lived experience of care (7).

The shape of the evidence

Some have suggested that person-centred approaches lack robust evidence (8). There remain concerns that subjective individual patient experiences cannot be extrapolated from (9). One of the main criticisms of stories is their anecdotal nature and the limitations of n=1 (10). This is justified through the universality of stories, which accounts for the heterogeneity of patients.

The scope of what constitutes evidence has narrowed due to the commonly held perception of the evidence hierarchy (11). This is further explored in Chapter 5. Even though some subtle changes have been made (12), this nuanced theory of evidence hierarchies has not yet fully translated into practice. Guidelines and funding decisions are often still oriented towards randomised controlled trials. In their paper on evidence-based medicine, Greenhalgh and colleagues reflect on the benefits of mixed-method narrative review over meta-analyses of randomised controlled trials particularly in complex or rapidly changing environments, quoting Ogilvie and colleagues' analogy of the need for dry stone walling rather than brick walls when building on mountainous terrain (13,14). Whereas bricks are the same size and shape, stones come in different sizes and shapes. This emphasis on different kinds of evidence promotes the inclusion of patient perspectives and priorities.

Throughout this chapter, we use the principles of evidence-based practice to explore the topic of patient perspectives and priorities, bringing together our own experiences and the full spectrum of evidence from patients' stories to formal research. We argue that it is the *integration* of these aspects that should underpin evidence-based practice.

This chapter explores three elements of care that we believe could be improved in generalist clinical practice and education: the intentions behind care (pseudo-person-centredness); behaviours (delving beyond 'just' communication skills); and power (of who judges if we achieve quality care, and the risks inherent with marking our own homework). Instead of exacerbating the differences between the patients, generalists and specialists, this chapter explores our shared common humanity and what matters to patients.

Intentional person-centred care

Approaches to person-centred care can be implemented for a wide variety of reasons. At the heart of these reasons is *intention*. In exploring the intentionality of person-centredness, we need to consider what we mean by person-centredness (Figure 3.1). In referring to person-centred care, instead of patient-centred care, we are not losing sight of the patients, but rather also including staff perspectives. Michael West

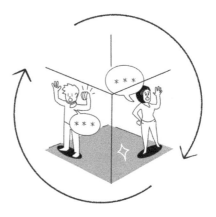

"We put patients at the centre"

Figure 3.1 Pseudo-patient-centred care. © National Voices. Drawn by Sandra Howgate, reproduced with permission

reminds us that the asset-based coaching approaches that are core to person-centred care are also considered best practices within clinical teams (15).

Simplicity and complexity

At its simplest, person-centred approaches are about human interactions, and as such, include all interactions between and amongst those providing and accessing services. Navigating the complexities of human interactions, however, requires a depth of skills, knowledge and judgement that continues to be learned through experience. Misaligned expectations, unfounded assumptions, limited time, resources and experience can all change the nature of the interaction.

The tension between this simultaneous simplicity and complexity is partly how pseudo-person-centredness can arise. If we make person-centred care too simple, by distilling it down to checklists, hashtags and buzzwords, we lose the depth of understanding required. If we make it too complex, we discourage professionals from routinely engaging in it. There is no one-size-fits-all rulebook for person-centred care. It is, instead, about applying values and principles to human interactions to help people feel seen, heard and respected. This chapter focuses on those individual conversations so that we engage more closely with patients' perspectives and priorities.

There are simplistic approaches to person-centred care. When these are done without the underpinning values, they risk losing intentionality and becoming pseudo-person-centred performative actions. We share some examples:

- Starting a clinical interaction with 'Hello, my name is …' but then barrelling on to the clinical content of the conversation without making space for the other person, continuing the conversation as you would have before. Through this, the underlying inherently lopsided power relationship is reinforced, ignoring the emphasis on shared power in a clinical encounter, as Kate Granger recognised and which motivated her to establish her campaign (16).
- Asking 'What matters to you?' without then acting on that information or using it to inform the ongoing conversation.
- Giving patients 'choice' about their care, but limiting this to a choice of treatment provider, rather than a range of interventions or a more nuanced shared decision to choose other options.

What matters to you …? (Fiona's story)

It was only day surgery but I was still scared. As the anaesthetic registrar walked me down to theatre, she suddenly said 'I forgot to ask, what matters to you?' At that moment all I could answer was 'not dying'. It wasn't why I was there, it wasn't the outcome I wanted or even the things in life that matter to me most. The answer was a product of the timing and environment, and, in that way, in that instance, it was meaningless.

Intentional person-centred approaches are based on principles and behaviours rather than a prescriptive methodology. It is worth noting that many of the system-prescribed measures for evaluating personalised care are system-centric, counting activities, rather than oriented towards patient priorities. This is perhaps one reason why we feel stuck in implementation. Don Berwick describes how we are sometimes guilty of 'hitting the target but missing the point' (17).

Person-centred care is deeply complex and judgement is required for it to feel intentional rather than performative. Specific examples using current 'buzzwords' help to illustrate this:

- **Social prescribing**
  Providing a leaflet about a community group to 'do' 'social prescribing', without consideration of what the person's goals are, how they prefer to receive information, their health literacy, or confidence to act on the information provided in the leaflet. This also ignores the significance of behaviour change and suggests a simplified understanding of 'I have said, therefore you shall do'.
- **Goal-setting**
  Setting goals *for* patients based on clinician or system priorities rather than what matters to patients, such as getting a clinical biomarker to within target in contrast to a more functional goal such as being able to play with grandchildren. By not establishing a patient's confidence to achieve the goal, we risk setting them up to fail when they perceive something as unachievable or unrealistic.
- **Self-management**
  Framing self-management as a reason for withdrawing support, penalising those patients who have developed knowledge, confidence and skills with reduced care, or encouraging it as a way to primarily reduce service utilisation rather than to improve a person's

quality of life (which might have secondary impacts on service utilisation).

- **Shared decision-making**
  Using shared decision-making to encourage less invasive options primarily to reduce service demands rather than support quality of life as the primary outcome (19); or limiting a person's choices to narrow medically defined options rather than applying the principles of Realistic Medicine which include the option of doing nothing (20).

What do you want to happen? (Fiona's story)

The consultant asked two questions: 'Why do you think you're here? What do you want to happen?' Over the following hour, this disarming simplicity let us (myself, my partner and the consultant) explore our hopes, fears and experience of living with the disease, and his clinical knowledge and experience. He talked us through treatment options, including 'do nothing', and made a recommendation based on what he had heard. He gave us time to decide what was the least worst option for us. At a difficult time, he gave us back some power and control over our circumstances.

Compassion fatigue versus work-related stress

In critiquing pseudo-person-centredness, there is an implicit assumption that intentional person-centred care is the 'right' way to deliver care. Although there are clear advantages, it is important to recognise some perceived disadvantages which include the time and resources required, and the personal demands on staff who might suffer from compassion fatigue (21). Empirical research, however, suggests that compassion fatigue is not caused by too much compassion; rather, it is an indication that a system is not taking adequate care of its staff (22). Notwithstanding time and money, more can be achieved through training and support for staff, including reflective practice, awareness, and acknowledgement of emotional labour through specific initiatives like Schwartz Rounds (23). Campaigns for more person-centred workforce initiatives such as flexible working for staff may help reduce burnout (24). As David Oliver says, it is difficult to ask staff to develop resilience without also increasing the resilience of the system within which they work (25). This multifactorial issue requires multifactorial solutions.

Value-based approaches

Some of these pseudo-person-centred actions could be seen as performative, with the impact lost. A common theme is how they are driven by service, rather than patient, needs. The *intention* is to meet service needs. So, part of pseudo-person-centred care lies in the difference between task-based and value-based approaches to care. While value-based recruitment is an excellent starting point, training post-recruitment should develop those values and equip staff or learners with the necessary behaviours. Similarly, within generalism, the role is by definition too broad to be task-focused, so a value-based approach gains additional importance.

What does a value-based approach look like? Similar to the pseudo-person-centred buzzwords listed above, 'value-based' is often used, without the depth of understanding required. The values and principles of person-centred care are well-established. From the extensive literature, there are four under-explored aspects that resonate with our own experience and we believe should be given more attention:

- **Curiosity** (26)
  Resisting the temptation to immediately give answers and taking the time to ask more, checking if there 'is something else?', showing an active interest, asking 'tell me more …', avoiding assumptions and relying on pattern recognition of 'I've seen this before …'
- **Individuality and diversity**
  Adapting to the person in front of you rather than following your own script or auto-pilot, recognising individual needs and preferences.
- **Hearing what is being said**
  Listening to understand rather than listening to respond, using what you hear to genuinely inform your care, creating the rapport and environment for the person to share what they really want to say.
- **Taking shared responsibility**
  Committing to what you say you will do, recognising the capabilities of everyone involved to take action, following up and taking a managed response, to help but not disempower: see NESTA guidance on good and bad help (27).

These distil person-centred care into something simple yet complex. They go beyond the rhetoric and semantics of dignity, and cannot be reduced to a checklist (which, we feel, is an indication itself of pseudo-person-centredness).

More than 'just' soft communication skills

Person-centred care has often been framed as a communication skill or a 'soft' skill (28,29). Studies exploring improvements in person-centred care consistently mention better communication, yet there is more to being person-centred than communicating better (30). Remaining person-centred in a clinical interaction is far more complex than asking rote-learned questions in an artificial setting with actors playing patients.

Before we unpick what is wrong with conflating person-centredness with good communication, we would like to be clear that communication does matter. In the UK in 2020–21, 13.5 per cent of reported written complaints about primary care focused on communication (31). An analysis of these complaints provides a detailed overview of how communication is linked to professionalism (32). Instead, we want to focus on what is needed to turn person-centred communication into person-centred care.

Framing person-centred care as more than 'just' soft communication skills highlights the following three assumptions and biases within healthcare and training cultures:

First, there is an assumption that clinicians will become person-centred if they are trained to be so. Although good communication skills are important, they are clearly not sufficient to ensure patient-centred care. If we frame person-centred care as a behaviour, the COM-B model (33) helps illustrate why there are recurrent themes of poor communication in patient experience surveys. The COM-B model (explored further in Chapter 17) states that a behaviour is based on motivation, capabilities and opportunities. Staff often come into healthcare with the *motivation* to be person-centred, although this may vary, and training can equip them with the *capabilities* (knowledge and skills). However, if they lack the *opportunity* to enact person-centred approaches amidst daily pressures and competing priorities, then this becomes a failure of the system, and not of training or willingness.

Secondly, where patient experiences are used to research perceptions of interactions and processes, some professionals critique or even dismiss the findings as subjective and unrelated to 'hard' outcomes. However, studies have shown that poor communication between staff, patients and their caregivers can also affect treatment outcomes (34). Moreover, subjective measures are often considered 'hard' outcomes in many forms of care, not least of all pain. Few would question the subjective relief of pain as a valid outcome of care.

Thirdly, we question the inherently dismissive way in which 'soft' non-technical skills are described in contrast to 'hard' technical skills, particularly within education and training. It is important to recognise that the way fixed diagnostic or treatment protocols are learned requires a relatively fixed educational approach, which will be different from that required for more complex person-centred behaviours. The difference should not imply a hierarchy – both are important. Indeed, person-centred skills can act as the oil to ensure our clinical tools work effectively (35). We also need to challenge the use of the word 'soft' – there is nothing soft about training for person-centred care.

We find ourselves returning to the balance of simple and complex, where good communication requires simple intentional approaches as well as complex judgements in response to individual needs. The range of situations and interactions encountered means personalised approaches become essential.

Describing person-centred behaviours

When engaging clinicians in training for person-centred care, we often need to start by rejecting the assumption of '*Oh, but we do it already*'; and one of the joys of facilitating is hearing post-session that participants can now see the difference between what they did before and what might be considered truly person-centred.

One way of distilling person-centred behaviours is the model commissioned by Health Education England in 2017 (36). This describes onion layers of enablers for person-centred approaches: starting with values; then core communication and relationship-building skills; then learning outcomes and behaviours relating to engagement, enablement and collaborative approaches to complexity; all nested within supportive organisations, systems and workforce development.

In 2020, a coalition of UK health and care charities launched an updated set of 'I Statements' (37) that aimed to outline what matters to people for health and care. These statements reflected on people's experiences of health and care services, as well as the pandemic-impacted circumstances of the time, but are relevant in thinking about what more than 'just' communication skills looks like:

1. I am listened to and what I say is acted on.
2. I make decisions that are respected, and I have rights that are protected.
3. I am given information that is relevant to me, in a way I understand.
4. I am supported to understand risks and uncertainties in my life.

5. I know how to talk to the person or team in charge of my care when I need to.
6. I know what to expect and that I am safe when I have treatment or care.
7. I am supported and kept informed while I wait for treatment or care.
8. I am not forgotten.

Some of these are fundamental to how we teach effective communication, while others feel more tangential. Some emphasise that it is not just about what happens in the interactions, but about the spaces in-between where people may feel poorly supported. To be meaningfully person-centred is to orient care around the patient; it is both the communication within individual interactions and the support and progress between interactions. This latter point is also provided through communication but it is complex, relationship-oriented communication that plays out in values, behaviour, and attitudes as much as the words spoken or written.

Developing person-centred behaviours

In asking how we learn person-centred behaviours, we need to recognise that formal teaching and training are not the only influences. There are also powerful 'informal' and 'hidden' curricula which, depending on the prevailing culture in the local service setting, might reinforce or contradict formalised training (38). The time trainees spend in formal training versus their exposure to the hidden curriculum is often skewed. Until person-centred care is fully embedded around learners, formal training sessions are likely to feel like a drop in the ocean. More subtly, other aspects of the formal curriculum might not be taught in a person-centred way, further increasing the difficulty for our colleagues in training to integrate person-centred approaches into their daily clinical practice. Training on person-centred approaches, however, can be cumulative over a career, but we need to manage our expectations of how a lifetime of professional habits can be broken in a 30-minute 'lunch and learn' session.

Not all professionals have such a gap, but we need to recognise the individual journey from where people are now to where they could be, and the time and development required for change. Within all this, there is the important involvement of patients and carers in designing, developing, contributing to, and leading training that develops these skills. We will unpick this further in the rest of this chapter.

Shared power and partnerships versus marking our own homework

This section focuses on the fundamental question of who judges whether care (or education/training) is person-centred. This is intrinsically linked to who our systems deem to have power, and who that power is shared with. We argue that a full spectrum of patient involvement is required. There is a risk of clinicians marking their own homework, whereby fellow professionals and colleagues give feedback and congratulate others on the nature of care provided, without knowing whether it felt genuinely person-centred to the recipient.

The spectrum of patient involvement

Patient feedback is necessary but not sufficient. The perspectives of patients are likely to differ from colleagues. While insights from colleagues may be helpful and learner-centred, we risk missing fundamental insights if we do not gather detailed feedback or facilitate meaningful involvement of patients in clinical practice and education.

There are a number of spectrums of involvement, including Health Canada's Public Involvement Continuum (39) and the International Association for Public Participation Spectrum (40). Elements of these have been combined to create Figure 3.2. This provides a framework for thinking about how insightful patient or carer feedback can be brought into training through genuine involvement. Collected feedback (listen) through surveys or complaints/compliments provides insight to make sense of specific issues affecting a particular service. Discussions with patients and carers, through meetings, focus groups or workshops can offer deeper clarity on themes arising from feedback surveys, and offer suggestions for improvements. In collaboration, patients and carers can be part of the team of trainers, developing and leading training. Crucially, involvement provides the opportunity for more dialogue than unidirectional feedback. The greater the opportunity for depth of insight, the greater the quality of teaching and learning opportunities.

Why shouldn't patients or carers be involved in training for person-centred care? We recognise the challenges inherent within this: how to do this well as trainers; psychological safety for participants; educational knowledge, skills and experience of patients or carers; and the time or resource cost – but we know these are not insurmountable. We all have our own lens and biases through which we see interactions; no one in

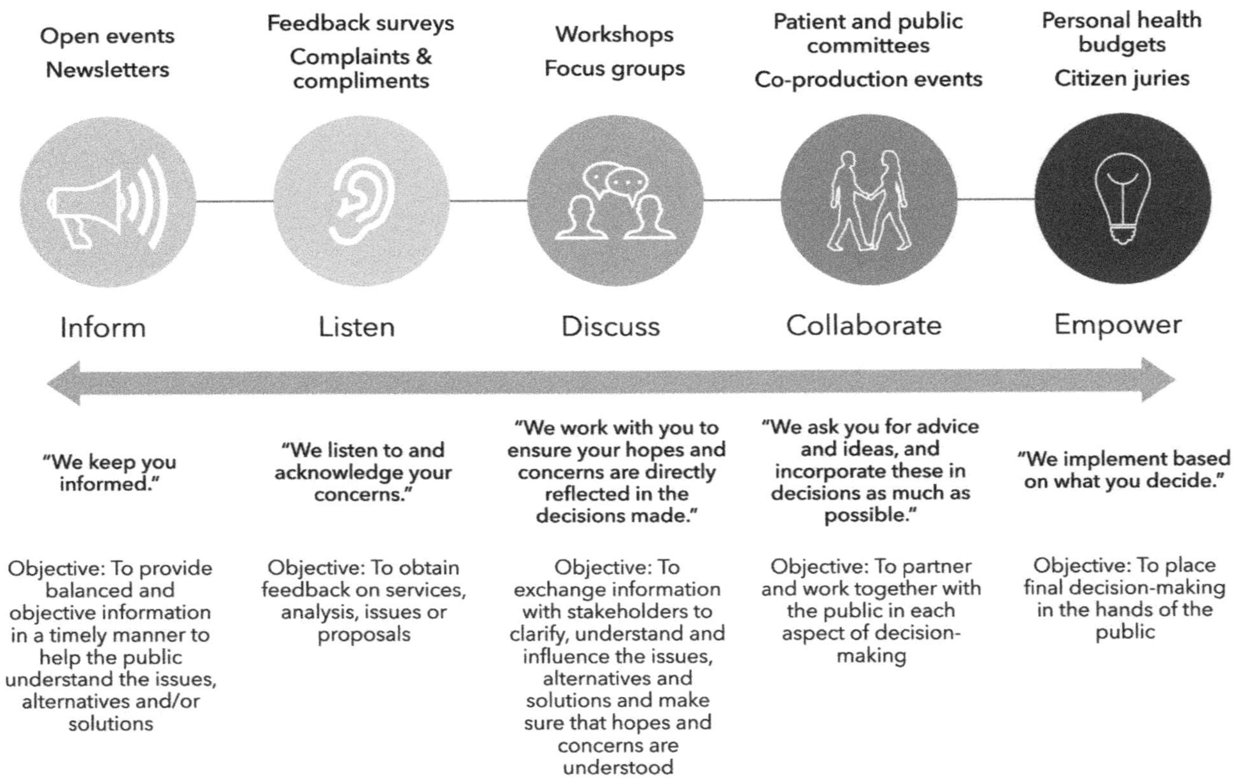

Inform

Open events
Newsletters

"We keep you informed."

Objective: To provide balanced and objective information in a timely manner to help the public understand the issues, alternatives and/or solutions

Listen

Feedback surveys
Complaints & compliments

"We listen to and acknowledge your concerns."

Objective: To obtain feedback on services, analysis, issues or proposals

Discuss

Workshops
Focus groups

"We work with you to ensure your hopes and concerns are directly reflected in the decisions made."

Objective: To exchange information with stakeholders to clarify, understand and influence the issues, alternatives and solutions and make sure that hopes and concerns are understood

Collaborate

Patient and public committees
Co-production events

"We ask you for advice and ideas, and incorporate these in decisions as much as possible."

Objective: To partner and work together with the public in each aspect of decision-making

Empower

Personal health budgets
Citizen juries

"We implement based on what you decide."

Objective: To place final decision-making in the hands of the public

Figure 3.2 Spectrum of involvement. © Fiona McKenzie. Based on elements of the Patterson Kirk Wallace Spectrum of Involvement and the International Association for Public Participation Spectrum

the triad of patient, generalist or specialist will have the universal truth, but missing one of these is like a three-legged stool losing a leg – it will fall over.

Involving patients in training for person-centred care

Patient and carer involvement in healthcare service delivery and quality improvement is well documented and the core set of principles is transferable, although related actions are context-specific (for additional discussion, see Chapter 12). The UK's Healthcare Quality Improvement Partnership (HQIP) have suggested the following seven principles of involvement: representation; inclusivity; early and continuous; transparency; clarity of purpose; cost-effectiveness; and feedback (41). David Gilbert articulates seven benefits: richer insights; potential solutions; changing relationships; individual benefits; better-quality decisions; changing practice; benefits beyond the project (42).

It is necessary to explicitly reference the impact of patients' involvement to meaningfully appraise the behaviours central to person-centred care. Patients should be the ones setting the grades when marking clinicians' work.

The involvement of patients and carers may provide richer insights through:

- The opportunity for more critical feedback;
- Greater moral weight and value for staff who are motivated to work in healthcare by patients.

If we only value encouraging or positive feedback, we may lose our ability to critique and improve. Training in a person-centred way for our colleagues means supporting growth through holistic appraisal.

In order to do this well, trainers need to be able to critically analyse communication skills. Our own experiences as humans are necessary but not sufficient. The ability to observe others' interactions and critique them is useful beyond clinical settings. Observers of interactions need to notice:

1. Elements of communication (verbal and non-verbal).
2. Specific communicative content, such as confidence-scaling, shared decision-making and shared agenda-setting.

How we train and teach for person-centred approaches/care

In order to work in a person-centred way, we need to think differently about how we train for this. Here, we share our thinking about **content**, **structure** and **approaches**.

The content

Person-centred and personalised care **content** has been well articulated in a national curriculum that was co-developed with patients from the Personalised Care Institute (44). Professional regulators in the UK such as the General Medical Council and the Health and Care Professions Council (45,46) have also stipulated person-centred requirements in the fulfilment of professional duties. For true validity, these curricula and standards need to be co-developed with patients and carers.

Much training for generalists will focus on the *what* we talk about in clinical interactions. There also needs to be the opportunity to focus on the *how*. We need to bring these two aspects together, to practise person-centred behaviours in conversations about referrals, prescriptions and symptoms. In the context of current developments in healthcare, the ability to master these skills in virtual consultations is essential, so any training should include practice in this (47). Furthermore, the clinical content and resources themselves can benefit from patient involvement, as evidenced in the BMJ Education series (48).

The structure

The content informs the **structure,** needing to reflect both the importance of person-centred approaches and its integration within all other aspects of clinical education. As in this book, it warrants its own chapter, while also being a thread woven throughout. The established practice of having person-centred approaches as a separate module might be part of the issue – compartmentalisation is necessary to some degree, but can one do quality improvement without underpinning core behaviours to build relationships and develop projects, for example? Being a partner in a general practice surgery or service manager requires all of this as well, so its relevance is not limited to clinical training but concerns any professional development. The structure of training should allow for:

- Time for learners to critically reflect before, during and after the training session, to develop the depth of learning required.
- Practice in day-to-day working life, essentially with the opportunity to follow up on the experience to further develop the skills.
- Sufficient intensity to keep the skills at the forefront of learners' minds when back in clinical practice between sessions, but spread out enough to allow sufficient breadth of experiences and opportunities to put the skills into practice.
- Going beyond 'classroom' experiences, to include initiatives such as paired mentorship across a joint shared learning environment (49).
- Including patients beyond clinical topics – for example, in debates around system issues of consumerism, access and choice to provide nuanced perspectives.
- Meaningful reflection on stories, using questions like:
  ○ When was the last time you heard a patient story in a training session?
  ○ How did it make you feel?
  ○ What difference did it make to your practice?
  ○ What could be done differently in training to maximise the potential of a patient story?

The approaches

The **approaches** we use need to reflect that behaviours are more than just transactional tasks – we need to give people time and opportunities in a value-based environment. This list is not exhaustive, but provides some examples:

- Teaching through modelling behaviours as facilitators, avoiding lecturing-style hierarchical dynamics, and building on what experiences and knowledge trainees might already have, both professionally and personally.

- Varied dynamics with different groups in the room (including patients and carers) to explore interactions and reflect one-to-one, and in pairs or groups.
- Observations, to provide specific feedback, when the observers have the skills and confidence to spot and articulate best practice and areas for improvement. The value of patients as observers in training settings is also significant.
- A flipped classroom, when time together is limited, so used for structured or facilitated reflection and discussion rather than delivery of information. This shift towards a more coaching approach mirrors person-centred approaches.
- Role play, as a way for facilitators/trainers to objectively analyse where people are at, and to create evidence to develop insight into practice. We recognise that role play can feel uncomfortable and unrealistic (50), and the clinical aspects of scenarios can distract but these approaches still serve a purpose within teaching.
- To develop role play, real play can be used, when participants use examples from their own lives, so they experience first-hand the benefits of this approach as often used when teaching coaching (51). One advantage is that it removes the medical context, orientating the conversation towards more of a human than clinical focus.
- Listen first. One way to reflect on how much this has been achieved is to think of the balance of who did the most talking in the conversation, and in particular how that balance played out at the start. How much do you think you let a patient talk before asking your own questions? Would you be surprised to hear that, on average, patients are interrupted within 11 seconds of their stories (52)? And why are you surprised? Is it because your practice feels very different from that? Do your patients 'feel' that difference?

To summarise, we need to train our colleagues to manage themselves as human beings interacting with other human beings, and not to lose that perspective when managing the clinical demands of being a generalist during interactions.

Conclusion

Simplified, this chapter comes down to the art of healthcare. Many other aspects of professional training predominantly consider the science. Once integrated, the art and science can interweave to create opportunities that are maximally focused and relevant to a person at that point in time. The art of healthcare is challenging, because of its subjectivity in contrast to the perceived objectivity of the science. However these challenges manifest, we should embrace this art of healthcare, in all its simplicity and complexity. This does, however, highlight an important difference in the way we train, and the learning preferences of our colleagues will naturally be suited to one way more than the other. Generally, because of the science-dominated approach, colleagues' learning preferences might often feel better suited to the science than the arts approach, so additional consideration should be given to supporting a new way of learning and knowing.

However important and well-done clinical practice and education are, we should recognise that behaviours take time to change, and it is the accumulation of training and experiences throughout a career that creates a clinician. How much feedback, in addition to other drivers, is needed to change a professional's behaviour? Although it might be the opening line of a TED talk, one bit of feedback is rarely pivotal to clinical or professional behaviours.

Person-centred care emphasises the perspective and role of people. Through their insights, stories, surveys, interactions and involvement, we have both lightbulb moments and ongoing opportunities for learning. As important as those lightbulb moments are, it is as much about what is slowly evolving. To sustain our motivation as educators, we need to be realistic. While we are turning on a lightbulb, there are multiple other circuits in professionals' hard-wiring that we can subtly influence. In modelling the principles of person-centred care, we also recognise that, as authors of this chapter, we do not have all the answers, but hope our approach to asking questions can help professionals generate their own solutions and answers with the people and communities they work with.

Further reading

From individuals

David Gilbert, *The Patient Revolution: How We Can Heal the Healthcare System* (Jessica Kingsley Publishers, 2019)

Havi Carell, *Illness: The Cry of the Flesh* (Routledge, 2018)

John Oldham (patient representative) What do patients want? Generalists versus specialists and the importance of continuity www.ncbi.nlm.nih.gov/pmc/articles/PMC6465842/

The Patient Patient blog (http://thepatientpatient2011.blogspot.com/)

My Heart Sisters https://myheartsisters.org/

Which me am I today? https://whichmeamitoday.wordpress.com/

From organisations

What Your Patient is Thinking series (BMJ)
National Voices
Patient Perspectives, BMJ Opinion series https://blogs.bmj.com/bmj/category/patient-perspectives/
The Richmond Group
Care Opinion
Schwartz Rounds
Point of Care Foundation
Personalised Care Institute
Peer Leadership Academy – NHS England
Personalised Care Group at NHS England and NHS Improvement
Alliance Scotland

References

1. Gilbert D. Paying the Price: The emotional labour of patient leadership. Future patient – musings on patient-led healthcare. 2015. Available from: https://futurepatientblog.wordpress.com/2015/04/26/paying-the-price-the-emotional-labour-of-patient-leadership/ (accessed 16 June 2023).
2. Tran VT, Barnes C, Montori VM, Falissard B, Ravaud P. Taxonomy of the burden of treatment: a multi-country web-based qualitative study of patients with chronic conditions. *BMC Med*. 2015;13(1):115.
3. Awwoc. Ageing | Ageing Well Without Children (AWWOC). Available from: www.awwoc.org (accessed 14 June 2023).
4. Ageing Without Children [@AWOCUK]. Important thread & discussion re #Ageing WithoutChildren & many of issues raised by #AWOC local groups & our website http://awoc.org.uk Also toolkit commissioned by @NCFCareForum on working with people #AWOC https://awwoc.org join the discussion! #MoreThanYouThink https://t.co/yO2FyuKuOY. Twitter. 2022. Available from: https://twitter.com/AWOCUK/status/1552560866058555392 (accessed 16 June 2023).
5. Speake J. When elephants fight, it is the grass that suffers. *The Oxford Dictionary of Proverbs*. Oxford University Press; 2015.
6. de Iongh A. Appointment day – the tip of an iceberg. *BMJ*. 2018;360:k430.
7. Gilburt H. Supporting integration through new roles and working across boundaries. The King's Fund; 2016. Available from: www.kingsfund.org.uk/sites/default/files/field/field_publication_file/Supporting_integration_web.pdf (accessed 29 February 2024).
8. Olsson LE, Jakobsson Ung E, Swedberg K, Ekman I. Efficacy of person-centred care as an intervention in controlled trials – a systematic review. *J Clin Nurs*. 2013;22(3–4):456–65.
9. Bull C, Byrnes J, Hettiarachchi R, Downes M. A systematic review of the validity and reliability of patient-reported experience measures. *Health Serv Res*. 2019;54(5):1023–35.
10. Riggare S, Unruh KT, Sturr J, Domingos J, Stamford JA, Svenningsson P, Hägglund M. Patient-driven N-of-1 in Parkinson's disease. Lessons learned from a placebo-controlled study of the effect of nicotine on dyskinesia. *Methods Inf Med*. 2018;56(99):e123–8.
11. Guyatt GH, Sackett DL, Sinclair JC, Hayward R, Cook DJ, Cook RJ, et al. Users' Guides to the Medical Literature: IX. A Method for Grading Health Care Recommendations. *JAMA*. 1995;274(22):1800–4.
12. Murad MH, Asi N, Alsawas M, Alahdab F. New evidence pyramid. *Evid Based Med*. 2016;21(4):125.
13. Greenhalgh T, Fisman D, Cane DJ, Oliver M, Macintyre, CR. Adapt or die: how the pandemic made the shift from EBM to EBM+ more urgent. *BMJ Evid-Based Med*. 2022;27(5):253.
14. Ogilvie D, Bauman A, Foley L, Guell C, Humphreys D, Panter J. Making sense of the evidence in population health intervention research: building a dry stone wall. *BMJ Glob Health*. 2020;5(12):e004017.
15. West M. NHS Leadership Academy. 2022. The key components of effective teamworking during the COVID-19 Crisis. Available from: https://learninghub.leadershipacademy.nhs.uk/teamworking/the-key-components-of-effective-teamworking-during-the-covid-19-crisis/ (accessed 16 June 2023).

16. Granger K, Granger C. Hello My Name Is | A campaign for more compassionate care. Available from: https://www.hellomynameis.org.uk/ (accessed 16 June 2023).

17. Berwick D. A promise to learn – a commitment to act: improving the safety of patients in England. National Advisory Group on the Safety of Patients in England. 2013 Aug. Available from:https://assets.publishing.service.gov.uk/government/uploads/system/uploads/attachment_data/file/226703/Berwick_Report.pdf (accessed 5 March 2024).

18. Sanders K. Hitting the target but completely missing the point? The King's Fund. 2012. Available from: www.kingsfund.org.uk/projects/point-care/staff-stories/hitting-target-completely-missing-point (accessed 16 June 2023).

19. Ford J, Gimson A, Toh CH. Clinical validation of waiting lists – we need to avoid worsening health inequalities. *The BMJ Opinion*. 2020. Available from: https://blogs.bmj.com/bmj/2020/10/28/clinical-validation-of-waiting-lists-we-need-to-avoid-worsening-health-inequalities/ (accessed 16 June 2023).

20. Realistic Medicine. Shared decision making, reducing harm, waste and tackling unwarranted variation. Available from: www.realisticmedicine.scot/ (accessed 16 June 2023).

21. Summer Meranius M, Holmström IK, Håkansson J, Breitholtz A, Moniri F, Skogevall S, et al. Paradoxes of person-centred care: A discussion paper. *Nurs Open*. 2020;7(5):1321–9.

22. Sinclair S, Raffin-Bouchal S, Venturato L, Mijovic-Kondejewski J, Smith-MacDonald L. Compassion fatigue: A meta-narrative review of the healthcare literature. *Int J Nurs Stud*. 2017;69:9–24.

23. Goodrich J. Supporting hospital staff to provide compassionate care: do Schwartz Center Rounds work in English hospitals? *J R Soc Med*. 2012;105(3):117–22.

24. Twitter. 2023. @FlexNHS ♥ (@FlexNHS) / Twitter. Available from: https://twitter.com/FlexNHS (accessed 16 June 2023).

25. Oliver D. When 'resilience' becomes a dirty word. *BMJ*. 2017;358:j3604.

26. Mannix K. *Listen: How to find the words for tender conversations*. London: William Collins; 2021.

27. Feldthusen C, Forsgren E, Wallström S, Jakobsson Ung E, Öhlén J. Person-centeredness and person-centred care in practice: an overview of reviews. *Int J Integr Care*. 2022;22(S1):32.

28. Levinson W, Lesser CS, Epstein RM. Developing physician communication skills for patient-centered care. *Health Aff (Millwood)*. 2010;29(7):1310–8.

29. Hower KI, Vennedey V, Hillen HA, Kuntz L, Stock S, Pfaff H, et al. Implementation of patient-centred care: which organisational determinants matter from decision maker's perspective? Results from a qualitative interview study across various health and social care organisations. *BMJ Open*. 2019;9(4):e027591.

30. The Health Foundation. Person-centred care made simple – What everyone should know about person-centred care. 2014. Available from: www.health.org.uk/publications/person-centred-care-made-simple (accessed 19 June 2023).

31. NHS England. NDRS. Data on Written Complaints in the NHS, 2020–21. 2022. Available from: https://digital.nhs.uk/data-and-information/publications/statistical/data-on-written-complaints-in-the-nhs/2020-21 (accessed 19 June 2023).

32. van Mook WNKA, Gorter SL, Kieboom W, Castermans MGTH, de Feijter J, de Grave WS, et al. Poor professionalism identified through investigation of unsolicited healthcare complaints. *Postgrad Med J*. 2012;88(1042):443–50.

33. Michie S, van Stralen MM, West R. The behaviour change wheel: a new method for characterising and designing behaviour change interventions. *Implement Sci*. 2011;6:42.

34. Pérez-Stable EJ, El-Toukhy S. Communicating with diverse patients: How patient and clinician factors affect disparities. *Patient Educ Couns*. 2018;101(12):2186–94.

35. de Iongh A. Oiling the wheels of occupational therapy. *OT News*, Royal College of Occupational Therapists. 29th ed. 2021 Mar 16;3.

36. Fagan P, de Longh A, Harden B, Wright C. Person-centred approaches: empowering people in their lives and communities to enable an upgrade in prevention, wellbeing, health, care and support. 2017. Available from: www.skillsforhealth.org.uk/wp-content/uploads/2021/01/Person-Centred-Approaches-Framework.pdf (accessed 5 March 2024).

37. National Voices. What we need now: what matters to people for health and care, during COVID-19 and beyond – new I statements 2020. 2020. Available from: www.nationalvoices.org.uk/what%20we%20need%20now (accessed 21 June 2023).

38. Hafferty FW. Beyond curriculum reform: confronting medicine's hidden curriculum. *Acad Med*. 1998;73(4):403–7.

39. Health Canada. Health Canada policy toolkit for public involvement in decision making. 2000. Available from: www.hc-sc.gc.ca/ahc-asc/alt_formats/pacrb-dgapcr/pdf/public-consult/2000decision-eng.pdf (accessed 5 March 2024).

40. International Association for Public Participation. Core Values, Ethics, Spectrum – The 3 Pillars of Public Participation. 2018. Available from: www.iap2.org/page/pillars (accessed 21 June 2023).

41. Healthcare Quality Improvement Partnership. A guide to patient and public involvement in quality improvement. HQIP; 2019. Available from: www.hqip.org.uk/resource/a-guide-to-patient-and-public-involvement-in-quality-improvement/ (accessed 22 June 2023).

42. Gilbert D. Seven things that patients bring: the benefits of patients as partners for change. *InHealth Associates*. 2015. Available from: www.inhealthassociates.co.uk/uncategorized/seven-things-that-patients-bring-the-benefits-of-patients-as-partners-for-change-2/ (accessed 22 June 2023).

43. Gilbert D. The Jewel Merchants – a parable for healthcare. *InHealth Associates*. 2017. Available from: www.inhealthassociates.co.uk/uncategorized/the-jewel-merchants-a-parable-for-healthcare/ (accessed 22 June 2023).

44. Personalised Care Institute. The Personalised Care Curriculum. 2020. Available from: www.personalisedcareinstitute.org.uk/wp-content/uploads/2021/06/The-personalised-care-curriculum.pdf (accessed 5 March 2024).

45. General Medical Council. Shared decision making is key to good patient care. 2020. Available from: www.gmc-uk.org/news/news-archive/shared-decision-making-is-key-to-good-patient-care---gmc-guidance (accessed 23 June 2023).

46. Health and Care Professions Council. Person-centred care. 2021. (Professional Standards). Available from: www.hcpc-uk.org/standards/meeting-our-standards/person-centred-care/ (accessed 23 June 2023).

47. National Voices. The Dr will Zoom you now: getting the most out of the virtual health and care experience. 2020. Available from: www.nationalvoices.org.uk/publications/our-publications/dr-will-zoom-you-now-getting-most-out-virtual-health-and-care (accessed 23 June 2023).

48. Richards T, Snow R, Schroter S. Logging The BMJ's 'patient journey'. *BMJ*. 2015;351:h4396.

49. The King's Fund. Building collaborative partnerships with patients and communities. 2016. Available from: www.kingsfund.org.uk/publications/leading-collaboratively-patients-communities-interview (accessed 23 June 2023).

50. Nestel D, Tierney T. Role-play for medical students learning about communication: guidelines for maximising benefits. *BMC Med Educ*. 2007;7(1):3.

51. Maini A, Fyfe M, Kumar S. Medical students as health coaches: adding value for patients and students. *BMC Med Educ*. 2020;20(1):182.

52. Singh Ospina N, Phillips KA, Rodriguez-Gutierrez R, Castaneda-Guarderas A, Gionfriddo MR, Branda ME, et al. Eliciting the patient's agenda – secondary analysis of recorded clinical encounters. *J Gen Intern Med*. 2019;34(1):36–40.

4
Researching generalism

Lindsey Pope, Helen Reid, Nigel Hart, Kay Leedham-Green, Emily Owen and Sophie Park

Introduction

This chapter examines a range of research approaches that maximise how we make visible generalist knowledge in healthcare and education research. We critically explore some of the dominant research paradigms in healthcare and use an example to advocate for the validity of a more expansive research base that is particular to clinical generalism. We include a range of practices to help prospective scholars enhance and reshape their research and consider ways this might inform exploration of generalist practice, teaching and learning.

How and what we research limits what it is possible to know. Perceptions vary about what evidence is useful and relevant to produce, access and utilise. These are conditional upon how we conceptualise professional practice (for example, as something fixed and standardised, or as something distributed and flexible) and the sorts of knowledge and interactions which become framed as legitimate or acceptable. Research is often assumed to 'uncover' existing truths or facts. This positions research as a detached process, free of influence from a researcher's values. Most research is in fact more complicated. It is a careful and lengthy negotiated process, constructing how and why we can claim 'to know' certain things, and the values that underpin what we choose to research. How we think about the 'thing' we want to research shapes how and what we can produce as a 'result' or 'knowledge claim'. Familiar research approaches used in clinical practice (for example, randomised controlled trials), tend to shape (and limit) the ways in which knowledge is formalised, codified and made explicit. These tend to compartmentalise and objectify knowledge and researchers, often positioning teaching, learning and clinical care as 'interventions' and research as measurement or comparison of their effectiveness. These approaches have focused, but inevitably constrained, what we are able to make visible, claim or 'know' about clinical practice and learning. These research preferences shape what and how it is possible to examine generalism at any one time and to what extent characteristic elements are made visible through the research process.

Let us consider how we can think about professional practice. One commonly held ideal for professional practice, espoused by the Australian Council of Professions, is that it is based upon a body of knowledge, agreed, codified, made explicit and practised by a 'disciplined group of individuals … who are prepared to apply this knowledge and exercise these skills in the interest of others' (1). This suggests a discrete and fixed set of knowledge, which can then be implemented in predetermined ways. This lends itself well to methods which compartmentalise and measure professional practice as something separate or discrete from the context in which it is done.

If we think about generalist professional practice differently, then relevant professional knowledge changes: utilising additional knowledge of people, places, context and use of ever-evolving theories of behaviour, cognition, values, psychology or social interactions. These would not be made visible using, for example, a randomised controlled trial, where context and human volition is perceived as a 'contaminator' (2). Wide-ranging knowledge forms are often more challenging to codify, particularly if applied in a variety of ways to adjust to local needs and contexts. These more expansive and distributed knowledge forms require a broad range of research methodologies. While it is desirable that a body of knowledge underpinning health professional practice should itself be built upon a credible and applicable evidence base, how an evidence base is built and curated matters. The evidence we produce to make the rich and detailed knowledge of generalism visible and explicit needs to reflect its complexity; be varied in nature; and attend to the breadth of possibilities for clinical practice and learning. Before continuing, we invite you to read the Example 4.1 and to use it to frame some of the abstract concepts that we introduce.

Example 4.1: Dr Ali (becoming a generalist researcher)

Medical school had taught Dr Ali to use evidence-based approaches to clinical decision-making and to make 'conscientious, explicit, and judicious use of the best evidence in making decisions about the care of individual patients'. On entering academic GP training, she joined a unit researching gender-based violence. Dr Ali wanted her research to provide evidence to help GPs in identifying people at risk of domestic violence during clinical consultations. Her initial plan was to conduct a robust randomised controlled trial, comparing two approaches to see which identified more cases: explicitly asking everyone in an 'at risk' category versus current practice (unknown).

Dr Ali's supervisors explored with her some of the potential pitfalls of this approach. What were its underlying assumptions, might there be unintended consequences, and how would any findings change future clinical practice or improve patient outcomes? They explored with her whether other types of knowledge, ways of knowing and methodological approaches might help her to take forward her research interests and address the knowledge gaps for approaches in clinical practice.

At her next supervisory meeting, Dr Ali discussed a recent patient encounter. The patient had initially brought symptoms of anxiety but on further exploration disclosed that they were experiencing domestic violence. Dr Ali was able to provide access to a crisis centre which provided emergency support and accommodation. Reflecting on this, she wondered how she, as a GP, could develop her skills to identify and support people better. Her supervisor suggested she go to this crisis centre and spend some time attentively listening and engaging with the staff and residents there to gain access to a diversity of views and perspectives. Dr Ali heard many heartbreaking narratives of attempted disclosures that had been ignored, but also inspirational stories where clinicians had spotted subtle signs and gone out of their way to help. She worked with them to create a research question that mattered to them, relating to barriers and facilitators to disclosure in primary care settings. After receiving the necessary approvals, she conducted a series of workshops for people with lived experience of domestic violence to articulate and reflect on stories of disclosure, and to collaboratively co-create future-oriented implications for practitioners. She shared and honed their recommendations at a local best practice meeting and worked with her clinical colleagues to implement and evaluate their recommendations in practice. She shared her findings at a national conference and was invited to create a training and evaluation pack to enhance a national safeguarding course. This wider evaluation demonstrated that GPs were indeed picking up more cases, and perhaps more importantly, that patients felt safe and heard when they disclosed.

Sharing and producing generalist knowledge

Dr Ali's final project involved making visible the tacit knowledge of people with lived experience of domestic violence. By aggregating, interpreting and sharing their knowledge, and combining it with the knowledge of practitioners, Dr Ali was able to create, evaluate and disseminate theoretically informed new practices that were adopted or adapted by other practitioners. We invite you to consider this as an example of how generalist knowledge is shared and produced more generally.

In real-world clinical practice, knowledge is often tacit or implicit (unspoken or indirectly implied). It may be that generalist clinical practice embodies knowledge and ways of doing that are more implicit than explicit. While tacit or implicit knowledge is not without value in an applied professional context, it requires the profession to embrace a broader range of knowledge approaches to enhance understanding of practice. The Nonaka-Takeuchi model (Figure 4.1) from the world of business provides an insight into how tacit knowledge can be converted to explicit knowledge, or vice versa, and how cycles of sharing and transferring knowledge help to create new knowledge (3). The Nonaka-Takeuchi model postulates four different modes of knowledge conversion:

- from tacit knowledge to tacit knowledge, through socialisation;
- from tacit knowledge to explicit knowledge, through externalisation;
- from explicit knowledge to explicit knowledge, by combination or synthesis; and
- from explicit knowledge to tacit knowledge, through internalisation.

This model illustrates the two-way links between tacit and explicit knowledge. Aligning with sociocultural learning theories, recognising that professional practice and learning does not occur in a vacuum, it proposes that knowledge can be enhanced and expanded through spaces for sharing, converting and creating knowledge (both explicit and tacit). Rather than knowledge being handed down from researchers to practitioners, it acknowledges that professional knowledge is often exchanged in more complex and sophisticated ways.

In generalist practice, dialogue between colleagues or between a teacher and learner might, for example, share 'how I did this and why'. This is the exchange of tacit knowledge through interaction (socialisation). This conversation might lead to the production of a case report or a practice standard operating procedure (SOP) which makes explicit how something is done (externalisation). A team, perhaps from a clinical or academic organisation, might then work to combine case studies

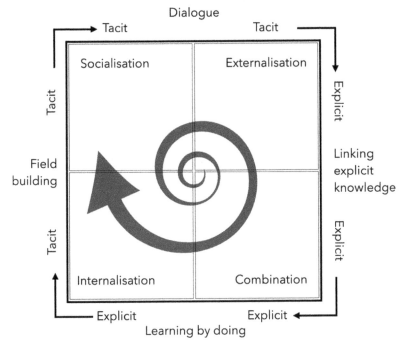

Figure 4.1 Exchange of tacit and explicit organisational knowledge.
© Sophie Park and Kay Leedham-Green, adapted from the SECI model
of knowledge dimensions (Nonaka and Takeuchi 1995)

and reports to form a collective document or consensus statement about
how something can or even should be done (combination). This document is then shared, used and adapted to inform new tacit practices
(internalisation).

Research about generalism therefore becomes more interesting,
inclusive and expansive if it not only examines exchange of explicit
knowledge, but also attends to how knowledge is shared, exchanged and
implemented in the workplace.

Paradigms of research

There is a wide range of approaches to research, summarised in Table 4.1.
Each 'paradigm' has different assumptions about reality (ontology, what
is knowable), knowledge (epistemology, how knowledge is created)
and values (axiology, what 'good' research is). We are not positioning
one paradigm over another, as each has advantages and challenges in
different contexts and for different types of research questions. We do,

Table 4.1 Research paradigms

Positivism
• Nature exists • Knowledge is objective, testable and generalisable • Experimental research, data tests hypotheses • Quality = p values, confidence intervals, reliability, validity *'Is learning to wash hands by e-learning as effective as face-to-face learning?'*
Realism – post-positivism / constructivism
• A real world exists, independent of how an individual perceives or constructs it (mind-independent reality) • Knowledge of a phenomenon will always remain partial, fallible and incomplete • An ongoing process of theory-building and testing is crucial for extending existing knowledge and advancing scientific research • Mixed methods (methodological eclecticism) • Quality = multiple perspectives, ontological depth, generative causation, explanatory insight, rigour, trustworthiness, transferability *'The use of e-learning in handwashing training: what works; for whom; and in what contexts?'*
Pragmatism
• It does not really matter whether nature exists or not • Knowledge is what you need to make an informed decision, context dependent • Action research, real-world imperfections in data • Quality = try and see if it works *'If I switch to e-learning handwashing training, do infection rates go up or down on my ward?'*
Social constructivism / interpretivism
• Nature exists through our perception, and is influenced by our sociocultural perspective • Knowledge is socially constructed (e.g. through interactions) and dynamic • Interpretive, qualitative methodologies, data is theory-generating • Quality = rigour, trustworthiness, resonance *'What are the factors influencing healthcare professionals' handwashing decisions?'*

(continued)

Table 4.1 (Cont.)

Critical theory
• Nature exists through our perception, and is influenced by our sociocultural perspective
• Knowledge construction is dominated by powerful elites at the expense of workers / women / minorities / environment, etc.
• Research is about disrupting and challenging the status quo
• Quality = impact, change
'The move from face-to-face to e-learning in handwashing training: in whose interests is this? managers, practitioners or patients?'

however, invite the reader to move beyond simple experimental designs when considering how to research complex social phenomena such as generalist education, interactions, systems and outcomes.

Positivist approaches assume a single reality that is objectively measurable, and researchers tend to adopt quasi-experimental designs. The legitimacy of the researcher is established through evidencing their detachment from the research process. Claims about rigour are made in relation to a researcher's objectivity, or absence of impact on data or analysis. This might be appropriate when comparing the impact of two drugs on a measurable outcome such as blood pressure. Within this approach, we assume that the outcomes that matter are objectively and reliably measurable. Measuring more complex constructs (anything that is shaped by human subjectivity, volition, reasoning and choice), however, is less straightforward. For example, if Dr Ali wanted to compare case findings in the two arms of her study, how might the research environment, the words that researchers use, their identity or subjective interpretations of 'violence' affect the results?

Realist approaches acknowledge imperfections in the objectivity of data. Within realist research, findings in one context are unlikely to be generalisable to all contexts (4). Realists ask research questions such as 'what is it about X that leads to Y?' and 'how does an intervention work, for whom, and in which circumstances?' (generative causation). Realists tend to combine data collection methods from qualitative and quantitative research approaches to explore a phenomenon across diverse contexts and from different perspectives (5). Transferability (rather than generalisability) is advocated in realism as this acknowledges the highly complex, dynamic and diverse influences of context. Although theories and findings may be relevant now, they may not be applicable (to interventions) in the future. Realist knowledge will need to be retested in different social, political and economic contexts and modified accordingly. An example of a realist approach might be comparing different types of domestic violence records for the same area (for example, clinical, police and crisis centre) to identify how different demographic groups disclose, followed by interviews to explore the underlying reasons why.

Social constructivism is a type of interpretivist discourse. This suggests that knowledge is constructed through social interactions and is therefore inherently subjective. Different constructions of the world might therefore elicit different responses and behaviours. Differences might emerge, for example, with research participants in different contexts, or in the ways researcher and participant interact. An example of a constructivist approach might be Dr Ali inviting residents at crisis centres to discuss their experiences of disclosing domestic violence as a group and to collectively make sense of their experiences and construct potential ways forward.

When using an interpretivist approach, 'critical reflexivity' becomes a core part of the research process and related knowledge claims. Reflexivity has been described by Gouldner (cited in (6)) as the 'analytic attention to the researcher's role in qualitative research'. It is both a process and a concept, embracing the positionality of the researcher and their ways of understanding the world. A helpful starting point, but also a false binary, is the concept of 'insider' versus 'outsider' research. A naïve assumption might be that to enhance rigour we simply ensure that an outsider is conducting the proposed study. This assumption suggests that positionality is simply defined by virtue of having (or not) a particular characteristic – e.g. being a GP or not being a GP. As a researcher, we may share some features with our participants, but be quite different in other ways. Both insiders and outsiders bring different values to the research being conducted. While an 'outsider' may bring a fresh curiosity and insights, an 'insider' may bring a more nuanced understanding or be more readily trusted by participants. Reflexivity, through its aforementioned 'analytical attention', requires the researcher to question and reflect on the inevitable relationship between them and their research. The rigour of the research is not established through the researcher's disconnectedness, but rather through their ability to reflect on and share insights about how their position shaped the production of the research findings.

If we are explicit and open about the range of possibilities for doing research, it becomes much easier to exchange conversations about the opportunities and challenges of using particular methods. Rather than these being hidden from view, they become part of a critical conversation about what particular studies are able to 'make visible', and how additional research might complement this to examine a topic or process from a different perspective, or in a different context. This moves our expectations of research from production of definitive 'facts', towards a more dialogic and iterative process of knowledge production and exchange, conditional upon the constraints of production and context of research implementation. In the words of Hafferty, such academic endeavours are often dynamic and contested, coming and going in 'windless waves of understanding' (7).

Cribb and Bignold argue that positivist discourses frame and justify research that tends to objectify, whereas interpretivist discourses focus more on humanising (8). Neither is right or wrong, but they forefront and limit how and what we can research in different ways. Clinical medicine and much of clinical education have tended to draw upon the same objectifying discourses that are helpful when researching biomedical sciences. This may cause dissonance when they are used to research what are essentially social practices: generalist practice and learning. Positivism positions elements of practice and learning as objects, minimising the ways in which we can understand or appreciate these as part of a vital, dynamic or interactive system. Interpretivist approaches, in contrast, focus much more on human and social aspects of practice, or the nature and value of interactions between people. In positivist research, counting or measuring is important to support research claims. In other paradigms, one instance of a story can form the central basis of an analysis. Here, it is not important to represent the views of all participants. Rather, analysis seeks to produce a new or contrasting idea, concept or perspective.

We are not asking readers to value one approach over another. Rather, we invite you to consider the limitations of every research approach and the need for multiple perspectives in research to understand and improve clinical practice and education.

Historically, we have a very limited empirical base for generalist practice, because of the dominance to date of positivist methods in this field. Increasingly, a wider range of methodologies has helped to make visible new insights and knowledge about how generalism is done and learned. Deciding on what to research, and how to research it, is a values-based process. In Chapter 5 our colleagues assert that how we research, limits what it is possible to know – that is, research can only answer the question(s) the study is designed to answer. In what may appear to be a paradox, it works both ways. We need also to consider 'what is knowable?' as that can constrain, or open, opportunities around what and how we research. A broader research paradigm opens up research avenues that may not be discretely packageable, but are nonetheless important to people and impact on their ability to participate in society. This might include researching the quality and experience of care for marginalised groups, health promotion, patient and carer engagement, strategies for self-care, collaborative working, and personalised and sustainable approaches to care.

Knowledge hierarchies and the challenge for generalism

The 'hierarchy of evidence' has become a heuristic that is embedded in the narrative underpinning decision-making for clinical practice. In 1995, Guyatt and colleagues wrote a paper in which they provided a 'method for grading health care recommendations' (9). The principle of appraising, ranking and applying evidence to clinical practice became well known through the 1990s and was soon embedded in clinical curricula and policy. This ranking of evidence led to descriptions of hierarchies and, through the work of organisations such as the Cochrane Collaboration, meta-analyses of randomised controlled trials found their way to the top of the hierarchy. Along the way, case reports, in-depth case studies and other forms of evidence lost currency and became devalued by the medical community.

In their influential 1996 editorial (10), Sackett and colleagues set out to describe evidence-based medicine – 'what it is and what it isn't'. They wrote that 'Evidence-based medicine is the conscientious, explicit, and judicious use of current best evidence in making decisions about the care of individual patients.' Helpfully, they expanded on this to say that 'The practice of evidence-based medicine means integrating individual clinical expertise with the best available external clinical evidence from systematic research.' However, the integration of individual clinical expertise has often been neglected along the way, alongside the recognition of the value of researching personalised patient-centred care.

This hierarchy of evidence became further enshrined through the establishment of guideline organisations. Around the turn of the millennium the GRADE (Grading of Recommendations Assessment, Development and Evaluation) approach was established by Guyatt and colleagues (11) and international guideline organisations started to evaluate and report on the quality and strength of evidence underpinning recommendations for healthcare interventions. GRADE would rate papers for their assessed validity of 'effect'. High-quality studies were those where there was 'a lot of confidence that the true effect lies close to that of the estimated effect'. Building on this, economic evaluations were added by some organisations further refining what was defined as best practice. This produces, however, a narrow view about both evidence and quality (see also Chapter 5).

The evidence hierarchy paradigm and the resultant guidelines, under the banner of evidence-based medicine (EBM), became the dominant arbiter of clinical practice, later referred to as evidence-based clinical practice (EBCP). 'Effect size', 'cost' and 'quality' (by virtue of position on the hierarchy) relating to a limited set of clinical conditions meant that other forms of evidence had limited legitimacy. Regrettably, the value of the integration of 'individual clinical expertise' heralded by Sackett and colleagues appeared to become mostly lost along the way. However, there was something of a departure from this dogma of guidelines being the ultimate arbiter of unquestionable best practice with the maxim 'Guidelines are guidelines not tramlines', a quote attributed to Sir Michael Rawlins, the first Chair of the UK's guideline organisation, NICE (as cited in (12)).

The development of EBCP and clinical guidelines (discussed further in Chapter 5) is not in itself problematic for generalism. Guidelines provide useful reference points for discussing a differential diagnosis or management action plan. The problem relates to the devaluing and, at worst, dismissal of research findings that do not find their way to the top of the hierarchy. Generalism, with its integrative, situated and holistic approach, risks losing connection with an evidence base that is relevant to its practices. A re-reading of the 1996 editorial of Sackett and colleagues (10) would suggest that the EBM movement led to an unintended consequence. As they state, 'Evidence based medicine is not restricted to randomised trials and meta-analyses. It involves tracking down the best external evidence with which to answer our clinical questions.'

As a result of the narrow range of research approaches dominating EBM, generalism has been relatively under-researched. Although many clinical decisions benefit from randomised controlled trials, there is an increasing acknowledgement that a broader range of methods is also necessary to inform the evidence base underpinning clinical practice. The increasing complexity of healthcare delivery requires multiple ways of knowing. Qualitative methods such as interviews, focus groups and observation, and methods that combine qualitative and quantitative approaches are therefore growing in popularity (13).

Quality considerations for generalist research

We argue that some widely held beliefs about research quality are situated in a positivist paradigm of knowledge and are not suited to the situated complexity of generalism. When these criteria are applied to generalist forms of research, dissonances can arise. For example, the concept of generalisability, or the extent to which findings of a study can be applied to other situations, is often mentioned when critiquing research findings. This term assumes that rigorous research findings reflect a universal truth – for example, claiming that findings from a study are rigorous if the results are replicable across different cultural and healthcare contexts, or that large studies must be conducted to root out contextual factors. Recently, our understanding of generalisability has become more nuanced, with consideration being given to how situated knowledge might be relevant to others beyond the particular circumstances researched (14). This could be through production of reusable insights or concepts, rather than specific or repeatable elements of practice. If the researcher provides sufficient contextual detail, the reader can select elements or concepts that might apply to their own contextualised practice. As a result, research can make visible situated ways of thinking or doing, enabling readers to engage in a critical and reflexive exploration of how things are, and how their own practice might shift or change.

There are many established quality criteria for clinical research, some of which depend on the researcher's paradigm and methodological approach. Such criteria include reliability, validity, trustworthiness, rigour and applicability. There are also ethical considerations relating to intentions, confidentiality, informed choice, minimisation of harms and maximisation of benefits. In addition to these, we argue that generalist research efforts aim to be:

- **participatory**: designed and conducted in collaboration with the intended beneficiaries and other stakeholders;
- **equitable and socially just**: paying active attention to whose voices are heard and ensuring decisions are made in ways that are fair and open;
- **reflexive**: so that external research agendas and the impacts of the researcher's identity, beliefs and positionality are made visible;
- **congruent**: so that the ways of thinking about research (methodologies) and the methods for collecting and analysing data are appropriate for the situational complexity of generalism and the knowledge claims being made;
- **oriented to generalism**: addressing an important generalist problem or unknown;
- **impactful**: insights produced have the potential to enhance generalist forms of care.

Research for generalism

Rather than explain every type of clinical research, we propose a set of research practices that are particularly suited to generalism. Unsurprisingly, these build on the philosophy and practices of generalism articulated in Chapter 1. Generalism is a complex and situated practice that connects multiple sources and types of knowledge, that values and needs participatory and collaborative approaches, and that implements knowledge in ways that are adaptive. These underlying principles invite approaches to research that are responsive to context, that are participatory and directed towards patient and public agendas, that give holistic attention to patient and population outcomes, and that pay attention to how new knowledge is integrated and adapted for future practice. We propose a set of research approaches that builds on these principles (Figure 4.2).

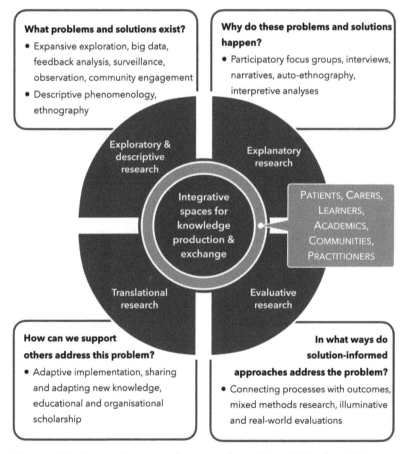

What problems and solutions exist?
- Expansive exploration, big data, feedback analysis, surveillance, observation, community engagement
- Descriptive phenomenology, ethnography

Why do these problems and solutions happen?
- Participatory focus groups, interviews, narratives, auto-ethnography, interpretive analyses

Exploratory & descriptive research

Explanatory research

Integrative spaces for knowledge production & exchange

PATIENTS, CARERS, LEARNERS, ACADEMICS, COMMUNITIES, PRACTITIONERS

Translational research

Evaluative research

How can we support others address this problem?
- Adaptive implementation, sharing and adapting new knowledge, educational and organisational scholarship

In what ways do solution-informed approaches address the problem?
- Connecting processes with outcomes, mixed methods research, illuminative and real-world evaluations

Figure 4.2 Generalist research approaches. © Sophie Park and Kay Leedham-Green

Exploratory and descriptive studies

Exploratory and descriptive studies help to ensure relevance to patient and population needs and are sometimes used to justify more focused explanatory or interventional studies. Exploratory approaches include exploring public health datasets to identify geographical or demographic clustering of risk factors or diseases, or archives of patient feedback to identify areas of practice that are working well or less well. Descriptive approaches might include describing a care pathway or system from the perspective of service users, or describing a phenomenon such as postnatal depression from the perspectives of the people it affects.

Within exploratory research, descriptive approaches are sometimes used as a precursor to quantitative methods – for example, to describe a phenomenon in depth before creating an instrument to explore its prevalence across different groups. An in-depth qualitative description of the characteristics of postnatal depression, for example, might be used to create and validate an instrument to identify and categorise cases. This instrument can then be used to explore regional and demographic variations.

The quantitative methodologies associated with this type of research include cross-sectional or cohort studies – for example, to determine the uptake of vaccines in an at-risk group, or regional variations in prescribing practices. Qualitative methodologies include ethnographic and phenomenographic studies – for example, to explore the culture and practices of a multidisciplinary healthcare team, or to characterise 'a good consultation' from the perspective of patients and carers. Survey, case study and narrative methods might be used to identify potential areas of excellence or concern – for example, through interviews or patient feedback. More statistical approaches might include using a validated measure to explore the association of a construct, such as 'feeling heard', with an outcome, such as adherence to treatment plans.

Explanatory research

Explanatory research might be conducted to explain the findings from a previous exploratory study – for example, to explain why certain demographics have different vaccine uptake rates, or to explain why higher levels of patient activation are associated with fewer hospitalisations. It can also be used to explain anomalous findings such as unusual or outlying results. Explanatory studies might also be conducted in conjunction with an interventional study, either beforehand to ensure the intervention is grounded in theoretical understanding, or afterwards to explain why the intervention did or did not provide value to its intended beneficiaries.

Theory generation through interpretation is a core aspect of explanatory research, and this is what makes it distinct from descriptive research. Explanatory research tries to answer questions such as 'why?' or 'how?' and therefore tends to have an interpretive emphasis. It is through a theoretical understanding of why or how something happens that interventions can be specifically targeted to address associated factors. Higgins and Moore describe how theory can be generated at multiple levels (15). Micro theory might explain why something happened during a specific instance – for example, identifying causal factors in a critical incident review and using these to theorise about wider implications. Meso theory integrates findings on a broader level to generate theory around a specific phenomenon – for example, why people who have survived a heart attack do not always take preventive medicines. This might involve, for example, interpreting from a thematic analysis across multiple case studies, documents, narratives, interviews or focus groups. Grand theory aims to build understanding that can be abstracted beyond a specific area of practice and that can be applied more generally – for example, behaviour-change theory or illness-perception theory – and often employs literature-based methodologies such as narrative synthesis and meta-ethnography. Charmaz describes approaches for building from data (16).

Evaluative research

Generalist approaches to interventional research are not only about 'proving the efficacy' of a particular medicine or intervention. Although quasi-experimental approaches are important, they are not included here as they are not specific to generalism. Because generalism is grounded in holistic approaches to patient and population outcomes and the complex link between approaches to care and those outcomes, generalist approaches to evaluative research tend to be more complex and to include 'real-world' and 'illuminative' approaches (17,18). A real-world evaluation of an intervention might include factors such as patient preference and the feasibility and acceptability of an intervention. An example of a real-world study might be evaluating the impacts of a diabetes intervention by looking at longitudinal data from wearable devices and comparing this to self-reported adherence to the intervention. Illuminative approaches focus on making processes as well as outcomes visible – for example, evaluating the factors that impact on engagement with the intervention. Illuminative approaches also aim to identify unintended consequences as well as intended outcomes. Such an approach might pick up the additional burden of an intervention, or indeed of benefits beyond the intended outcomes – for example, feelings of validation and belonging experienced by people attending a group intervention. Generalist evaluations are often mixed-methods, partly because not all outcomes that matter to people are countable, but also as a form of additional or complementary exploration or explanation. Are the identified outcomes related to the intervention or to some other factor?

Generalism invites participatory approaches to evaluation that take into consideration structural inequalities. Focusing on the outcomes that matter to people is important. For example, an evaluation of an intervention supporting engagement with people's families and communities. Or an evaluation focusing on sustainability, comparing the human, carbon and economic resource implications of two effective clinical pathways.

Translational research

The focus of generalism on holistic patient and population outcomes means that the creation of new knowledge is not the end point of research: research impact is enhanced through efforts to translate findings into tangible improvements to people's lives. Generalism is not a static practice, but constantly evolving in response to patient and population needs; therefore, practitioners need opportunities to absorb and learn from research efforts. Efforts to disseminate knowledge and translate knowledge into action might be written up into project reports and shared at conferences or in journals, and these reports are used to create meta-knowledge about how knowledge is effectively shared and translated. Translational research is closely related to organisational and educational scholarship, and includes innovation and improvement methodologies, implementation science, behavioural and cognitive science, and theories of leadership, teamworking, change and action. These are discussed further in Chapter 5 (implementing generalist knowledge), Chapter 6 (educational approaches), Chapter 13 (sustainable healthcare) and Chapter 14 (quality improvement and innovation).

Strengthening the generalist evidence base

The previous sections have set out perspectives on ways of knowing and of producing knowledge and the dominance associated with particular lenses and knowledge hierarchies informing and directing clinical practice. Example 4.1 (Dr Ali) shows how the dominant hierarchy of EBM might not maximise the visibility of generalist knowledge. Reflecting on the knowledge and perspectives needed to meet the challenges of a day's caseload in clinical generalism offers up many insights into the tacit and implicit knowledge being called upon and the inadequacies of the dominant hierarchies in providing or exchanging this. How should a clinical generalist approach meeting the needs of a grieving mother whose son has died by suicide, or school refusal in a 13-year-old male with an autistic spectrum diagnosis who is navigating the emotional turbulence of puberty, or how to identify those at risk of homelessness to facilitate a morbidity-reducing harm prevention, or a clinical consultation about symptoms that are likely to originate from poly-substance use in managing pain? While many of these examples may, at face value, appear isolated and unique, it is likely that many clinical generalists can relate to these clinical dilemmas, and empirical examination (for example, through ethnography or mixed-methods approaches) could identify some useful principles or insights to inform practice elsewhere, or enhance generalist learning.

Many clinical generalists may have, through experience, arrived at a bespoke and personal tacit knowledge base that orientates their approach with such clinical dilemmas, but this knowledge may not have been made explicit for the benefit of other clinicians or learners. Arguably, this knowledge can and should be made explicit, shared and built upon in order to contribute to evidence gaps that characterise a generalist approach. Selecting the tools to do this well, however, requires careful and expansive thought. For the generalist base to strengthen, structural factors around funding and ethics also need to be addressed so that interpretivist discourses are included in addition to hypothetic-deductive research approaches.

Acknowledging the constraints and limitations of generalist research

Earlier in this chapter, and in Chapter 5, we refer to the situated complexity of generalist approaches to care and, in turn, the evidence base that is needed to underpin such approaches. Generalist research, however, also has limitations in being able to provide a concrete evidence base for many granular questions important in clinical practice – for example, which dose of drug A resolves the presence of condition B? The integrative complexity of the evidence base it would seek to establish constrains its suitability for synopsis into explicit guidelines, certainly of the style and form that is typical in the current EBM guideline paradigm. However, it is perhaps because such an evidence base is absent that guidelines fail to embrace the affordances of generalist knowledge. It will perhaps only be when generalist approaches to evidence generation gain greater recognition that the affordances are seen as equal in measure to the constraints and limitations. Learners and clinicians can then integrate and move between these knowledge forms to support practice.

Conclusion

It is hoped that, through reading this chapter, you have been challenged to think expansively and creatively when considering how to produce knowledge that is relevant to generalist practice. We have presented our view that to explore generalist practice we need to recognise and embrace a broad range of methods as legitimate. In so doing, we aim not for reproducibility but for useful insights about how and why we might choose to work with a patient or a system in a particular way.

Research paradigms such as realism, constructivism and critical theory can provide new 'entry points' to examining generalist practice, producing evidence to support learners' reading, use and creation of generalist knowledge. This chapter has included a range of examples to enhance and reshape future research about generalist teaching and learning. It is equally important to consider how study design and research questions constrain what can be known as a result of a particular study. With research recognised as production of new knowledge or insights, it is beholden on every researcher to consider both the strengths and limitations of their work and how their knowledge might impact on clinical practice. Furthermore, to meet future population needs, we need further investment in the academic discipline of generalism alongside research funding aligned with generalist practice and priorities.

References

1. Australian Council of Professions (ACoP). What is a Profession? 2003. Available from: www.professions.org.au/what-is-a-professional/ (accessed 13 June 2023).
2. Pawson R. Evidence-Based Policy: A realist perspective. 2006. Available from: https://uk.sagepub.com/en-gb/eur/evidence-based-policy/book227875 (accessed 7 March 2024).
3. Nonaka I, Takeuchi H. *The Knowledge-Creating Company: How Japanese companies create the dynamics of innovation*. New York: Oxford University Press; 1995.
4. Pawson R, Tilley N. *Realistic Evaluation*. London: SAGE; 1997. pp. xvii, 235.
5. Jagosh J. Realist synthesis for public health: building an ontologically deep understanding of how programs work, for whom, and in which contexts. *Annu Rev Public Health*. 2019;40(1):361–72.
6. Dowling M. Approaches to reflexivity in qualitative research. *Nurse Res*. 2006;13(3).
7. Hafferty F. Reconfiguring the sociology of medical education: emerging topics and pressing issues. In: Bird C, Conrad P, Fremont A, eds. *Handbook of Medical Sociology*. 5th ed. Upper Saddle River, NJ: Prentice Hall; 2000. pp. 238–57.
8. Cribb A, Bignold S. Towards the reflexive medical school: The hidden curriculum and medical education research. *Stud High Educ*. 1999;24(2):195–209.
9. Guyatt GH, Sackett DL, Sinclair JC, Hayward R, Cook DJ, Cook RJ, et al. Users' guides to the medical literature: IX. A method for grading health care recommendations. *JAMA*. 1995;274(22):1800–4.
10. Sackett DL, Rosenberg WM, Gray JM, Haynes RB, Richardson WS. Evidence based medicine: what it is and what it isn't. *BMJ*. 1996;312(7023):71–2.
11. Guyatt GH, Oxman AD, Vist GE, Kunz R, Falck-Ytter Y, Alonso-Coello P, et al. GRADE: an emerging consensus on rating quality of evidence and strength of recommendations. *BMJ*. 2008;336(7650):924.
12. Kelly MP, Atkins L, Littleford C, Leng G, Michie S. Evidence-based medicine meets democracy: the role of evidence-based public health guidelines in local government. *J Public Health*. 2017;39(4):678–84.
13. Shorten A, Smith J. Mixed methods research: expanding the evidence base. *Evid Based Nurs*. 2017;20(3):74.
14. Carminati L. Generalizability in qualitative research: a tale of two traditions. *Qual Health Res*. 2018;28(13):2094–101.
15. Higgins PA, Moore SM. Levels of theoretical thinking in nursing. *Nurs Outlook*. 2000;48(4):179–83.
16. Charmaz K. *Constructing Grounded Theory*. SAGE; 2014.
17. Gray DE. *Doing Research in the Real World*. 3rd ed. London: SAGE; 2014.
18. Stufflebeam DL, Shinkfield AJ. Illuminative evaluation: the holistic approach. In: *Systematic Evaluation: A self-instructional guide to theory and practice*. Dordrecht: Springer Netherlands; 1985. pp. 285–310.

5

Implementing generalist knowledge

Sophie Park, Claire Duddy and Kamal Mahtani

Introduction

Clinicians are familiar with – and often comforted by – the concept of evidence-based or evidence-informed practice. It suggests that, where clinical dilemmas exist, we can reach for the experience and wisdom of others to locate an answer. This process gives us a sense that, although potentially alone in the consultation room or clinic, we are part of an interconnected network of professionals: that what we plan to do and action is within the norms and boundaries of what is considered to be good and acceptable. In reality, this process is more complex: sometimes the connections between available evidence and other important factors are unclear; often evidence is not directly relevant to a particular patient context; perhaps a patient has multiple conditions with potentially conflicting guidance; or the questions we need addressed have yet to be answered in ways we find useful.

We sometimes refer to these possibilities for selection and use of evidence as 'clinical judgement'. Most clinicians can describe situations where there was no available 'right' answer or linear pathway. These dilemma-moments can feel like personal failure or deficiency. They are often hidden from explicit public and professional conversations, yet they are a routine and normal part of generalist clinical practice. The problem is not that these moments exist, but that we have not yet found a common language to share these experiences and elements of work, nor ways to feedback our learning and expertise about how to integrate these into more collective professional bodies of knowledge. This chapter acknowledges, explores and celebrates situations where we face the unknown, why they can be so unsettling, but also how we can negotiate them so that clinician and patient can not only act, but flourish.

To do this, we need to acknowledge how we are making sense of the world around us. We all have a familiar or favourite lens through which we perceive the world. It governs how we prefer to notice, value and attend to certain things (such as resources or institutions) as important or valuable; why we think in particular ways; and how we speak, act and produce. Sometimes this lens becomes so familiar and normal to us that we fail to recognise that it is only one (partial and limited) way in which to perceive and make sense of the world. We therefore select approaches which align with our lens, and regard others as wrong or less worthwhile.

This lens-partiality can affect clinical practice by informing our decision-making and range of possible judgements. For example, if we prefer a biomedical lens, we might focus on locating or excluding disease; utilising research which examines objects as separate from their context; measuring items we can reduce or compartmentalise in order to count; valuing progress, action and development in relation to change in those measures. Our rationale for a legitimate path is then created by bringing together pieces of evidence or artefacts which fit within this lens, disregarding everything else as irrelevant.

What if you could change your preferred lens and view things differently? – the range of evidence you are able to draw upon as legitimate or valuable shifts. You can build your scaffolding and rationale for action differently. An experiential lens, for example, allows you to notice elements of your patient–clinician interaction, perhaps an expression of emotion, or a story about an experience (see Chapter 15). This scaffolding is just as limited and constrained as the biomedical one, but different. Connect these different perspectives together, utilising the strengths and weaknesses of each, and you broaden the range of 'relevant evidence', rationale and possibilities for action. This also enables a more informed and varied dialogue between clinician and patient or colleague about what matters most at this moment, informing what to do next.

Before reading on, consider the kind of evidence and knowledge you regularly observe or use in clinical practice. Perhaps you see guidelines, professional or expert panel consensus statements, qualitative and quantitative research, or patient surveys. Think about the relative value you attribute to each, their perceived strengths and weaknesses, and how they inform your clinical practice. How might you prioritise one piece of evidence above another? When does use of evidence feel straightforward to you, your patient or both? And how might you deal with potentially contrasting or conflicting pieces of evidence?

What do we mean by evidence?

As outlined in Chapter 4, the evidence-based medicine (EBM) movement arose in the early 1990s and has heavily influenced how clinicians value the relevance of certain information and knowledge as legitimate to inform clinical practice, and what comprises 'good practice' (1). EBM includes a triad of factors informing clinical care: evidence, judgement and values. Many, however, only associate EBM with what Guyatt, Sackett and colleagues proposed as a *hierarchy of evidence* (2). This idea that some evidence is better than others still strongly influences how clinicians often perceive, value, use and dismiss certain forms of evidence and ways of knowing. This positions different methodologies as more or less reliable and valuable. Research questions, for example, that examine intervention effectiveness (for example, randomised controlled trials (RCTs), meta-analyses, systematic reviews) are situated as the pinnacle of knowing, a gold standard (3).

How we value each type of evidence (and whether we even consider it as evidence) is conditional upon the lens(es) we choose to use. RCTs, for example, work extremely well to assess effectiveness where an intervention or object is relatively discrete (see Figure 5.1). However, the premise of this approach is that an element of practice (for example, an object or intervention) can be isolated so that its effectiveness can be tested against a placebo or control group. This is not always possible – there can be ethical limitations on control groups, or perhaps the circumstances in which an intervention is used are key to its success – meaning

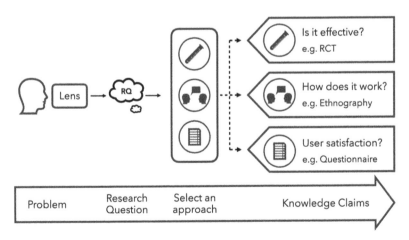

Figure 5.1 How research approaches shape knowledge claims.
© Sophie Park

that RCT-derived evidence may be limited, absent or inappropriate. Depending on your lens, this might lead you to conclude that something does not work, or to dismiss it as 'not evidence-based', simply because it has not been possible to demonstrate comparative effectiveness through RCT methodology. In other words, the lens you have adopted makes it easier for you to assume limitations in the practice or therapy, and harder for you to acknowledge the limitations of the methods used to evaluate it. Figure 5.1 shows how evidence is focused (and limited) by: (1) particular ways of framing something as 'a problem' to (2) address certain research questions and (3) produce particular knowledge claims.

A lens focused on this hierarchy (with RCTs and meta-analyses at the pinnacle) views generalist clinical practice as something of a 'wicked problem': one that is difficult or impossible to explain because of incomplete, contradictory and changing characteristics. Generalist practice becomes positioned as 'not evidence-based' and so minimal attention is given to studies on generalism, which often employ methods 'low' on Guyatt, Sackett and colleagues' hierarchy of evidence.

Generalism is about the situated implementation of care, the nuance of context and circumstance being key to its application and excellence. Generalists must identify and select suitable evidence where needed, to address a particular problem or question (4). How we do so is shaped by reflexive use of judgement and values.

Implementing knowledge in generalist practice requires us to use a range of evidence. This includes experiential 'bottom up' extrapolation of learning (from patients, our own practice, or others) about application and implementation of evidence in particular patient circumstances (sometimes referred to as 'clinical expertise'). Application of this evidence in future or elsewhere then draws upon this expertise and ability to use evidence. Our knowledge might need to be adapted; connected with a different set of knowledge; reframed; or re-chunked to make it relevant and useful to a different situation or patient. Evidence which produces theoretical insights about detailed and rich descriptive research, for example, can inform how we think and approach other situations. Similarly, case studies can equip us with a suite of evidence and possibilities from which to select and adapt practical 'know how'. We might integrate evidence with other knowledge about a particular patient and their preferences, shaping which evidence we select and how we use it to inform practice. This process is more than reproduction or 'knowledge retelling' and involves an active process of knowledge transformation or reconfiguration, to select, adapt and use evidence elsewhere. Rather than simple replication or reproduction, this requires active participation by the evidence user to critically engage in decision-making about which evidence to use, how and when (see also Figure 4.2).

Choosing evidence

We tend to think of evidence as unambiguous and definitive facts that inform good practice, national guidelines and patient pathways. However, whether or not a particular piece of evidence is useful right now depends on two things: the *nature* of the evidence and its 'internal validity' (how was this evidence constructed? – for example, the quality, research question scope, rigour with respect to methodological boundaries, funder) and its *relevance* or 'external validity': is it right for *this* patient *today*? (including patient population (mis)match, and provenance – for example, clinic setting).

Internal validity (how well was this study conducted?)

The *nature* of evidence concerns how and why it was produced. Ask yourself: were the methods used fitting for the questions being asked? Were the methods performed rigorously (within the methodological rules or norms of the approach used)? Are the knowledge claims a sensible fit for the approach taken (for example, effectiveness claims using a comparator)? Who produced the evidence and what were their motivating factors (for example, who funded the work)? What is the provenance of the evidence? Much the same as asking in a restaurant where the ingredients were sourced: does the provenance meet the practical, moral and ethical needs for this situation? So, for example, was the evidence sponsored or supported by a pharmaceutical company with a particular interest in promoting a certain condition as 'a problem', or in promoting their medication as a suitable 'solution' (5,6)? This may be declared in the 'conflicts of interest' or 'funder' sections of papers, but not always. How have the authors chosen to present the results to communicate a conservative or dramatic message, for example, have potential effects of treatment been amplified through presentation as 'relative risk', rather than 'absolute risk' figures (7,8)? 'Quality appraisal' assessments are typically built into decisions about inclusion in systematic reviews and practice guidelines. However, it is important to examine how such decisions were made. Many inclusion decisions are method-driven, reflecting Guyatt, Sackett and colleagues' hierarchy of what counts as 'legitimate' evidence to make effectiveness claims. Were they inclusive enough to inform your practice-based decision?

External validity (how applicable is this evidence to my patient or scenario)?

The second factor to consider is *situational relevance*. We often think of evidence as providing us with objective truth. However, its relevance and importance to your decision-making within clinical care is dependent upon how (or not) the evidence aligns with your particular clinical situation or question. To whom do the results of this trial apply (9)? Ask yourself about the relevance of the patient context to your situation. Is this evidence, for example, based upon the super-selection of a niche set of patients in tertiary care, or has the study been done within a population or primary care setting? How might the outcomes or recommendations be different depending on these factors and do the outcomes measured matter to the person in front of you?

Decisions about relevance can be quite complex. For example, a patient describes symptoms to you as a clinician which *could* represent a common, mild and self-limiting condition, but *could* represent a life-threatening event. You are likely to share with the patient the potential risks of investigation for the life-threatening event, but frame these as potentially worthwhile, given the risk of not detecting this condition (for example, chest pain being possible indigestion or myocardial infarction). If, however, the patient characteristics align only loosely with the available evidence about the prevalence of the life-threatening condition (for example, in a young non-smoker), a clinician may feel more reluctant to recommend exposure to potentially inconvenient or harmful medical intervention. These sorts of decisions involve inherent risk (what if I miss x?), but also potentially reduce risk for a patient through minimising exposure to invasive tests (complications, side effects, impact on missing work and so on).

Limiting scope: navigating overdiagnosis and over-investigation

Some conditions can present with vague or undifferentiated symptoms. Most patients presenting with such symptoms in a primary care setting are unlikely to have a particular disease. In the context of a tertiary clinic, this prevalence shifts – more patients are likely to have the disease. Retrospectively, it can seem obvious to the clinician and patient in tertiary care that earlier 'screening' or 'investigation' might have identified this condition sooner. The relevance of the evidence here is crucial, as the nature of the population in these two clinical settings is different. The side effects of screening an entire primary care patient population with similar vague symptoms are often collectively not worthwhile for the patients involved. This decision is based not only on resource allocation but also concerns about over-medicalisation and its short- and longer-term effects (for example, patients who have been investigated for one set of 'vague symptoms' are more likely to feel anxious about and present for investigation of subsequent similar symptoms (10)). Embarking on multiple sets of investigations without clinical imperative is unlikely to benefit the patient concerned (11).

There are multiple examples of an imperfect application of medicine to a population who *might* have a disease. Ductal carcinoma in situ (DCIS) of the breast is a common outcome detected during breast screening (12). The benefits of 'treating' this condition are contested, and tension arises here between individual and population-based decisions. At an individual level, a patient may feel that DCIS having been detected, should be removed (given the very small but potential risk of malignancy). A clinician, similarly, may have personal experience of seeing DCIS develop and so recommend lumpectomy to a patient. At a population level, however, the available evidence has been interpreted in different ways to justify or refute collective action for detected DCIS (13,14). Screening programmes can have both potential advantages and disadvantages. Evidence informing how something is done (or not), when, where and with whom, might vary depending upon how claims about 'effectiveness', 'success' or 'cancer' (for example, whether DCIS should be considered cancer in all sub-populations) are all defined and positioned within the research. Each might produce different thresholds for medicalising or treating certain patients with particular clinical features.

Interpretation of evidence involves value judgements. For example, lowering the diagnostic threshold for hypertension, chronic kidney disease (CKD) or diabetes. While there might be some potential benefits if examined through a particular set of circumstances (e.g. context of a stroke clinic), the benefits may be less clear-cut in a primary care context. Here, the patient might present more readily with short-term side effects and avoidance of medication due to polypharmacy, or falls and faints due to hypotensive episodes, or depression triggered by anxieties around mortality and being a burden to carers. The 'fact' becomes conditional in relation to its relevance to the particular circumstance of this patient at this point in time.

Working between the known and the unknown

Some clinicians (and patients) become very attached to the existence of evidence. In essence, if the evidence to support something does not exist (or is not available in a form familiar and accepted by them) then they do not wish to acknowledge the problem (or potential solutions) (15). It is important for clinicians to be critically reflexive about this ambiguous space. This space is dependent upon time and the nature of evidence the research community has thus far chosen or been able to gather (depending for example, on limitations of funding, feasibility or acceptability of methods). If 'no evidence' is said to currently exist to support particular claims, the clinician and patient are faced with decisions: could this be pattern x, which has been reported elsewhere but is not currently recognised by some, as no RCTs exist for this as a 'disease' (for example, chronic fatigue syndrome); might evidence in future suggest that this is a disease, or support particular management; or might this pattern of symptoms remain a set of symptoms with no identifiable cause (nevertheless causing discomfort or distress to the patient involved)? In order to work productively with patients in this space, clinicians need to be critically reflexive (16), have open discussions with patients about the limitations of the available evidence, and be willing to think creatively with patients about ways to tackle situations where little or no evidence is available, without dismissing the existence of a patient's symptoms ('because there is no evidence'). This conversation needs to be balanced to avoid over-medicalisation, but recognise the potential of a clinician to 'hold' symptoms *with* a patient and attempt to address these wherever possible, regardless of cause.

Using familiar evidence versus finding new evidence

Some evidence is used repeatedly as part of a clinician's regular repertoire of clinical practice, perhaps to inform a conversation about the pros and cons of statins, or the impact of diet on reducing diabetes. Other evidence might feel less embedded in the clinicians' tacit knowledge, and require clarification or checking each time it is used or encountered. For both, it can be useful to re-check or confirm that no new relevant or contrasting evidence exists. This requires us to see evidence production and engagement as an ongoing and routine part of clinical practice. Searching for evidence can be a useful tool to integrate into discussions with some patients (or to share as a resource after a discussion).

The nature of evidence used may vary between clinicians or patient/carer audiences. Selecting something to inform a discussion which is accessible, rigorous and reliable can be challenging. Often secondary sources of evidence might be used which summarise information, rather than sharing or using primary sources. This process of summarising involves interpretation, and it is important to ensure you are happy with the way in which this has been done, before sharing a link with others.

This process might require some background work to become familiar with certain narratives about the value of a particular piece of evidence to inform practice, but also with a range of ways and resources to share this information (17).

Navigating uncertainty

Uncertainty is an important part of clinical practice and learning. Uncertainty can be positioned as a knowledge deficit (for example, as mentioned earlier in relation to missing or incomplete evidence) and therefore experienced as discomfort, inadequacy or tension. Uncertainty can, however, be a productive and creative space. Within EBM, this is where clinical expertise, patient values and good humanistic judgement come in. A clinician can navigate and implement knowledge to adapt to the particular situation in front of them: a particular patient, situation or unanticipated challenge. This requires individual-level, real-time adaptations and adjustments within practice in the face of partial, incomplete or multiple forms of knowledge. It involves recognising, appreciating and balancing available knowledge; recognising the existence of gaps; and maximising opportunities to make suitable connections between what is known and the current situation. This process is situated and therefore not fixed, and not possible to predict in advance. It can, however, be informed by particular sets of prepared values or moral accountability (18): a commitment, for example, to work towards achieving what appears at that time to be in the best interests of a patient, within the bounds of current possibilities.

While there has been much research on and many analytic models of how learners experience uncertainty (e.g. 19,20,21,22,23,24), a central theme has been the shift from individual defeatism or 'lackism' of the novice learner towards a position of expertise where the individual is part of a connected network or web of knowledge. The clinician can begin to decipher what they do not know; has confidence to focus where in the network to explore; then shares possibilities for action with the patient, based on the (potentially incomplete) knowledge they are able to ascertain. There is therefore expertise related to not only knowing (or not) about a particular knowledge topic or content, but also in knowing how to position oneself within wider networks and communities of knowledge, keeping connected and up to date with new developments and changes.

The generalist is at the intersection between their professional web of knowledge and a web of knowledge about *this* patient, acquired perhaps through continuity and care of their family and community. This familiarity with the personal situation and experiences of the individual patient shapes, for example, the clinician's confidence in their account and a nuanced application of professional knowledge to this patient's situation. Both professional and patient webs of knowledge have limits, and the clinician requires trust and self-compassion to have the confidence to acknowledge something is unknown (by self or the community); to distinguish between self and community uncertainties; and to recognise, accept and act in the face of uncertainty.

One important tool to tackle this challenge is curiosity. An openness within clinical practice enables clinicians to actively listen to patients, to recognise and utilise the knowledge(s) they bring, and to collectively act together with what available knowledge(s) they have. A second tool is critical reflexivity, encouraging the clinician to sustain and use a questioning approach in their practice: to avoid assumptions, or at least to be aware when they are making assumptions, and to use this same criticality in their engagement with others (peers, patients and so on). Thirdly, the clinician can actively embrace a range of knowledge forms, moving fluidly and dynamically between different knowledge lenses or paradigms. So, while an area may remain an 'unknown unknown' using one particular lens (for example, biomedical), it is possible to identify, explore and address it using a different lens or approach.

Applying evidence in practice

Integrating different forms of knowledge (for example, biomedical and biographical) extends from the initial problem-setting with a patient (see Chapter 1) into the implementation stage of the clinical interaction: selecting what is relevant to this situation, for this patient, at this point in time. Here we find that the problem to solve (and hence the solution to it) are not predefined but often enmeshed, complex, incomplete or unknown. There is considerable intellectual movement and work done within the patient–clinician interaction to draw upon and integrate a range of potential knowledge. This includes how problems have been constructed or deconstructed; the overlap or conflict between identified problems; differing thresholds for naming something as a problem; identified priorities; and alignment (or dissonance) between experiential values and biomedical or standardised guideline approaches. While this complex intellectual activity can be invisible to the observer, it becomes vividly available to those actively involved in and adopting responsibility within clinical interactions (25).

To illustrate this, let's take an assumption of linear healthcare: that, provided a clinician can identify the relevant evidence or guideline, it will tell them exactly what to do for this patient. Predetermined healthcare pathways are relevant in their entirety in some circumstances. We will use an example (see also Example 18.1).

Example 5.1: Mrs Joper

Mrs Joper attends a follow-up appointment to discuss her X-ray report. It shows no evidence of fracture, but mentions osteopenic (bone-thinning) changes and recommends further investigation for possible osteoporosis. Mrs Joper is a carer for her husband and doesn't drive, so is reluctant to travel to the hospital for appointments. She knows her mother had osteoporosis and is keen to minimise her future risk of fracture (primary prevention). The clinician can see two available UK-based guidelines written by NICE (English National Institute for Health and Care Excellence) and SIGN (Scottish Intercollegiate Guidelines Network). Their recommendations for how to identify osteoporosis (for example, using a fracture online risk assessment tool, or DEXA – dual energy X-ray absorption – bone scan) differ. So too do the recommended thresholds for treatment and length of treatment. Mrs Joper and the clinician reflect upon the values shaping each guideline: NICE is using a measure of cost-effectiveness to determine what to prioritise and the recommended action, whereas SIGN is prioritising patient outcomes. Mrs Joper is not keen to attend hospital for a bone scan. They use the Qfracture online risk tool as this definitely has her ethnic group included in the data. Her risk score is 10 per cent, which puts her into the NICE risk category. Mrs Joper decides that, based on their discussions, she will try medication (bisphosphonates), but if she experiences side effects (for example, heartburn) then she will stop the tablets and opt for a DEXA scan to inform next steps.

Why wasn't there one outcome or answer? NICE or SIGN make their recommendations using *different value systems*, in this case cost-effectiveness versus patient outcomes. These value judgements are based on serving 'populations' rather than individuals, often as a way of rationing or allocating finite resources within a healthcare system. At the time of writing, the research community has yet to conduct a perfect study to inform practice and, indeed, such a study may not even be possible: Mrs Joper is not a 'textbook' case (if such a case exists) where rules are clear and straightforward. Instead, clinicians must be able to judge and adapt available evidence to meet the particular needs of the patient in front of them, bringing together areas of relevant knowledge, while also acknowledging gaps and uncertainty.

The collective claims of a research study can never be comprehensive or universally relevant: researchers must focus on specific questions and outcomes, and select only certain members of the population to take part. For example, a study might limit the inclusion of patients to those with a single known clinical condition (avoiding those with multiple diseases), or only recruit patient groups who speak and read one language. The result is that the people included in the studies are not necessarily representative of wider groups; they are often younger and healthier, and participation is limited for patients from particular ethnic and cultural groups or those with learning difficulties or disabilities. The evidence is inevitably conditional, but often gives an illusion of collective truth: 'we know x about patients who have condition y'. Similarly, it might not be clear how to resolve a tension or contradiction between guidance about how to manage two co-existing conditions experienced by the same patient.

In generalist practice, we are constantly responding to the identified needs of each patient so that we can apply available knowledge in an acceptable, relevant way. This means that we must dispel the idea of 'standardised practice', because it omits much of the complex decision-making of how and when we apply appropriate rules and knowledge. One result of this is a paradox whereby the patient (and society more generally) expects all patients should have access to the same care, while individually wanting their care to be adapted to their context and needs. In other words, there is an expectation of *equality* (same care for all) but, in fact, most want *equity* – that is, equal opportunity to reach the same outcome by different means, or to reach a different, but more suitable outcome.

Informing collective practice through sharing situated knowledge

Guidelines and standards are not wrong (26) and can be extremely helpful in informing clinical practice, as a starting point, a reference or an aide-mémoire. However, recognising their limitations is crucial to sustainable, person-centred clinical care. To share the dilemmas clinicians encounter when faced with incomplete knowledge requires a safe space where they can express a vulnerability with trusted individuals who will judge these elements of practice within a broader frame of the acceptable limits of clinical practice and learning. To articulate these dilemmas, clinicians need a language that is regarded by the community as legitimate within professional boundaries. They require professionals to act with moral principles which prioritise the flourishing of patients, self and society. These cannot be standardised as they will differ for every patient a clinician meets. To use this moral compass to inform practice requires individuals and society to place trust in clinicians. We cannot remove this need for trust through attempts at standardising practice. Rather, governance approaches can either attempt to make these dilemmas invisible, or produce spaces to make them explicitly visible and explore them creatively and collectively (Table 5.1).

Table 5.1 Approaches to clinical practice and learning where use of evidence is ambiguous

Generalist Capability	Example
Curiosity and Open Mindset Being inclusive about different lenses (e.g. biomedical, experiential) which hold value at particular times as most relevant and important. This lens preference informs what evidence options appear good or legitimate.	If a clinician approaches a clinical dilemma using a lens of person-centredness to approach care, they will likely use factors most important to the person to inform their decision. In contrast, if the clinician uses a biomedical lens, they will utilise disease-based facts and knowledge to judge what appears to be the best possible course of action. These are often not mutually exclusive, but might require discussion if there are potential contradictions or tensions.
Critical Reflexivity Noticing what forms of knowledge and evidence we are particularly drawn towards or attached to. Are we preferencing one above another, and if so why? Can we move between these flexibly to adjust to the needs of the patient in front of us?	Put 10 clinicians in a consultation with a patient and all would likely do something slightly different. This is fine, but we need to safety net this flexibility with an ongoing self-critique about how and why we draw upon certain evidence or knowledge in particular ways. This 'second head' (27) helps question how we feel and think, and how this informs and shapes what we do. Once we are able to articulate these for ourselves, we can become curious about and appreciate how others think, feel or make sense of a situation.

(continued)

Table 5.1 (Cont.)

Generalist Capability	Example
	This process is essential if we are moving between and using a variety of evidence and knowledge forms. While each is different (i.e. cannot be directly compared), we need each time to consider its suitability and relevance to inform decision-making. How and why are we doing this? How might this impact patient care? How is this informing or limiting the ways in which we and others make sense of a situation? Might additional forms of knowledge or evidence strengthen our approach?
Agile movement between knowledge and evidence forms We move between, across and configure different forms of evidence, akin to making a jigsaw (28). This helps produce new insights, questions or reframing of problems. A gap or 'wicked problem' through one lens might appear different through another. This agility can help us find and agree a management plan now, while agreeing safety nets and future review.	If something feels unsolvable or unknown (at least in part) using one approach, we might reframe the issue through a different lens. This makes visible new opportunities or challenges and makes available different evidence or knowledge to help us to unpick or reframe problems in different or complementary ways. Each time, we evaluate the relevance of the evidence or knowledge to the current situation and select a way forward, drawing upon what appears to be most rigorous in its relevance and applicability to this interaction at this point in time. This requires us to explore and consider different forms of evidence which are not comparable, but potentially important in different ways (e.g. RCT and patient experience). We need to consider both, appraise the value and limitations of each, and use what is helpful in relation to the present situation or dilemma. This ability supports consideration of more than one form of evidence at one point in time, including review of its utility and relevance over time.

Rather than using a single (for example, biomedical) lens, governance groups could discuss a range of lenses, perhaps explaining why they might do things differently in different circumstances. They could still produce a document on good practice, but it would no longer be a hierarchy; instead you would see a selection of case studies which articulate different ways in which a problem might be approached, with contextual factors describing how and when to utilise each.

You can now imagine a practitioner is reaching for some guidance on how to tackle a particular clinical problem. There are no explicit guidelines, but there is a consensus document. It may take longer to read through and digest case studies than it does the bullet list of generalised recommendations for a given condition. However, case studies can allow patient and clinician to discuss the range of options the experts share, selecting those elements which appear most relevant to this patient and present situation. This can build trust and confidence to both recognise gaps and implement the available evidence. The outcome achieved might be similar to a generalised recommendation, but could be very different. Either way, the process and experience of patient and clinician will differ: one approach reinforcing a clinician's deficiencies, and another their capabilities.

Conclusion

In this chapter we have talked about what knowledge is, and how certain types of that knowledge are regularly valued over others. This hegemony contributes to making many important aspects of generalist practice invisible in standards and/or governance documents. As a result, the clinical community has tended to limit its focus towards research which objectifies and reduces practice, seeking to make generalisable or comparative claims. While these studies have a role, they do not represent the full array of clinical judgement regularly required to adapt evidence to the individual context of patients in practice. This creates a dissonance for clinicians seeking to fulfil standardised aspirations of care, while having to limit application and use of these forms of knowledge in practice. Similarly, it produces challenges for clinicians and patients attempting to integrate a range of knowledge to inform clinical care.

If we can be more inclusive in our appreciation of knowledge relevant to clinical practice, embracing some of the more agile, flexible and elastic aspects of knowledge application in practice, this will support clinicians to legitimise and develop ways to adapt evidence for local contexts. Furthermore, an inclusive approach to knowledge might also encourage production of evidence which examines a fuller range and breadth of clinical practice to include some of the more situated aspects of care. If we can learn to feed this knowledge about how situated care is done back into collective professional knowledge systems, then we can further develop generalist practice. This could utilise a broader, relevant field of evidence and create more agile, responsive learning systems to inform clinical practice.

References

1. Greenhalgh T. *How to Read a Paper: The basics of evidence-based medicine*. John Wiley & Sons; 2014.
2. Guyatt GH, Sackett DL, Sinclair JC, Hayward R, Cook DJ, Cook RJ, et al. Users' guides to the medical literature: IX. A method for grading health care recommendations. *JAMA*. 1995;274(22):1800–4.
3. Guyatt GH, Oxman AD, Vist GE, Kunz R, Falck-Ytter Y, Alonso-Coello P, et al. GRADE: an emerging consensus on rating quality of evidence and strength of recommendations. *BMJ*. 2008;336(7650):924.
4. Masic I, Miokovic M, Muhamedagic B. Evidence based medicine – new approaches and challenges. *Acta Inform Medica AIM J Soc Med Inform Bosnia Herzeg Cas Drustva Za Med Inform BiH*. 2008;16(4):219–25.
5. Moynihan R, Heath I, Henry D. Selling sickness: the pharmaceutical industry and disease mongering. *BMJ*. 2002;324(7342):886.
6. Heath I. Overdiagnosis: when good intentions meet vested interests – an essay by Iona Heath. *BMJ*. 2013;347.
7. Byrne P, Cullinan J, Smith SM. Statins for primary prevention of cardiovascular disease. *BMJ*. 2019;367.
8. Gigerenzer G, Wegwarth O, Feufel M. Misleading communication of risk. *BMJ*. 2010;341.
9. Rothwell PM. External validity of randomised controlled trials: 'to whom do the results of this trial apply?' *The Lancet*. 2005;365(9453):82–93.
10. Salmon P, Humphris GM, Ring A, Davies JC, Dowrick CF. Primary care consultations about medically unexplained symptoms: patient presentations and doctor responses that influence the probability of somatic intervention. *Psychosom Med*. 2007;69(6):571–7.
11. Bass C, Mayou R. Chest pain. *BMJ*. 2002;325(7364):588.
12. McCartney M, Armstrong N, Martin G, Nunan D, Richards O, Sullivan F. 'Delicate diagnosis': avoiding harms in difficult, disputed, and desired diagnoses. *Br J Gen Pract*. 2022;72(725):580–1.
13. Maxwell AJ, Hilton B, Clements K, Dodwell D, Dulson-Cox J, Kearins O, et al. Unresected screen-detected ductal carcinoma in situ: Outcomes of 311 women in the Forget-Me-Not 2 study. *The Breast*. 2022;61:145–55.
14. Barratt A. Overdiagnosis in mammography screening: a 45 year journey from shadowy idea to acknowledged reality. *BMJ*. 2015;350:h867.
15. Greenhalgh T. Miasmas, mental models and preventive public health: some philosophical reflections on science in the COVID-19 pandemic. *Interface Focus*. 2021;11(6):20210017.
16. Park S, Bansal A, Owen EC. Well-being, burnout and value fulfilment: Let us situate individuals within systems. *Med Educ*. 2023;57(3):208–10.
17. MacWalter G, McKay J, Bowie P. Utilisation of internet resources for continuing professional development: a cross-sectional survey of general practitioners in Scotland. *BMC Med Educ*. 2016;16(1):24.
18. Bansal A, Greenley S, Mitchell C, Park S, Shearn K, Reeve J. Optimising planned medical education strategies to develop learners' person-centredness: a realist review. *Med Educ*. 2022;56(5):489–503.
19. Fox RG. Training for uncertainty. In: *The Student-Physician: Introductory studies in the sociology of medical education*. Harvard University Press; 1957. pp. 207–42.

20. Simpson DE, Dalgaard KA, O'Brien DK. Student and faculty assumptions about the nature of uncertainty in medicine and medical education. *J Fam Pr*. 1986;23(5):468–72.

21. Beresford EB. Uncertainty and the shaping of medical decisions. *Hastings Cent Rep*. 1991;21(4):6–11.

22. Pilpel D, Schor R, Benbassat J. Barriers to acceptance of medical error: the case for a teaching programme. *Med Educ*. 1998;32(1):3–7.

23. Lingard L, Garwood K, Schryer CF, Spafford MM. A certain art of uncertainty: case presentation and the development of professional identity. *Soc Sci Med*. 2003;56(3):603–16.

24. Park S. Embracing uncertainty within medical education. In: Giardino AP, Giardino ER, editors. *Medical Education: Global perspectives, challenges and future directions*. Nova Science Publishers. 2013. pp. 288–313.

25. Atkinson P. In cold blood: bedside teaching in a medical school. In: Chanan Gabriel, Delamont S, editors. *Frontiers of Classroom Research*. NFER; 1975. pp. 163–182.

26. Gabbay J, May A le. Evidence based guidelines or collectively constructed 'mindlines?' Ethnographic study of knowledge management in primary care. *BMJ*. 2004;329(7473):1013.

27. Neighbour R. *The Inner Consultation: How to develop an effective and intuitive consulting style*. Radcliffe Publishing; 2005.

28. Gough D, Oliver S, Thomas J. *An Introduction to Systematic Reviews*. SAGE; 2012.

Part II: Educational approaches

The second part of this book (Chapters 6 and 7) explores generalist approaches to clinical education. The clinical knowledge of a generalist is, by its very nature, dynamic and responsive. In this part, therefore, we consider how the principles of generalism articulated in Chapter 1 can be taught, learned and assessed, and how these principles inform approaches to education.

6
Education for clinical generalism

Sophie Park, Kay Leedham-Green and Ben Jackson

Introduction

In Chapter 1, we looked at generalism as a philosophy of practice. We began to explore how generalist knowledge is not fixed, but alive and dynamic: responsive and adaptive to current identified needs. We described in Chapter 2 how generalists work successfully within this unboundaried knowledge space to address all types of problems at all stages of life, working collaboratively and drawing on external expertise as needed. In Chapters 4 and 5 we explored how the implementation of generalist knowledge within clinical practice is often not a linear process, but one with multiple possible pathways, co-constructed between the patient and their healthcare professional according to individual needs and preferences.

There are of course parallels between approaches in generalist practice and the approaches that support learning about generalism, as these are underpinned by the same philosophy. Generalist principles to education apply at all educational stages of a clinician's career arc as the emphasis gradually shifts from full-time learning, to service provision, to leadership and teaching.

We argue that generalist learning is optimally facilitated through holistic clinical workplace-based experiences and patient-based learning. Clinical debrief and 'critical reflexivity' are employed to explore unmet patient needs and co-construct learners' educational needs (1). Learning *through* practice is supplemented by responsive study and adaptive strategies for addressing personal learning goals so that the relevant knowledge necessary to optimise clinical outcomes is *connected* with dynamic patient and population needs. Learners are engaged as partners in, rather than as recipients of, education.

We begin by thinking about the nature of generalist knowledge (what is being learned) and how educational systems enable or inhibit how that knowledge is shared, communicated or exchanged (the process of learning). Although we touch on assessment, this is covered in more detail in Chapter 7. Whether you are a teacher, learner or clinician (or perhaps all three), we hope this chapter will enable you to consider opportunities for sharing and building generalist knowledge and suggest strategies to mitigate and overcome any challenges.

Learning is sometimes thought to be a unidirectional and didactic transfer of pre-existing knowledge from teacher to learner ('telling'). Similarly, knowledge is sometimes presented as a 'universal truth', to be learned. These perspectives create discrete power dynamics between 'the knower' and 'the receiver' of knowledge. This can disempower the learner as a passive observer or recipient, rather than as an active contributor to the production of knowledge. Similarly, we tend to think about apprenticeship learning as a linear progression, with novices at one end and experts at the other. These 'pre-set', hierarchical perspectives on learning often suggest that there is one right way to acquire knowledge and a pre-defined, ideal outcome at the end of the learning process.

We invite you to think differently: to imagine knowledge and learning as dynamic and flexible. First, knowledge is often 'situated'; either adapted, or unique to a particular social or physical setting. Second, knowledge is 'interactional'; co-produced locally through exchanges between people. These perspectives open up a whole set of possibilities for thinking about what knowledge is; where it is located; how it is produced; and how it is shared and developed. It also moves our view of learners from being positioned within pre-set levels towards a more fluid appreciation of expertise dependent on the situation and individual and system requirements.

Within this dynamic view of learning, knowledge becomes 'distributed' between those involved in its co-production. Learning becomes participatory and dependent upon the learner, their teacher, the patient and the environment in which they are interacting (2,3).

Knowledge content: what is to be learned?

Some forms of knowledge are explicit and easy to categorise. As discussed in Chapter 4, these are sometimes referred to as 'codified' knowledge (4). An example of codified knowledge might be which childhood vaccinations are recommended for which ages? This knowledge is clearly defined by current guidelines and relatively easy to describe and assess. In clinical practice, however, knowledge is often broader, more complex and conditional upon the circumstances in which it is used. It therefore needs to be adapted to meet those particular circumstances. For example, negotiating childhood vaccinations with hesitant parents. Here, required knowledge might include knowing which health visitor is best to ask for advice (situated), what approaches work best when engaging in conversation about previous experiences of side effects (experiential and narrative), approaches to negotiation and inclusion (interactional), and how health beliefs might be understood or challenged (theoretical). Generalist solutions to problems are therefore seldom fully codified because every person and situation is different, and there are likely to be competing theoretical understandings. Generalist expertise involves implementing codified (e.g. biomedical) knowledge *alongside* other expertise.

Roger Kneebone, in his essay on crossing knowledge paradigms (5), talks about some of the difficulties learners (and indeed educators) may encounter when moving from a fixed idea of knowledge to a more unboundaried concept of what needs to be learned. This disorientation happens when learners and educators begin to recognise the 'complex amalgam of factual knowledge, personal experience, anecdote and empathy, played out against a background of professionalism and underpinned by a sense of care and compassion' that is involved in clinical practice. It also involves recognising that many so-called testable 'facts' and indeed 'competencies' are not fixed but socially constructed: for example, competing clinical guidelines based on different social or economic values (6), or competency-based assessments that do not reflect the complexities of practice (7).

Generalist knowledge and ways of knowing and practising are expansive. There are multiple available forms of knowledge (for example, biomedical, experiential, relational, experimental, procedural, social, behavioural, political, narrative) for the clinician to recognise or use. The process of implementing knowledge is interpretative and adaptive, informed by theories, values and frameworks, and there is therefore not 'one truth'. A patient rarely comes with a predefined condition and leaves with a quick-fix solution to that problem. Rather, their symptoms and concerns are interpreted in relation to causal factors, their environment and concurrent concerns and conditions, as well as future potential concerns. Attending to the psychosocial does not mean ignoring biomedical aspects of the presentation, nor does attending to the biomedical mean rejecting the psychosocial. Rather, the generalist considers additional and complementary approaches and interprets each in the light of the other.

Once we acknowledge that knowledge comes in multiple shapes and sizes, we can embrace the idea that valuable knowledge will be located across different settings and individuals. For example, patients or carers might become recognised as educators, able to share their expertise about living with a condition or their experience of care. A learning conversation moves from 'delivery of information' to an exchange which recognises the pre-existing knowledge of the learner, as well as the fallibility and ongoing learning needs of the teacher. Knowledge becomes ever-developing, rather than an end point. The process of learning moves from acquisition of 'the right answer' to inviting a dialogue or exchange of mutual learning that acknowledges different perspectives. This shifts the desired or expected outcome of a clinical learning event from memorising guidelines towards achieving an appropriate solution for unique conditions, priorities and circumstances.

The work of generalists involves integrating biomedical knowledge with other complex ways of knowing. These include negotiation of:

- What might work for this person in this context (for example, particular circumstance or situation, consideration of gaps)?
- What has worked for similar people in similar contexts (for example, previous experience of self or other)?
- What frameworks might inform our approach to their problem (for example, how we value or position one thing as more important over another)?

After exploring challenges to generalist learning, we discuss potential opportunities and strategies.

Challenges to generalist learning

The elevation of biomedical knowledge

Medicine has a long-established and persistent division between 'preclinical' (scientific) and 'clinical' (practical) knowledge. This shapes dominant and persisting approaches to medical education, including the ways institutions locate certain knowledge in particular settings and people (for example, university or clinical placement). This division is attributed to Flexner (8), who in the early 1900s proposed a model for medical training, comprising two years 'pre-clinical' training in biomedical sciences such as anatomy and physiology, followed by at least two years of clinical experiences. This divide of university-based and clinic-based knowledge has permeated medical curricula internationally for over a century. This maintains that learners must become sufficiently familiar with biomedical knowledge, before they can learn how to apply this in practice with patients. This perspective suggests that relevant knowledge is learned separately from patients, and then applied (or done) to them. We argue that this is a counterproductive source of polarisation and separation that perpetuates the Cartesian split between mind and body. We propose a more collaborative, integrative approach between places of knowledge production, places of learning and places of clinical practice.

Compartmentalised learning

Within clinical education, the 'pre-clinical years' tend to be compartmentalised around body (dys)functions (for example, physiology, pharmacology, pathology) or body systems (for example, cardiology, neurology). Similarly, clinical experiences tend to rotate through a series of discrete specialty placements, with sequential assessment about each discipline at the end of each placement or year. Almost exclusively, these rotations have tended to focus on hospital-based experiences (and their expertise around diseases or body parts) rather than community or primary care (and their expertise in universal and comprehensive patient care). Annemarie Mol argues that, from an early stage, learners are taught to see patients through the lens of compartmentalised disciplines, organs or diseases (9). Other knowledge becomes less visible to the learner: for example, learning about a patient's journey across health and illness, the interactions between diseases they experience, or their movement between clinical services. Isabel Menzies Lyth describes the dissonance this creates for staff in caring for an individual as a holistic whole. She argues that compartmentalisation of patients and practices into components or tasks can be construed as a mitigation against the potential anxiety arising from, or emotional work related to, personal and subjective connections between practitioner and patient (10).

The relegation of experiential knowledge of illness

This compartmentalisation within learning and practice raises questions. If learners become familiar with a set of predefined knowledge before, rather than alongside, their interactions with patients, this can shape their long-term use and preference for certain forms of knowledge over others. Some associate this separation with paternalistic, protocolised approaches to clinical practice, policy and research with the delegitimisation of more person-centred approaches (11). For example, teaching learners to focus exclusively on anatomy, physiology, pathology and pharmacology at the beginning of their studies can make it harder for them to notice, acknowledge and respond to other forms of knowledge, which might be equally, if not more, important to the patient. If the biomedical lens is only part of the potentially relevant knowledge that informs clinical practice, then it is perhaps counterproductive to forefront this incomplete knowledge in isolation so early in a clinical learner's education.

Combine this focus on disease-based knowledge with assessments that encourage early learners to preference fixed notions of knowledge – for example, through single-best-answer questions – and we create the conditions for learners to develop a very limited, deductive engagement with patients. The developing clinician focuses on knowledge they have been told is most legitimate (pharmacology, pathology, protocols and so on) and uses this to frame their attention during their patient interactions. Forms of knowledge that do not fit their assessment paradigm, such as the humanities, communication and social sciences, become deprioritised. Elevating biomedical ways of knowing can produce a power discrepancy between clinicians and their patients, dismissing other knowledge – for example, the knowledge brought by the patient, the knowledge that is co-constructed during the encounter, and the theories that might inform the interaction – as less important.

Insulating learners from the hidden work of generalists

There is an educational tension between the delivery of discrete codified, accessible 'pots' of knowledge and the need to integrate, connect, transform and implement knowledge in practice. An assumption within the Flexnerian model is that learners can develop a series of knowledge 'pots', and then work out how to connect and apply them: which pot to use when, and how the pots might relate to one another. This produces challenges when a patient brings undifferentiated symptoms such as 'tired all the time' or 'out of sorts', or when people have multiple complex conditions or enduring symptoms or disabilities (see Chapter 18 on multimorbidity). Sometimes clinical educators attempt to protect learners from these complex and potentially overwhelming 'presentations' by preselecting or limiting the focus of a learner–patient interaction – for example, by triaging less complex patients for learners, or focusing on a specific curriculum topic, or detaching the learner from the clinical management process.

These attempts to predefine the learning encounter position the clinical teacher as 'the knower' in relation to the learner, and the patients' symptoms become a puzzle to be correctly solved through some advance preparation. While these more concrete and discrete ways of teaching can provide a sense of incremental growth and control, they can also produce a counterproductive illusion of simplicity, or devalue the situated nature of illness and disease, effectively hiding the complexity of generalism: 'I have already seen a case of COPD, so don't need to see another', or 'that patient isn't relevant to my learning, as they don't have a formal disease diagnosis'. At worst it can promote a situation where people presenting with real suffering that is difficult to codify are dismissed as irrelevant or peripheral to clinical education priorities, perpetuating the problem for future patient interactions. Similarly, separating diagnosis from management can insulate learners from complex challenges around the suitability and clinical need for treatment and referral beyond simple guidelines and referral pathways.

Before proposing generalist solutions to some of these challenges, we share an example of a generalist community of learning based in primary care.

Example 6.1: The Village Practice (an educational community of practice in primary care)

The Village Practice has four general practitioners, two practice nurses, a link worker, an apprentice healthcare assistant, a practice manager and several administrators. The local university sends four undergraduate medical students who come every Tuesday for a year, and two graduate doctors in training who rotate every six months. The university provides teacher development and an annual educational conference.

The four undergraduate medical students have broad learning outcomes specified by their university, as well as project work and 'sign-offs', but the university is flexible as to how these outcomes are achieved. Each pair of medical students sees two or three patients from that day's list who have agreed to longer 'teaching appointments' at booking. The students spend up to 40 minutes with each patient before inviting their GP supervisor to debrief with the patient and check any clinical decisions. At the end of the session, they reflect together and agree on personal learning goals. For the rest of the day, they work in pairs on a 'community action project', or see one of their 'longitudinal patients'. These patients are people with multimorbidity who have agreed to share their experiences with students. The students visit them at home several times over the year, helping them identify an achievable change that might make a difference, and supporting them in making it happen. Students debrief with their supervisor after each visit and sometimes act as the patient's advocate with the social prescribing link worker. Their community action projects are adapted from a list of university suggestions: one pair is evaluating a local walking group; the other is doing an inhaler recycling project. Their project posters will be assessed at the university's annual teacher conference and presented at the practice learning group.

The two graduate doctors have seven clinics and three education sessions each week. Each clinic is three hours long and they see around 12 patients followed by a GP-led debrief where they collaboratively review decisions, discuss any unmet patient needs, and identify knowledge gaps and learning goals. Evidence of engagement and progress towards learning goals is stored in their e-portfolio. One of their education sessions is at the local university with other trainees; the other two are self-directed. They are currently practising for an upcoming 'simulated consultation assessment' (see Chapter 7) so they analyse their most interesting or challenging consultations together.

The apprentice healthcare assistant is being trained by the practice nurse in phlebotomy, vaccination, ECGs, spirometry, anticoagulation and routine monitoring. They are currently learning how to support the chronic condition reviews that happen before personalised care-planning appointments (see Chapter 18). Once their 18-month apprenticeship period is over, they intend to stay on at the practice.

The practice manager organises a fortnightly practice learning group over an extended lunch break. Everyone attends, including their patient participation group. Anyone can suggest a topic for learning or improvement and upvote the topics that interest them. Recent topics have included: continuity of care, trauma-informed care, the appointment booking system, shared decision-making, responding to feedback, social prescribing, advances in smoking cessation, and responding to mental health crises. After each meeting, everyone commits to an action which is reviewed at subsequent meetings. They finish by agreeing on the next topic and an educational strategy: perhaps an article or video for discussion, a learner-led workshop, or inviting patients and carers to share their experiences and co-design improvements.

Reflective questions

We invite you to reflect on how the principles of generalism are enacted in this example. What diverse knowledge forms are included? How is new knowledge co-created in ways that are responsive and agile to clinical needs? How are collaborative practices and distributed expertise reflected? How are research, practice, patients and learning connected? From an educational perspective, what structures support effortful learning, meaningful feedback and personalised approaches to learning? How are teachers and learners developing together?

Opportunities and strategies for generalist learning

We now discuss some of the potential strategies for enabling learning that support authentic generalist approaches to clinical practice. Generalism is a situated practice, informed by and connected with scholarly resources and evidence. This includes knowledge about people, places and local systems as well as the biomedical, social and behavioural sciences. It is key, therefore, that learning about generalism includes a close and integrated connection between clinical practice (service delivery) and learning.

Assessments that support generalist learning

John Biggs reminds us that educators often start by defining what is to be learned, then design associated teaching strategies, and last of all, create assessments to check what has been learned (12). Learners, on the other hand, tend to focus on what is to be assessed. They see their assessments *as* the curriculum, and focus their learning activities accordingly. The trick, then, is to create assessments that align with the knowledge and competencies that patients, experts and other stakeholders need learners to acquire and use (3): assessment *for* learning, rather than simply *of* learning.

Nowhere is the divide between expansive generalist knowledge and boundaried biomedical teaching made more obvious than within assessment practices. When assessing clinical learning, written papers for high-stakes examinations are increasingly machine-marked formats such as multiple-choice, or single-best-answer (13), implying an objective single-best approach to patient problems. Practical examinations test isolated procedures, such as examining an abdomen, with objective structured mark sheets, implying a right or wrong (rather than responsive) way of practising. High-stakes examinations, such as the UK Medical Licensing Assessment (MLA), specify the types of patient problems and procedures that might appear in the assessment (14), implying a finite amount of knowledge that means one is 'prepared for practice'. What does this assessment paradigm say about how we value critical thinking about different approaches to clinical practice? Or adaptive approaches to meet patient needs or context? Or working safely when the answer is uncertain? Or team-based practice? Or relationship-based care? These assessment challenges are further explored in Chapter 7.

Positivistic approaches to assessment can convey dissonant messages to learners and teachers about the value of 'top-down' knowledge standards (for example, being able to recall management guidelines) versus 'bottom-up' experiential learning through patient encounters (for example, being able to implement guidelines with a patient where the diagnosis is currently uncertain, or where the patient has other complex needs). There is a risk that assessments drive learners to focus on rote memorisation and repetitive practising of decontextualised skills where, for example, the abdominal examination becomes a performance rather than a genuine diagnostic tool. Brian Hodges reminds us to be critically aware of the dominant discourses that frame our approaches to assessment. Poorly aligned assessments might create the illusion of competence but may risk inadvertently driving incompetence (7). The purpose of assessment is not just to assess simple description or reproduction of learning. Rather, assessment can drive meaningful learning through stimulating knowledge transformation or consolidation.

Immersive workplace-based learning

Generalism invites an authentic approach to learning through clinical interactions so that learning is responsive to patient needs. Paul Atkinson describes the distinction between learner–patient encounters which are filtered (which he calls 'cold') and encounters which are contemporaneous with a patient's clinical care and healthcare journey (which he calls 'hot') (15) – see Figure 6.1. Cold learning is predetermined, producing an impression of certainty or 'the right answer' to be uncovered. Hot learning, for us, is workplace-based learning at its best. A learner meets with a patient early in their clinical care, rather than 'clerking' them after they have been 'processed'. This maximises opportunities for active engagement in the clinical process and learner contributions to care (supported according to their capabilities). A learner can explore diagnostic possibilities and uncertainties, while considering a wider range of diverse patient needs.

Facilitated debrief and reflection about the patient encounter can stimulate further self-directed learning. The learner can become familiar with a broad range of reasons for attendance, not all of which fit the 'diagnose, treat, cure' paradigm of textbooks. Such interactions with patients may address disease-oriented needs, but are also likely to include consideration of social and psychological complexities, symptoms that never reach a point of diagnosis, living with chronic conditions, and even complaints or requests for second opinions. This affords opportunities for learners to implement their current knowledge (how to elicit, filter, prioritise, select and focus), to construct new knowledge through social interactions, and to purposefully expand their knowledge

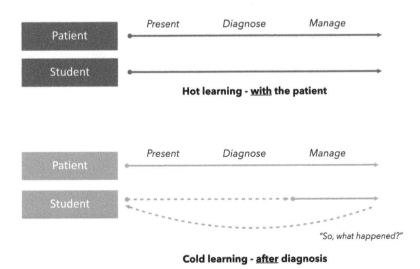

Figure 6.1   Hot and cold clinical learning. © Sophie Park, based on description in Atkinson, 1975

around identified gaps. The disease label or absence/presence of disease no longer becomes the sole learning focus or end point, as learning has arisen through the process of patient engagement. Learners also learn to manage uncertainty from the outset, and how to navigate the ethical and social dilemmas encountered within clinical care. Learning becomes shaped towards both topic-based knowledge *and* the capabilities to implement and adapt that knowledge content to situated patient care.

Learning in partnership with patients

Generalist learning happens in participation with patients, who need to be recognised as a legitimate and expected part of learning conversations (see also Chapter 2). This means sharing the learning process with patients, including whether the learner wants feedback on a specific aspect of the encounter so that they can contribute fully to the learner's development. It also means checking in with the patient during the learning encounter or inviting them to debrief or provide feedback afterwards, so that patient experiences inform the future organisation and delivery of clinical learning.

Patients may need support and guidance on how they can contribute to a learning encounter (16–18). This can be done through some basic groundwork, which can be negotiated by the supervisor on behalf of the learner, or by the learner during the encounter. Service and teaching are often integrated within clinical organisations. It is, however, important wherever possible to ensure that people contributing to service-based learning are comfortable. This includes consent (ideally before entering a clinical space) and iterative checkpoints as the interaction evolves (17). This helps to orientate and set expectations. This includes sharing:

- Information about the learner and their course or placement (for example, 'I am Rehan, training to be an Advanced Clinical Practitioner; I have a background as a paramedic').
- What the learner is currently working on, and how this interaction fits in (for example, 'I am working on exploring people's concerns. My supervisor will join us after our conversation, and help plan next steps together …').
- Explicit confidentiality assurance and repeated iterative consent at different stages of the interaction for discussion, examination, deliberation with a colleague and so on (for example, 'First, can we have a conversation? Now, is it OK if I examine you?').

- Nature of the planned patient–student interaction and feedback opportunities (for example, 'I will try to summarise our discussion to my supervisor – would you mind letting me know how my summary sounds?').
- What the student knows and would like to learn, and any additional learning established through the encounter (for example, 'I haven't met many people with x yet; could you tell me about how you were first diagnosed and what you've found helpful since then?').
- How the patient–learner interaction will contribute to the patient's care (for example, 'Let's try to come up with a plan together, but this will need to be checked by my supervisor before you go').
- Any ground rules such as mutual respect and time out if either feels discomfort.

Learning *through practice* provides opportunities for learner–patient interactions that actually contribute to the care process rather than simply being a 'dummy' parallel process. Establishing safe ways in which this might happen can give the learner a sense of responsibility and provide recognition that the knowledge they acquire and implement is 'live'. Feedback from a patient that their story and concerns have been accurately summarised, for example, can provide encouragement for even the earliest learners that they are developing useful skills for generalist care.

Supporting learners to work safely with uncertainty

An important part of establishing a sense of safety before patient interactions is for both the learner and teacher to discuss how uncertainty should be managed: not *if* it occurs, but when and how. Should uncertainty be explored with the patient present as an observer or partner in the conversation, or should this be discussed in the next room? Is it safe to wait until after the patient has left? The teacher may also want to clarify whether, when and how the learner is expected to try to address their own uncertainties. Should this be done with the patient? Should this be done immediately, or noted for later discussion? How might the learner develop independent strategies for addressing their own knowledge gaps (for example, by consulting online guidelines, or discussing with peers)? Or should they ask their teacher first? How and when will the teacher respond to the learner's uncertainties, and will they share their own uncertainties and model their own strategies for dealing with them?

Supporting learners to engage in deliberate and scholarly work

Although immersion in the clinical workplace is important, it is not enough *in itself*. We need to develop expert practitioners who engage with generalism's research-informed practices and complex evidence base. Anders Ericsson talked about the concept of 'deliberate practice' in the development of expertise (19,20). He observed that the most effective learners were constantly pushing the boundaries of what they could do, guided by experts, studying the practices of others, identifying their own weaknesses and purposefully practising around them. Social engagement ('being immersed') is not enough. Learners also need to be cognitively engaged: identifying gaps in their knowledge through expert guidance, reflection and feedback, and effortfully and purposefully addressing those gaps.

Scholarly engagement with the diverse knowledge that underpins generalism may be straightforward if innate curiosity motivates learners to explore. This intellectual engagement is, however, hard work. This therefore needs encouragement, guidance and structural support. It is important to build expectations and opportunities for learning into the clinical learning environment; and to align activities, assignments and assessments so that they drive engagement with generalist knowledge forms. Learners can then begin to access and experience the connection between clinical practice and learning approaches, and their scholarly or intellectual underpinnings. Helping learners to develop their own approaches to developing and sustaining scholarly informed practice is key.

Engaging learners in a connected curriculum for generalism

Dilly Fung, in her book *A Connected Curriculum for Higher Education*, argues that attempts to standardise clinical education have led to it becoming disconnected from the evolving needs of patients and society, as well as from research and innovation (21). Fung argues for a more dynamic curriculum that is built on two-way connections and the construction of new knowledge between all the stakeholders: learners, clinical teachers, academic faculty, leadership, administration, patients and communities. In this form of connected curriculum, learners require regular points of dialogue to help frame, bound or expand understanding about a particular clinical experience from other sources.

Examples of connections from the primary care-based Example 6.1 include responsive learning goals identified through debrief after clinical encounters; the postgraduate trainees bringing research-informed ways of practising from the university to the team; the students' community-based projects being shared with both the team and the university via the teaching conference; and the practice learning group which has a dynamic rather than fixed curriculum that is multiprofessional, involves patients, and brings historically separated areas of knowledge together. In this way, service-based learning activities and the needs of patients and learners *inform and are informed by* curricular goals or outcomes, which also *inform and are informed by,* for example, research and policy (21). These two-way connections allow learners and teachers to attend not only to what is known and experienced, but also to what is not (22): enabling them to articulate and address the unmet needs of patients and society and their own unmet educational goals, as well as ensuring learning is research-informed.

There is a multitude of ways to create and use curricula in more dynamic and connected ways. The key to supporting generalist learning is to ensure that the process supports 'hot' or 'bottom-up' learning: from and through practice. The temptation to predefine topics and areas for learning is huge, shifting autonomy and control towards the governing institution rather than the learner. Trust and agility are required, but so are structures that enable inclusive points of connection, such as the practice learning group in Example 6.1. Curriculum space and learning effort then become more agile and responsive to learner and patient needs and to new research.

Creating a supportive learning environment

Participating in new communities of practice is not easy for learners and must be dynamically negotiated (23). Most professional groups or communities will, over time, develop unique words, rituals and meanings which they attribute to particular ideas, processes or objects (2). These might be simple things like whether to 'wear' a stethoscope, whether to use first names, or who sits where around a meeting table. Communities of practice that use complex knowledge also tend to develop a particular language as theories and ideas are given shorthand labels: for example, 'concordance' or 'functional'. Language, artefacts, rituals and attributed meanings, however, can feel impenetrable to a novice and produce a barrier between a learner's position as 'outsider' and their desired position as 'insider' or 'knower'. If a learner is used to being in a hospital clinical setting, they might feel very unsettled if their position shifts from insider and 'knower' to peripheral member and 'partial knower' within an unfamiliar primary care context, or vice versa.

The positioning of a learner within a new community of practice needs to be carefully managed. Learners need to feel welcomed and invited, and trust their seniors and near-peers not to humiliate or ostracise them for 'not knowing', but rather celebrate their curiosity. This 'insider–outsider' tension can present at any transition between clinical learning environments (24), and even after a period of absence when terminology and associated meanings might have shifted. If novices feel welcomed and invited to share their curiosity, this has broader advantages for that community. Their 'fresh eyes' can invoke critical curiosity about what words mean, and how and why things are done in certain ways. This can help clinical teams to recognise the value (and occasionally the absurdity) of established ways of working (25).

It is also important from a patient-safety perspective for learners to feel safe to discuss their ideas, questions and concerns, and to say when they are unsure and to focus with curiosity and openness on what they do not know, rather than retreat to what they do. This requires an environment that fosters a growth mindset (26) and a sense of psychological safety (27). A learner-led multiprofessional exploration of psychological safety in generalist learning environments (28) found a sense of safety was inhibited by hierarchical and boundaried working and fear of ridicule for 'not knowing'. Conversely, safety was engendered through a variety of modifiable mechanisms: educational supervisors and team leaders who created a safe and inclusive learning culture; strong interpersonal relationships supported through extended or longitudinal placements; peer-to-peer support through small-group learning (hence in our example undergraduate learners worked in pairs); and opportunities for open and inclusive dialogue across hierarchies and silos, often supported by a 'boundary spanner' who creates spaces for conversations that might not otherwise happen (in our example, the 'boundary spanner' was the practice manager who convened the practice learning group).

Learners require a safe place to think (often aloud), to listen and challenge, to explore and try things out, and a trusting dialogue with those providing support and guidance. A sense of safety and trust supports the learner to stretch themselves further towards the limits of their capability and maximises the extent to which a teacher or organisation will position a learner as an active participant in the clinical environment.

Personalising educational approaches

Dewey and, more recently, Freire have challenged the idea dominating many educational models where learning has become a standardised and industrial process to produce 'outputs' on exiting a course with repro-ducible and replicable traits and behaviours (29,30). In contrast, they propose a model of education which enables each learner to be treated as an individual. Learning therefore becomes more focused on professional development needs, with each individual having their own trajectory, dependent on their evolving role, patient and societal needs, and contex-tual constraints. Forefronting the aim of learning as personal growth and engagement in clinical practice (in addition to reaching a standardised or pre-set competency) positions learners in the driving seat and allows them greater agency over their own learning journey.

Conceptualising a more dynamic approach to clinical learning requires a dynamic curricular map. E-portfolios are an important and potentially dynamic tool in highly distributed learning environments such as the clinical workplace, where learners might be attached to different clin-ical teachers across many different sites, or rotate between sites. A dynamic e-portfolio can enable educational institutions to share their desired 'top-down' outcomes with teachers and learners, but with flexible personalisa-tion as to how and when those outcomes are achieved. Administrators and accrediting bodies can connect with learners and their supervisors via the e-portfolio so that all are clear on progress towards accreditation stand-ards and any additional evidence needed. A dynamic portfolio of learn-ing can also help learners and their educational supervisors to keep track of 'bottom-up' personal learning goals, generated in response to clinical encounters, which can be handed forward to new supervisors or mentors, providing a purposeful focus for learning effort. Learners and supervisors can see what has been learned, so, rather than duplicate prior learning, effort can be focused on areas for improvement. As learners progress from novice to practising professional, personalised education becomes increas-ingly important as learners bring more and more prior professional knowl-edge and develop increasingly unique professional journeys. Learners can also showcase additional projects or learning that they have undertaken in areas of personal or professional interest.

If clinical learning changes from a top-down curriculum to a more connected 'real-world' curriculum that reflects both regulatory priorities *and* clinical care 'as practised', students are likely to find themselves moving into the spaces where care actually happens. Training might follow actual patient pathways, thereby embracing a wider range of health and social care knowledge and producing graduates who are genuinely prepared for practice. Of course, clinical learners need to function within a certain agreed range of norms and regulatory standards. Personalised approaches, however, acknowledge that norms and standards are constantly changing (sometimes slowly, sometimes – as in the case of the COVID-19 pandemic – rapidly). Equipping clinicians with the ability not just to follow pre-set rules and rehearse pre-set routines, but to question how and when they might need to be applied or adjusted, enables clinicians to adapt their knowledge to the ever-changing demands of patient care. It also enables learners to develop a professional identity that feels personally congruent rather than imposed, supporting their future wellbeing (31).

Promoting clinical reasoning and critical reflexivity through debrief

Feedback can take many forms. It might be corrective – for example, if a learner has prescribed an incorrect dose. It can be directive – for example, if a learner has failed to follow guidelines or consider important possibilities. Feedback can also help a learner judge whether something was good or bad from a particular perspective – for example, whether the patient felt listened to. Generalist learning, however, requires feedback to both embrace and move beyond corrective, directive or judgemental forms, towards connecting what was done with outcomes, so that it not only supports safe effective consultation outcomes, but also stimulates collaborative meaning-making, critical reflexivity and transferable learning about how those outcomes were met. If debrief is purely corrective – attending only to 'right or wrong' outcomes, or even the 'teacher' effectively doing the learner's consultations again for them – then limited transferable learning happens. If, however, it attends to processes (for example, 'what were your thoughts at this stage?', 'at what point did you realise you were uncertain?', 'how else could you have managed that uncertainty?') then feed-forward learning is more likely to happen. As Suzanne Kurtz and colleagues remind us, there is no 'right or wrong' form of communication, only whether it served its intended purpose (32). We use the term 'debrief' for this richer form of feedback.

Debrief after a clinical encounter is an opportunity to develop shared meaning-making and to highlight areas and potential strategies for personal development. Debrief can happen between learner and teacher, peer-to-peer, or in small groups but should happen as soon as possible after the learning encounter (hence, in our Example 6.1, after each session for graduate doctors, and after each patient for undergraduate learners). Teachers can also model their learning processes by debriefing their own consultations with learners. A debrief need not start with what was done right or wrong – rather, with a rich description of what happened (explicit), what participants were trying to achieve (implicit), followed by collaborative meaning-making and co-creation (and sometimes rehearsal) of alternative solutions. Where a learner is unsure whether they had missed something, attention and connections can be drawn to relevant models, theory or knowledge sources.

Debrief can also help to make explicit the implicit steps within a generalist clinical interaction (Table 6.1), thereby enabling learners to critique their own consultation processes, clinical reasoning and approach to uncertainty over time. With continuity, the process of debrief (Table 6.2) can support learners in developing a reflexive repertoire of internally available processes, questions and safety nets so that they become able to question their own clinical reasoning processes (for example, what is this likely to be, what does my patient think is going on, what else is possible or easily missed, what do I need to exclude now, what can wait, what might be unsaid? (33)).

Table 6.1 A generalist model of clinical interactions

Steps (not always linear)	Clinical focus (implicit aim)	Associated practices (how it might be achieved)	Potential debrief questions (open, probing or direct)
Connect	Bringing prior information forward. Ensuring people feel welcomed and accepted. Eliciting their story and concerns.	Checking notes. Welcoming, connecting, listening, observing, attending to emotions. Noting cues, clues, metaphors, concerns and gaps.	How did/could you prepare? How have they been since last reviewed? How did they seem when they first came in? What was their main concern? Do you feel you gave them enough time to talk? What emotions were expressed?
Forage (inductive)	Building a picture. Not trying to 'diagnose'–aiming to approach a shared understanding of the issue(s).	Dialogue to probe, clarify and explore contextual information.	What were you most curious about? How did you explore that? What else might be relevant? (e.g. abuse, poverty, preventive measures, chronic care needs, etc.)

(continued)

Table 6.1 (Cont.)

Steps (not always linear)	Clinical focus (implicit aim)	Associated practices (how it might be achieved)	Potential debrief questions (open, probing or direct)
Problem-set	Together, negotiate how to frame and prioritise the current focus, noting anything important but not urgent to return to.	Trying different lenses (is this part of a wider issue, ongoing problem, contextual factors?), framing, negotiating.	Taking all this into consideration, what are the potential issues? How did you agree where to start?
Sort and seek (deductive-inductive loops)	Clinical reasoning. Exploring together the likely possibilities, causal factors, potential impacts. Testing ideas. Exploring red flags, potential implications. Considering what might be unsaid.	Sorting knowledge gained from patient. Sharing own thinking. Seeking new knowledge where needed (e.g. focused questioning, focused examination, external sources of knowledge).	Talk me through the possibilities. What is likely/ urgent/important/ easily missed? What would help you to sort them? What other information did you need? What did you find? Was that sufficient? Where else could you look/ask?
Integrate	Collaboratively configuring jigsaw pieces, acknowledging gaps, and negotiating next steps.	Sharing and inviting understanding. Agreeing how this shared understanding might inform next steps.	How did you bring all this together? What was your patient's analysis? How did you resolve any differences / agree unknowns?

(continued)

Table 6.1 (Cont.)

Steps (not always linear)	Clinical focus (implicit aim)	Associated practices (how it might be achieved)	Potential debrief questions (open, probing or direct)
Plan	Together, agreeing a personalised plan based on joint understanding, safety net, and confirming if/ when to connect together and/or with others.	Exploring ideas for what might help. Agreeing and reviewing the plan. Creating a mitigation and review plan (what to do if ...).	What guidelines might be useful here? What ideas or preferences did your patient have? How did you agree on next steps / resolve differences? How did you confirm understanding and safety net? How did you hand over to the patient / another professional / the next consultation?
Review	Active and critical reflection. Record-keeping. Self-care and preparation for next patient.	Writing in the notes. Noting areas for reflection or debrief. Taking a 'breath' before the next patient.	Talk me through your record-keeping / prescribing / referrals. How do you feel that encounter went? Why? Were there any unmet patient needs? Is there need for additional follow-up, referral or ongoing conversation? What do you need to work on?

Table 6.2 A clinical debrief for generalist learning

Check in: acknowledge feelings, attend to immediate wellbeing	
Agree expectations: time constraints, priorities for feedback, privacy, etc.	
In parallel …	
Learner summarises …	Teacher (or colleague) opens notes and considers …

• **Clinical summary:**
  ○ Summary of the patient's concerns and symptoms
  ○ What the learner explored, any examination findings
  ○ What the learner thinks might be going on, and why
  ○ What next steps were agreed with patient/carer, and reasoning.
• **Consultation processes:**
  ○ What happened in the consultation including any consultation difficulties
  ○ What did not happen but should have ('what I knew but didn't do').
	• **Problem-framing:** How was the problem framed? Might a different lens be helpful? How did the learner integrate future/past considerations and contextual information?
	• **Patient perspective:** In what ways were the patient's perspectives and priorities integrated, and how were differences resolved?
	• **Gaps:** What (if any) are the gaps? e.g. additional potential diagnoses or factors that need considering
	• **Uncertainty and safety:** How were serious causes considered (red flags)? How was uncertainty navigated (safety netting)? How were clinical guidelines used?
	• **Housekeeping:** How were the notes written and coded, and referrals/prescriptions done?

Collaboratively, and with critical reflexivity:
• Discussion on why the consultation went as it did, including areas of excellence and missed opportunities
• Plan for addressing any unmet patient needs
  ○ Is there a need for additional follow-up, referral or ongoing conversation?
• Plan to address learners' educational needs
  ○ Strategies, frameworks, guidelines, theories, areas of understanding, consultation areas to work on
  ○ Agreed and recorded for follow-up (e.g. in e-portfolio)	

Conclusion

There are strong parallels between generalist approaches to education and clinical practice. Characteristics include being learner-centred, relationship-based, expansive and adaptive, positioning learners as active partners and participants in a learning ecosystem, and drawing dynamically upon different forms of knowledge to address what learning is needed for a particular situation or circumstance. Learning moves from something finite to something infinite: an incremental process that informs meaningful ways by which professionals enhance their clinical practice. In order to integrate clinical practice and learning, we need to articulate and make explicit the knowledge we use, and how we use it. Because the nature of generalist knowledge is complex and distributed, so too are the approaches to teach, learn and assess this knowledge. The content and approaches of generalist clinical practice and learning are both experiential and scholarly, and it is the ongoing connection between these which enables clinicians and clinical learners to adapt, re-form and apply their knowledge in previously unknown or unencountered circumstances.

References

1. Eve R. *PUNs and DENs: Discovering learning needs in general practice*. Radcliffe Publishing; 2003.
2. Wenger E. *Communities of Practice: Learning, meaning, and identity*. Cambridge University Press; 1998.
3. Biggs J. What the student does: teaching for enhanced learning. *High Educ Res Dev*. 1999;18(1):57–75.
4. Eraut M. Transfer of knowledge between education and workplace settings. In: *Knowledge, Values and Educational Policy*. Routledge; 2012. pp. 75–94.
5. Kneebone R. Total internal reflection: an essay on paradigms. *Med Educ*. 2002;36(6):514–18.
6. White J, Paton JY, Niven R, Pinnock H. Guidelines for the diagnosis and management of asthma: a look at the key differences between BTS/SIGN and NICE. *Thorax*. 2018;73(3):293–7.
7. Hodges B. Medical education and the maintenance of incompetence. *Med Teach*. 2006;28(8):690–6.
8. Flexner A. *Medical Education in the United States and Canada*. The Carnegie Foundation for the Advancement of Teaching; 1910.
9. Mol A. *The Logic of Care: Health and the problem of patient choice*. Routledge; 2008.
10. Menzies Lyth I. Social systems as a defence against anxiety: an empirical study of the nursing service of a general hospital. *Hum Relat*. 1960;13(2):95–121.
11. McCormack B, van Dulmen S, Eide H, Skovdahl K, Eide T. Person-centredness in healthcare policy, practice and research. *Pers Healthc Res*. 2017;3–17.
12. Biggs JB, Tang CS. *Teaching for Quality Learning at University: What the student does*. 4th ed. Open University Press; 2011.
13. Swanson DB, Roberts TE. Trends in national licensing examinations in medicine. *Med Educ*. 2016;50(1):101–14.
14. General Medical Council. MLA Content Map. 2021. Available from: www.gmc-uk.org/education/medical-licensing-assessment/mla-content-map (accessed 16 March 2023).
15. Atkinson P. In cold blood: bedside teaching in a medical school. In: Chanan Gabriel, Delamont S, editors. *Frontiers of Classroom Research*. NFER; 1975. pp. 163–182.

16. Park S, Khan NF, Hampshire M, Knox R, Malpass A, Thomas J, et al. A BEME systematic review of UK undergraduate medical education in the general practice setting: BEME Guide No. 32. *Med Teach*. 2015;37(7):611–30.
17. Park S, Khan N, Stevenson F, Malpass A. Patient and public involvement (PPI) in evidence synthesis: how the PatMed study approached embedding audience responses into the expression of a meta-ethnography. *BMC Med Res Methodol*. 2020;20(1):29.
18. Park SE, Allfrey C, Jones MM, Chana J, Abbott C, Faircloth S, et al. Patient participation in general practice based undergraduate teaching: a focus group study of patient perspectives. *Br J Gen Pract*. 2017;67(657):e260.
19. Ericsson KA. Deliberate practice and the acquisition and maintenance of expert performance in medicine and related domains. *Acad Med*. 2004;79(10):S70–81.
20. Ericsson KA. Acquisition and maintenance of medical expertise: a perspective from the expert-performance approach with deliberate practice. *Acad Med*. 2015;90(11):1471–86.
21. Fung D. *A Connected Curriculum for Higher Education*. UCL Press; 2017.
22. Luft J, Ingham H. The johari window. *Hum Relat Train News*. 1961;5(1):6–7.
23. Chen MX, Newman M, Park S. Becoming a member of a nursing community of practice: negotiating performance competence and identity. *J Vocat Educ Train*. 2021;76(1):164–78.
24. Young Y, Leedham-Green K, Jensen-Martin J. Improving transitions between clinical placements. *Clin Teach*. 2023;20(4):e13580.
25. Leedham-Green KE, Knight A, Iedema R. Intra- and interprofessional practices through fresh eyes: a qualitative analysis of medical students' early workplace experiences. *BMC Med Educ*. 2019;19(1):287.
26. Dweck CS. Motivational processes affecting learning. *Am Psychol*. 1986;41(10):1040–8.
27. Edmondson AC. *The Fearless Organization: Creating psychological safety in the workplace for learning, innovation, and growth*. John Wiley & Sons; 2018.
28. Remtulla R, Hagana A, Houbby N, Ruparell K, Aojula N, Menon A, et al. Exploring the barriers and facilitators of psychological safety in primary care teams: a qualitative study. *BMC Health Serv Res*. 2021;21(1):269.
29. Dewey J. My pedagogic creed. *Sch J*. 1897;54:77–80.
30. Freire P. *Pedagogy of Freedom: Ethics, democracy, and civic courage*. Rowman & Littlefield; 2000. Available from: https://books.google.co.uk/books?id=Hdl4AAAAQBAJ (accessed 10 March 2024).
31. Leedham-Green K, Knight A, Iedema R. Developing professional identity in health professional students. In: Nestel D, Reedy G, McKenna L, Gough S, editors. *Clinical Education for Health Professional Practice*. Springer Nature Singapore; 2020.
32. Kurtz SM, Silverman DJ, Draper J. *Teaching and Learning Communication Skills in Medicine*. 2nd ed. Radcliffe Publishing; 2005.
33. Murtagh J. Common problems: a safe diagnostic strategy. *Aust Fam Physician*. 1990;19(5):733–4.

7
Generalism and assessment

Eleanor Hothersall and Eliot Rees

Introduction

In this chapter we focus on assessment, building upon Chapter 6 which describes the ways that generalism can be taught and learned. We draw on examples from medicine, but there are many relevant parallels across clinical education. Inevitably, in order to demonstrate that learning has been achieved, some form of assessment must follow. In this chapter we explore how assessment is traditionally viewed, highlighting how the standard approaches to assessment have developed, with a particular emphasis on summative assessment – where information is used to determine whether a learner has reached a sufficient standard to progress (or to maintain current status, as with processes like revalidation). We discuss how the generalist perspective and the associated values of holism and embracing uncertainty bring particular challenges to assessment, and look at some attempts to address this which are currently in use. Finally, we pose some challenges which are in urgent need of being addressed.

Somewhere in the journey from early schooling to working as a professional our perspective on assessment shifts. In part, this comes from the acceptance that assessment in some format is needed to demonstrate understanding and capability (often referred to as competence, as discussed below) and in part realisation that assessment is more than just dreaded exams.

Consequently, here we discuss assessment in its widest sense, described by Fenton (1) as 'the collection of relevant information that may be relied on for making decisions'. We can think of this as any process for determining the learning, understanding, ability and/or skill of a learner. Assessment in the context of education for healthcare professionals can be carried out to:

- Determine whether a learner is ready to progress to the next level of training, or to finish training (for example, exit exams).
- Determine whether candidates meet a minimum standard (for example, licensure exams).
- Distinguish between candidates, and predict future performance (for example, determining Honours, or guiding selection decisions).
- Diagnose gaps in learning or teaching (for example, an end-of-module quiz to assess understanding).
- Compare institutions or training programmes (for example, national exit exams).

This chapter outlines the essential role of assessment in ensuring learners are competent and safe to provide healthcare to patients. We highlight the challenges posed as the elements valued in clinical education, particularly for doctors, are brought into contrast with the paradigms of the generalist perspective, including the ways of teaching and learning outlined in Chapter 6. We demonstrate that current assessment practices are not always well aligned with a generalist approach, concluding with an exploration of ways in which educators can employ assessment practices that value generalism, and highlighting the challenges which still need to be addressed.

Purposes of assessment

It is often thought that assessment and exams are synonyms, but there are many purposes of assessment beyond the exam. Assessments have many functions, which may be the sole purpose of the assessment, or may have additional roles which can be intentional or have unintended consequences (this can be part of the hidden curriculum as described by Hafferty (2)). Examples of these are:

- Quality assurance or benchmarking – for example, ensuring that all learners have had sufficient time and opportunity to learn what has been deemed key (an additional function) or, in the case of primary school assessments in England and Scotland, measuring the performance of the cohort not the individual (main function).

- Feedback to learners on progress – this can be structured through practice tests or 'mocks', or can provide wider-ranging feedback, for example through simulation exercises or workplace-based assessment.
- Ensuring patient safety – for example, assessing learner prescribing or behaviour in a simulated setting. It is argued below, however, that this is a somewhat reductionist view of safety.
- Driving the learning behaviours that we seek – where, for example, an assessment emphasises biomedical knowledge over empathy, we encourage learners to spend more time with books, and less time with patients. Norcini and colleagues (3) describe assessment as having a 'catalytic effect', and Harden warns that changes to assessment can bring about significant changes to whole curricula, while students may change their entire approach to learning (4).

Assessments are commonly divided into two broad categories, referred to as 'summative' and 'formative'. Summative assessments are those where a decision is made about progression or success – exams are the most obvious example. This is often referred to as 'assessment *of* learning'. Formative assessment in contrast is 'assessment *for* learning'. Formative assessments can be less structured, and less obvious. As an example, when learning to drive, each lesson contains elements of formative assessment as your instructor looks at your technique performing manoeuvres, and provides feedback on how to improve. When you are deemed ready, you then sit the summative assessment of the driving test, and if you pass that, you are ready to progress to being an independent driver.

Standards

In Chapter 6, the power dynamic was highlighted which can put the learner in a disadvantaged position. This is most evident in the case of assessment, where the learner is 'judged' either by themselves or another (or others). All assessments include some form of 'standard'. The most common and obvious example of this is the 'pass mark', but reflect for a moment on other assessments you may have experienced in the past: whether a portfolio assessment or revalidation, assessments include within them some notion of 'good enough'. This returns us to the concept of assessment as gathering evidence for decision-making referred to above. In the case of these unscored assessments, the portfolio submitted must reach a certain standard to be judged sufficient, and if insufficient there are consequences, such as requiring extra work or an extension to training. Even self-assessment requires that the learner have an opportunity to consider correct or model answers to be effective. It is the process of validation or judgement which defines assessment.

With formative assessment, the application of a standard can be less obvious, but will still ultimately link back to the concept of 'good enough'. However, where that concept is not clearly articulated it can be difficult to provide appropriate feedback, and confusion may arise. As an example, if during a ward round a supervisor wishes to provide a doctor in training with formative feedback relating to their approach to patient-centred care, they will need to have a clear understanding of what are the most important elements to emphasise. Using structured debriefing tools can be a helpful way of ensuring that the feedback given is tailored to meet the learner's needs (5,6).

Pass marks are probably the most commonly understood standards (commonly a percentage score). The application and interpretation of standards is highly context-specific, and care needs to be taken to ensure standards are set and used appropriately. This is particularly relevant where different perspectives of the same assessment may be taken (for example, a national licensing exam which is also used as an institution's assessment). In contrast, in formative assessment, pass marks may be wholly inappropriate. Indeed, in this setting, they may reinforce a positivist perception of a pass/fail outcome, when in fact the important element will be to identify areas of strength and weakness to target future learning and teaching.

Where numeric standards, or 'cut scores' are used, these should also vary according to purpose (for a good summary of this, see Ben-David (7)) and the value placed on passing the assessment, either by the institution or more widely. Commonly used standard-setting methods usually make an attempt to adjust the cut score for each iteration of an assessment to take into account the (usually small) differences between exams, but standard-setting methods are not particularly consistent across institutions (8), and as discussed later, may be an area where the generalist perspective could bring some changes in the future.

Assessment data can also be used for quality assurance and monitoring within training programmes (undergraduate and postgraduate): where a question or subject area performs poorly this can be an early signal of changes to teaching or experience making previously core topics harder to access. The challenge then is that, since learning and assessment are intertwined, it can be difficult to identify the source of the difficulty.

Drivers of assessment

The different possible drivers of assessment mean that no single assessment, or indeed assessment method, can meet all the requirements for either learner or assessor. For example, formative assessment to identify gaps in learning should allow learners access to model answers (as highlighted in previous chapters, and discussed below, the idea of a single correct answer is in itself worthy of challenge), and also offer opportunities for feedback. In contrast, in summative assessments learners are effectively penalised for gaps in knowledge, and feedback often comes in a limited format, if at all. It is thus helpful to understand the driver of a given assessment or assessments, in order to determine which functions and qualities should be emphasised. Without this clarity, conflicts can arise. Assessment can be a positive trigger for learning, facilitating transformation, development or implementation of knowledge rather than simple recall. For example, an essay question which stimulates learners to reframe and apply their understanding of the literature, and select, consider and appraise relevant evidence to inform their critically reflexive arguments.

Stakeholders in assessment

Institutional priorities dominate current assessment approaches, making them exam- rather than education- or practice-focused. A generalist approach requires us to consider the perspectives of additional stakeholders (such as patients and learners) and integrate them more meaningfully into our assessments. For example, integrating person-centred language, or even engaging students in assessment question-writing to highlight to them the constraints of knowledge possible to assess within particular assessment approaches. Norcini and colleagues (9) identified a number of stakeholders who influence the purpose and design of assessments. These include:

- learners;
- teachers and institutions;
- patients; and
- healthcare systems and regulators (and by extension, governments).

Involving patients in the *design* of assessment may be a way to mitigate concerns of bias expressed when patients are directly involved with exams (see below), but at present, this happens rarely (10,11) and there are significant concerns about the introduction of bias. This could be a very fruitful area for development, to increase the holistic perspective and social accountability of assessments in the future.

Where assessments can include regulators and institutions among their stakeholders, these are likely to be an additional complication within the design of an assessment, as such organisations must be able to demonstrate fairness across assessments, in order to be able to defend themselves against appeals. As such, the use of 'objective' measures such as checklists and rigid scoring systems tends to proliferate. This is of course to the detriment of any consideration of nuance or context that might be valued in a generalist view of assessment.

The tension between standardisation and authenticity

As members of the public, we want to be reassured that our healthcare practitioners are 'safe', and that our regulators are fulfilling their function to ensure that this is the case. Meanwhile, as healthcare practitioners, we want an assessment of our ability (and thus safety) that is as close to our real-life experience as possible. Furthermore, the very concept of safety may be challenging: a skilled practitioner should be able to identify when following a guideline is not the most appropriate course of action, for example, although an assessment may be guideline-based. This section outlines how the different purposes of assessment emphasise very different values, and thus bring the paradigms into conflict.

Validity

Core to this conflict is the concept of 'validity'. For most people, this term is reasonably self-explanatory, and relates to an understanding of how well an assessment feels like a fair reflection of the material taught (or learned) and the purpose of the assessment. As an example, an exam to determine progression into the next year of study which covers a wide range of topics covered in a teaching programme and has an achievable pass mark might be considered 'fair', and thus valid, while an exam which only covers a small amount of the taught curriculum, with a high pass mark might seem unfair. However, in assessment 'validity' is a technical term, used to describe a number of different ways in which assessment performance and design can be analysed to determine different more specialised ways of considering assessments. Kane in 2006 (12) described these as scoring, generalisation, extrapolation and implications, and these have been applied to the requirements of assessment in medical education by Cook and colleagues in 2015 (13). Institutions in general tend to concentrate their efforts on demonstrating the first three dimensions of validity of assessment, while the learner being assessed tends to be far more concerned with the implications. Furthermore, it is important to note that assessment methods are highly context-specific, meaning that all have limitations, and should be revalidated if used in a different context.

Quality of assessment

It goes without saying that all participants in assessment wish for high quality. However, Norcini and colleagues, when describing both individual assessments and programmes of assessment, emphasised that the assessments need to be valid in order to be considered high quality (3,9). Given that validity varies according to the beholder, this again creates a challenge. Moreover, this entire perspective of assessment brings with it the implication that assessments can only be 'pass or fail', emphasising the positivist, even binary, approach, and leaving little room for formative or iterative assessments. Furthermore, this summary does not capture the complexity of equating or balancing different assessment methods, which may all be useful but have different levels of acceptability or trust. In particular, where pass/fail or progression decisions are made, assessments which could be considered subject to bias (such as vivas) can be subject to numerous appeals and challenges. Combining several assessment modalities into one summary mark or grade can also be problematic, as they inevitably include value judgements: if a portfolio makes equal contribution to the final mark as a large exam, that says something very different from a situation where a portfolio contributes 10 per cent of the final mark. This corresponds with the observation made by Apple that we use the curriculum, including assessment, to demonstrate what knowledge is 'of most worth' (14, p. vii).

The needs of institutions

Schools for undergraduate clinical programmes (for example, medical schools), postgraduate training providers and regulators all have an important role to play as gatekeepers of clinical education. They need to be able to demonstrate that they have created assessments which will ensure that the learner has proved that they have learned whatever has been deemed necessary for that point in training. Here we encounter something of a potential conflict of interest, as progression is determined by institutions, who also (usually) set the standards. To counter this, the concept of 'minimum competency' has been introduced (although the term is unpopular). While this is rarely explicitly expressed, it has a significant impact on standard setting in summative assessment (as, for example, is the commonly used phrase 'what percentage of just passing students would get this question right?', which is used in the Angoff or modified Angoff method of standard setting, common in medical school assessments (15)).

In turn, the idea that all learners must demonstrate attainment of a minimum standard within healthcare means there is a push for standardised, national exams (such as the new Medical Licensing Assessment or 'MLA' in the UK, or the Medical Licensing Examination in the USA). If all learners sit the same exam, with the pass mark derived in the same way each time, there should be confidence that whatever route the learner took to get to the assessment, if they manage to pass, they have reached the same desired outcome.

However, introducing such exams is highly controversial, as in such assessments there is a significant challenge in balancing the needs and perception of validity by the public (future and current patients), and the regulator, compared with the profession and the learner. At the same time, it is often thought that having a national, standardised exam makes it easier to compare performance across institutions, although the data are far more nuanced than is obvious to the casual observer. In particular, differences in admissions processes mean there are justifiable and indeed desirable differences between learners in different medical schools (16). It does, however, mean that there is pressure on the institution and learner to perform as well as possible, even 'gaming' the system. This can have a dramatic effect on curricula, meaning any aspect which is not included in the national assessment blueprint is deemed less important, and thus squeezed out (4,14), pushing schools to increase standardisation of content and lose the ability to respond to local needs: a significant form of top-down control.

Creating national exams can also mean that standardisation comes ahead of what is termed 'content validity', which is to say whether the material being assessed truly reflects what should be the priorities of an assessment at that time. It is common for assessments to cover what can be assessed easily, rather than what might be truly important. As an example, the new UK MLA blueprint covers a wide range of clinical topics, but a very small percentage of questions cover ethics, psychology, sociology, population health, and research methods, even though these topics are highly emphasised within the national required learning outcomes for newly qualified doctors (17). That is both because of the relative 'value' placed on those topics by assessors (compared with, for example, the ability to differentiate a Gram negative from a Gram positive cause of meningitis), but also because questions in those topics are difficult to fit into the standard format of the exam (18).

It is vital that, when considering the form and content of an assessment, it reinforces the desired behaviours and outcomes. As an example, where an assessment focuses heavily on book learning, the learner may then focus on this over clinical teaching (19). Newble commented in 1998 (20) that '[i]n many institutions assessment practices misdirect student learning activities in ways that may seriously undermine the aims of the curriculum'. The requirements for acceptably standardised assessments thus undermine attempts to introduce flexible, responsive and generalist curricula.

The needs of learners

In contrast with institutions' need to create standardisation and reproducibility, learners need assessment methods that support and reinforce the teaching that they experience, a process known as constructive alignment (21). This is achieved by ensuring that the assessment content matches the taught content. If the learner is seeking a generalist, holistic education, then the assessment should mirror this. However, as mentioned above, if the assessment is to be tightly controlled and mapped to predefined content, then the learner will also seek taught content which matches this.

Assuming, however, that a compromise between intended outcomes and taught content can be found, authenticity is also important to a learner's perception of validity. By this, we mean that an assessment must feel like both the content and the format are a close match to the real-world applications where the assessed material might be used. As an example, multiple-choice questions (MCQs), discussed in more detail below, are thought of as fairly inauthentic, as patients do not offer a range of options for their diagnosis or management. In contrast, although there are time limits and the environment can be artificial, the OSCE is generally considered by learners to be a more authentic type of assessment (22) – presumably because they can see the direct applicability of the format.

Finally, learners also need feedback from all assessments, including summative (23). This is particularly true for those who have not met the standard, in order to help the learner identify weaknesses to prepare for a repeat attempt, but is also valuable for those who have passed. As an example, structured feedback formats that encourage discursive meaning-making, such as the Diamond debrief tool (5), can help to develop a culture of feedback, creating environments which offer learners more opportunities to reflect on their learning.

State of play

The present approach to assessment in clinical education is to require learners to undergo a series of different types of assessment during their education. This is an attempt to address the problem already described above, that no one assessment can cover all relevant areas of learning, and meet all requirements of stakeholders. These assessments consequently tend to be somewhat siloed, with a range of assessments across programmes aimed at assessing discrete domains or capabilities which are considered important within individual areas or specialties. These tend to be simplified relative to the broad scope of learning outlined in Chapter 6. For example, when assessing knowledge, assessments focus on codified knowledge (usually exclusively biomedical): facts learned, and application of those facts, rather than the wider sense outlined previously. For summative assessments in particular, the components (or competencies) assessed tend to be compartmentalised into domains of knowledge, clinical skills, or professional values and behaviours (as outlined, for example, in the UK General Medical Council's Outcomes for Graduates (17)), with different assessment formats usually chosen depending on the domain intended to be assessed. This is in itself an extension of the framework for clinical assessment outlined by Miller in 1990 (24), adapted in Figure 7.1. As with learning and teaching, this has the effect of legitimising one aspect or domain, often to the detriment of others. Often these assessments are 'pass/fail', which reflects a very positivist, even absolutist, lens of assessment.

We will outline some of the common assessment modalities in use currently and highlight some of the threats to generalist practice that they pose. We have divided these into modalities that are predominantly used for summative assessments (high stakes, assessments *of* learning) and those predominantly used for formative assessment (low stakes, assessments *for* learning). We recognise this dichotomy is not perfect and that some of these modalities are used for both in different circumstances.

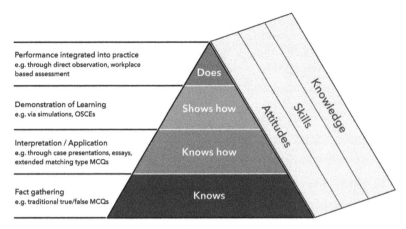

Figure 7.1 Miller's triangle with its alignment to common current assessment domains. © Eleanor Hothersall, adapted from Miller's Triangle

Summative assessments

Knowledge assessments

Despite the challenges posed in Chapter 6 to the very concept of what it means to 'know' something, when assessments are constructed they tend to be based on the premise that there are facts to be learned and applied, and there are consequently answers which can be construed as either 'right' or 'wrong' (or possibly 'partially right').

Current assessments of knowledge usually take the form of written assessments, although oral exams or 'vivas' are still used in some areas. Written assessments can either be free text (short answer or essay questions) or fixed response (multiple-choice questions, MCQs). Each of these has strengths and limitations. Essay questions are considered better for providing evidence of the construction of an argument and demonstrating reason. Timed, closed-book essays allow learners to demonstrate recall and related topics, while open-book essays or assignments can give learners the opportunity to demonstrate a wide range of skills including literature searching in addition to core knowledge. It is comparatively quick and simple to write an essay-based assessment. However, they are resource-intensive to mark, have challenges regarding content validity (you can only sample a limited number of content areas using essays, so too few questions mean not enough content is assessed, too many and the exam is unreasonably long) and inter-rater reliability (markers do not always agree). Beyond a simple re-statement of facts, essay-type assignments are inherently subjective in their marking, which can lead to accusations of unfairness and inconsistency.

In order to achieve acceptable levels of reliability and content validity, written assessments require many items sampled from across the full range of topics in the curriculum. Using multiple-choice questions (MCQs) enables this. Common multiple-choice formats include true or false, single best answer (SBA), or extended matching questions. They are also able to be computer-marked which makes them less resource-intensive. Consequently, MCQs now account for the majority of so-called written assessments (25). Well-designed MCQs will test both knowledge and application to a clinical scenario. However, creating such questions is highly challenging and labour-intensive, and many questions are not of such a high standard. Many MCQs are limited to testing discrete items of knowledge (26). This is a challenge to both authenticity and generalism. It is also difficult not to 'cue' the answer within multiple-choice questions – for example, by having distractors which are all related to managing the same condition, or from the same class of drugs. Equally, such scenarios can lead to oversimplification of complex scenarios, such as a patient with headache, who may need support for a change in lifestyle to reduce his blood pressure, screening for risk of stroke, *and* pharmacological management of his headache. Best practice in writing MCQs is to have the options as homogenous as possible, meaning that the options in this case might be five different analgesics, thereby obscuring the need for the other interventions. Fundamentally, MCQs do not generally permit the assessment of nuance. A 'single best answer' MCQ, by definition, has one correct answer. By extension, this means that the other answers are wrong. In contrast, personalised care invites practitioners to co-construct ways forward with their patients, meaning that the true correct answer to many questions is 'it depends'.

Another aspect worth noting is that the breadth of questions included in this type of exam means that a detailed form of 'blueprinting' is needed, to demonstrate the content validity of the assessment. This again leads to excessive compartmentalisation – for example, a question on unexplained backache may not fit neatly enough into any category, and so be omitted. Such blueprints can be subject to considerable scrutiny, both from worried learners who wish to ensure they have covered the appropriate learning points, and from subject experts keen to ensure their particular interests are represented. Given the risk to the institutions carrying out the assessments in the event of appeals or challenges to decisions, it is perhaps understandable that the process tends to favour the clearly defined over the nuanced.

A recent innovation is the development of very short answer questions (VSAQs) (27). This format asks similar questions to single-best-answer items but without giving fixed response options. Candidates are instructed to give short answers (typically one or two words). Responses can be mostly computer-marked. Despite this form of assessment being more challenging, candidates felt they were more authentic (28), although it could be countered that the fundamental flaw of the MCQ – that of oversimplification – persists. From a generalist perspective, the key limitation of these assessments of knowledge is that, as we increasingly ask learners to 'manage uncertainty' (17,29), it seems counterproductive to have such reliance on a system of assessment which forces the selection of one single correct answer.

Another significant challenge to generalism is how standards are derived in knowledge-based assessments. The most common form of standard setting for such assessments is currently the modified Angoff process (30), although this is variably applied in different institutions (8). Although standard setters view themselves as objective, their own experience has a profound influence on their concept of question difficulty (8). Where learners are more able, standards tend to be higher (15). Furthermore, such methods tend to require subject experts and curriculum experts to provide a cut score based on their expectations of a 'just passing' candidate, which are then averaged together. It is far from clear whether the average score of a number of subject specialists is equivalent to the scores that might be provided by a generalist, and indeed there is evidence to suggest that, where raters are unfamiliar with a topic, they tend to consider it artificially difficult, thus lowering the overall cut score (31). This may also bias the generalist, who may be less familiar with unusual presentations or rare phenomena, even though they may be commonly taught. Moving to statistical definitions of cut scores, using item response theory (32) to identify and measure performance at the borderline may bring greater precision as the subjective element can be removed, but is complex, and lacks the transparency of the current methods. Ultimately a pass/fail decision can only be as good as the assessment it is based on.

Clinical skills assessments

Several different forms of clinical skills assessments exist. These include long case examinations, Objective Long Case Examination

Records (OSLERs), Objective Structured Clinical Examinations (OSCEs) and Objective Structured Assessments of Technical Skills (OSATS). Long case examinations were historically used in both undergraduate and postgraduate assessment of medical students and doctors. They involve a candidate performing a history and examination (unobserved) on a real patient before presenting their findings to an examiner(s) and being questioned. These have high face validity (in other words, they feel authentic and realistic to both examiners and learners), but raise concerns about inter-rater reliability and context specificity: what seems like a 'pass' to one examiner might not do so to another, and doing well in one exam (for example, a surgical long case) might not translate to equivalent ability elsewhere (33). If a candidate's outcome is dependent on only one or two examiners and only one or two clinical cases, then the effects of strong opinions of examiners can become significant and content areas are insufficiently sampled. Equally, the assessment of communication skills and shared decision-making is based on the outcome of a process that was unobserved.

A more structured version of the long case, the OSLER has been implemented in some medical schools to try to reduce the variability outlined, through the introduction of direct observation of the clinical interactions, and using a structured rating scale. However, the issue of context specificity remains and at least ten separate encounters are required in order to achieve reliable measurements (34).

Currently, the predominantly used clinical skills assessment is the OSCE which consists of a timed circuit of objectively marked clinical and professional skills stations. Developed by Harden and colleagues in 1975 (35), OSCEs have been demonstrated to have higher reliability due to having multiple independent judgements and wider case sampling; and they assess discrete aspects of consultations (for example, history taking, examination, breaking bad news, information giving). The OSATS is similar but restricted to technical skills (36). These types of assessment are thus intended to provide a holistic assessment of a range of clinical skills but are still limited to a small range of acceptable actions within the time constraints of the station. Many clinical skills assessments still rely on checklists, with the implication that there is a specific path to follow, and asking a patient more questions gains more points, regardless of how much use the candidate makes of the answers given. Moving from a checklist approach to a domain-based assessment (for example, including patient-centredness and confidence as domains to be scored) is an increasingly common way to allow examiners to score learners more holistically, but this comes at the expense of the objectivity afforded by a checklist. From a generalist perspective, this is no bad thing, but institutions need to guard against accusations of bias, and so the pendulum continues to swing.

Clinical skills assessments tend to be extremely expensive for institutions to run but are valued for their high quality and authenticity (22). However, Hodges (37) argues that clinical skills assessments, particularly the OSCE, cannot genuinely demonstrate reliability because 'the test itself creates the reality it is designed to assess'. As he explains, given that the format of the exam has been explicitly used by institutions to change the nature of professional behaviour, it is then disingenuous to use performance in the same exam to measure those behaviours: '[A]n examination result may be considered valid if it reflects accurately performance in "real life" outside the exam. But if the exam itself contributes to changes in the external performance then it is no longer a truly objective measure of it' (37, p. 252).

That said, it is an enormous challenge in clinical education to demonstrate safety and competence in vital clinical areas, with minimal risk to patients or the public, and so some variant of clinical skills assessment is likely to remain for the foreseeable future. Setting aside the issues of objectivity, it could be argued that the specifics of the clinical skills assessment are less important than the fact that the assessment takes place, with our own experience being that learners who have gained extensive experience in the genuine clinical setting (thus developing procedural and experiential knowledge as outlined in Chapter 6) perform better in these types of assessments, regardless of precise marking format. A useful development in this area would be to increase the use of clinical skills assessment in a formative setting, such as ward or clinic simulation exercises, or the Safe and Effective Clinical Outcomes (SECO) clinics (38), discussed below.

Professional values and behaviours

Professional values and behaviours are arguably the most challenging domain to assess summatively, and historically less time and effort has been put into assessing this domain (39). Some would, in fact, argue that assessment of values or elements of 'professional identity' are rather problematic, constraining or even suppressing the potential range of 'being human' as a clinician. To some extent, professional values and behaviours are observed in other assessments – for example, observing interactions with patients in clinical assessments (where behaviours can be included in domain-based marking or specific behaviours can be included in a checklist), or essays can offer learners the opportunity to demonstrate ethical reasoning. However, there is also a range of assessment modalities designed specifically for these competencies. These primarily include multisource feedback (MSF), patient and carer feedback, portfolio assessments (which can include components from any other format) and situational judgement tests (SJTs), which are scored and thus can be given a 'cut score'.

Multisource feedback assessments involve inviting a number (usually 10–15) of multidisciplinary colleagues to provide anonymous feedback on a learner's professional behaviours (see for example (40)). These responses are then collated and normally fed back by a supervisor or appraiser. They can provide valid assessments of teamworking and other professional behaviours, but depending on the setting are unlikely to reflect a clinician's interactions with patients. For example, in a general practice or hospital outpatient clinic, the doctor–patient interaction is unlikely to be observed by colleagues. The MSF can also be manipulated – for example, by only including colleagues with whom one has a good working relationship. Finally, although normally anonymised, it is difficult to provide feedback to the learner in a way which is meaningful without also being identifiable.

Patient satisfaction surveys may overcome this challenge, and provide unique insights into healthcare professional behaviour. These can also be combined with other measures to derive wider process measures of quality of interaction (see for example the CQI-2 tool (41)). It is, however, important to note that patient expectations may not be well aligned with current understandings of good practice (for example, appropriate prescribing of antibiotics) so will always have some distortion. Moreover, the question of whether experience can be reduced to a numerical value or metric remains challenging, despite these tools, but some compromise between ease of use and quality of content is probably inevitable.

Situational judgement tests (SJTs) are intended to assess professional behaviours, typically for the purposes of selection. They present hypothetical role-relevant scenarios and assess candidates' responses. They can be either fixed response or essay style. The fixed response formats, unlike knowledge assessments, do not ask for a single best answer. Rather, they require the selection of appropriate responses or ranking of the appropriateness of response options (see Example 7.1).

Example 7.1: SJT from the UK Foundation Programme practice paper (42)

Note: items marked with * have definitions provided at the beginning of the exam.

At your morning handover/briefing you are reminded by Infection Control* that all hospital staff should wear shirts with short sleeves. When wearing long sleeves, they must be rolled up and secured, particularly when having clinical interaction with patients. During your shift, you notice that your FY1 colleague always has her long sleeves down.

Rank in order the appropriateness of the following actions in response to this situation (1= Most appropriate; 5= Least appropriate).

A. Tell Infection Control that your colleague is not complying with their policy
B. Speak directly to your FY1 colleague about your observation
C. Raise your observation with the nurse in charge of the ward
D. Do not say anything immediately but monitor the situation over the course of the next few days
E. Discuss the situation with your specialty trainee*

Answer: BCEDA

Rationale: This question is looking at your communication with team members and patient focus. All doctors have a duty to raise concerns where they believe that patient safety is being compromised by the practice of colleagues. However, doctors strive to provide the best care possible to their patients and this situation may have arisen out of some misunderstanding. It is best therefore to speak directly to your colleague to explore the issue (B). Infection control is the responsibility not just of doctors but of the whole team of staff and indeed the organisation. The nurse in charge of the ward, although not a direct line manager, will have a key role in ensuring standards are met and so would be a sensible person to alert (C). Your specialty trainee may be able to help address this situation, though this option is less likely to explain directly the reason for your colleague keeping her sleeves down (E). Monitoring the situation (D) is less appropriate as it does not immediately address the problem. However, it is more appropriate than involving Infection Control at this stage (A) as this would risk damaging your professional relationship with your colleague and does not explore the cause of the problem.

SJTs are not without controversy. While they have been demonstrated to be a moderate predictor of subsequent measures of interpersonal skills (43), in the UK a national retrospective cohort study of administrative data found no association between SJT score and later disciplinary action by the General Medical Council (44). In other words, they may not even detect the lack of professionalism for which they purport to be designed. The standard-setting process for SJTs is also difficult, as even experienced clinicians can disagree about the most appropriate course of action in some situations (45). Similarly, scoring can seem discriminatory to both ethnicity and country of origin (45,46). Recent controversy surrounding the use of the SJT for allocation of choice of first posts immediately following qualification in the UK has led to the proposal that the assessment be abandoned for this purpose (47,48).

A commonly used form of assessment of professional values and behaviours is the professional portfolio. Here a number of different types of work can be presented, perhaps with a narrative or cross-referencing system, to allow an assessor to consider a body of work and determine whether it meets the standard needed to demonstrate sufficient understanding of, or engagement with, the topics. This is commonly used in postgraduate assessment, for example in the Annual Review of Competency Progression of UK medical trainee doctors (49), and in revalidation of senior doctors. Portfolio assessments can be highly subjective, depending on how much autonomy is granted to the assessor. Cook et al. argued in 2016 that methodology from qualitative research could be applied to written work, particularly portfolios, to make assessment methods more defensible, but as yet there is little evidence of this having been applied (50). Generally, there is an element of 'checklist' to a portfolio, with the first barrier to success being determining whether all the required items have been included, prior to making a judgement on the quality of the contents. A well-designed portfolio assessment, however, can allow a personalised and contextualised understanding of a learner's progress, and with good feedback can permit useful discussion about progression and development.

Systems of summative assessment

Historically, medical schools and postgraduate training programmes would assess learners using a selection of different assessments, aimed at these different domains. If learners performed satisfactorily on each of the individual assessments then they could progress in their training. This approach, however, inadequately accounts for the importance of integration of these individual skills and capabilities. If we return to the example of learning to drive, in many countries there is a knowledge-based assessment relating to the legislation and safety when driving. Some countries have an assessment of mechanical skills, such as changing a tyre or checking oil pressure. There may be a simulated element, where the learner can demonstrate that they know how to operate a car technically, using the controls in an artificial environment. However, without an assessment of how a learner driver integrates these competencies and applies them in practice, would this feel like an adequate assessment of a learner's ability to actually drive? Yet many programmes of assessment fall into just this pattern, in the expectation that the sum of the parts of the assessment is somehow greater than the whole. Furthermore, these assessments need to reflect authentic clinical practice, striving for the 'does' of Miller's pyramid (24).

This approach, using multiple assessments to assess different domains in a programme of assessment, is currently considered to be 'best practice' in assessment. The current move to programmatic assessment (where many assessments are combined to make progression decisions, with no one assessment determining the outcome (51)) makes considerable progress towards eliminating the binary element of the pass/fail decision, but without review of assessment content and purpose, it will not make further progress towards a generalist perspective. While this produces a multidimensional sum of assessments, it is a considerable leap to argue that this is equivalent to the holistic level of assessment that is needed for a truly generalist approach. The inclusion of MSF, patient feedback and workplace-based assessments (see below) may help to redress this, but for assessment to be truly holistic, more development is needed.

Formative assessments

Formative assessment takes a variety of formats, although there can be a significant difference between the educators' meaning of formative assessment (which can be wide-ranging and include verbal feedback in any educational setting) and the learners' meaning, which tends to focus more on practice exams and indicative marks (52). Any of the assessment types described can be used in a formative format if they are not used to make progression decisions and are primarily aimed at providing feedback for learners to improve their future performance. However, workplace-based assessments are designed specifically for feedback on performance. While summative decisions may be made on the basis of a range of workplace-based assessments, each individual assessment should be low-stakes. This section also explores developments in simulation which may help to create safe assessment spaces for feedback and development and finally considers ways in which self-assessment can be used to direct learning.

Workplace-based assessments

Assessments of authentic, integrated, workplace performance attempt to overcome the limitations of the aforementioned siloed assessments. Common workplace-based assessments currently used in the UK include case-based discussions (CBDs), mini-clinical evaluation exercises (mini-CEX), directly observed procedural skills (DOPS) and the acute care assessment tool (ACAT).

Workplace-based assessments provide a real opportunity for assessment of generalist practice. However, they too have their challenges, perhaps the most troublesome of which is the phenomenon of 'failure to fail'. Here assessors give passing grades to learners who are insufficiently competent. This arises either through a lack of recognition (that is, due to insufficient direct observation) or through an unwillingness to report for fear of repercussions (53,54). This is a pervasive issue in clinical education and one which requires significant investment in staff development to address, as it is, in essence, a failure to provide sufficient feedback to allow the learner to develop appropriately.

Simulation

Simulation is used in a formative setting to allow learners the chance to explore authentic work-like settings but with no risk to patient safety. This can be in the format of a ward or clinical simulation (for example, for final-year medical students to give them a taste of 'real life' after graduation). One format that has shown promise is the Safe and Effective Clinical Outcomes (SECO) clinic (39). These provide learners with the opportunity to run a simulated clinic, undertaking authentic whole consultations with simulated patients which are assessed based on whether the outcomes of the consultation are safe and effective.

Learners are provided with feedback based on the notes they document from the consultations, the management plans generated, and their communication skills by the simulated patients (55).

Interestingly, although there is plenty of published evidence demonstrating the validity and utility of examinations for the assessment of knowledge, synthesis and judgement, and of OSCEs for the assessment of clinical skills, there is less evidence in support of simulations and workplace-based assessment (9). Simulation is well-used (56), but hard to produce consistently, is resource-intensive and not tested across a range of areas, but is well evaluated when it is used.

Self-assessment

Self-assessment tools are often not considered with other assessments, presumably because by definition they do not include an external assessor. The challenge, though, is that there is some mistrust of self-assessment, with a number of weaknesses identified (57):

- Learners may not understand what is expected of them.
- Self-deception – learners may over- or under-estimate their competence, or score potential or ideal (rather than actual) performance.
- Learners may score for effort rather than achievement.

However, the information provided from the self-assessment process can provide very valuable information for the learner, and enable them through reflection to determine which areas of their learning or practice need further work, and which are satisfactory. Indeed, elements such as patient feedback outlined above can play a significant role in the learner's self-assessment, although it may not always be articulated in such a way. Conscious self-assessment is a valuable part of lifelong learning (57). Future developments of well-designed self-assessment tools, prompting reflection and clear guidance towards next steps, could permit genuine integration of codified knowledge ('do I know the pathophysiology of this condition?') and broader contextual knowledge ('how might this condition impact aspects of a patient's life?', 'what might influence a patient's decision to consider radical or conservative management of this condition?', 'where might this patient get extra support?'). Another area which is worth exploring is the possibility of developing 'self-monitoring' tools, which are intended to be quicker and easier to use, allowing micro-reflections 'in the moment' (58).

Assessing with a generalist lens

Given the drive towards developing more generalist clinicians, we need to move towards assessing with a more generalist lens. Accepting that it is unlikely that summative assessment will be abolished any time soon, it is vital to consider whether current assessments are able to adapt to a generalist perspective, or whether some problems are insoluble without designing entirely new formats of assessment. Some positive changes have already been highlighted, and will not be rehearsed here (see Table 7.1 where changes that have been made, or could be made, are summarised). Instead this section will highlight additional developments and finally lay down the gauntlet for developing assessment in the future. The focus will be on summative assessment, but with an expectation that formative assessments will be easier to develop along similar lines since challenges such as defensibility are less prominent (see Figure 7.2).

Table 7.1   Current and developing assessments, current issues, and how to bring a more generalist perspective

Modality	Issues	How to make it more generalist
Assessing knowledge		
Multiple-choice questions (MCQ) and very short answer questions (VSAQ)	Question selection and standard setting tends to come from specialist perspective Difficult to capture nuance, e.g. patient perspective	Include generalists in blueprinting, question selection and standard setting by generalists (as experts in generalism) Patient involvement in writing questions VSAQ may permit wider range of questions
Structured essay questions	Short structure and time pressures can mean emphasis on facts over broader perspectives Generalism may be restricted to a single question, suggesting it is peripheral	Increase integrated and cross-disciplinary knowledge in questions Involve generalists in question design

(continued)

Table 7.1 (Cont.)

Essays and case discussions	Risk of superficiality Restricting to one subject (e.g. General Practice) may imply it is optional elsewhere	Range of markers and/or tasks Integration of reflective element to emphasise applicability
Assessing skills		
Clinical skills exams (e.g. OSCE)	Checklists may give artificial weighting to inappropriate elements Students may game the system Risk of superficiality	Domain-based marking can increase value placed on key attributes, e.g. shared decision-making and communication Include generalists in blueprinting, station design and examination Include patients in station design and marking
Clinical/ward simulation	Expensive and difficult to standardise	Consider community-based simulations Include patients in design Include post-hoc reflection
Entrustable professional activities (EPAs)	Potential to be over-prescriptive Risk of bias	Write EPAs from generalist perspective Emphasise core skills and capabilities Emphasise role of context for learner and patient Involve patients in writing
Workplace-based assessments	'Failure to fail' Insufficient direct observation of clinical work Potentially time-consuming	Emphasise need for feedback for learning Emphasise role of context for learner and assessors Include patients in design and delivery
Assessing reasoning		
Situational Judgement Tests	'Black box' standard setting Allegations of cultural bias	Emphasise context and communication in questions
Viva/Long case	Subjective/bias common	Include reactive and contextual elements Involve patient as assessor

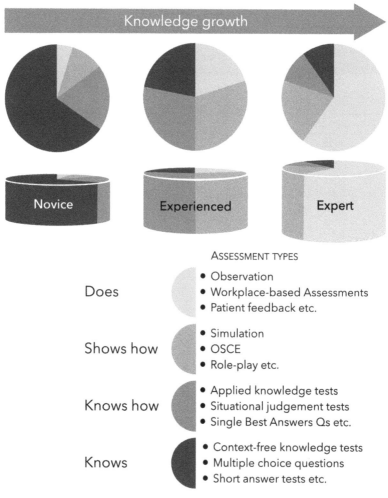

Figure 7.2 Towards an integrated generalist assessment. © Sophie Park and Kay Leedham-Green

Developing existing assessments

As outlined above, current summative assessments are constructed mostly from panels of experts each creating their own items. These assessments, therefore, end up testing a broad range of specialist areas, rather than those which are interconnected or interdependent. Knowledge of individual conditions is typically assessed in separate items, and the highly complex or nuanced is generally overlooked in favour of the concrete. However, as clinical curricula include more complex learning outcomes, the onus is on assessors to develop ways to assess. One example is the inclusion of topics such as leadership and patient-centred decision-making into the UK undergraduate medical curriculum (29), which has then necessitated the creation of assessment items to include in the new national licensing exam (59). However, past experience is that some topics are not easily included in this assessment framework, despite the best efforts of question writers (18).

Redefining what needs to be assessed: the problem with 'competencies'

Both individual assessments and systems of assessment must strive to ensure they reflect authentic clinical practice. This involves taking a holistic approach to patients' wellbeing, adopting a biopsychosocial model of care, and considering the interplay of comorbidities. Within clinical education, these now tend to be referred to as 'competencies'. The concept of competencies was introduced in medical education in the early twenty-first century, and was something of a revolution (60,61): remember that previously most educational milestones in medicine were defined by 'time served', with little objective measurement of the process. In contrast, this new approach outlined first the desired final outcomes of the educational process; then competencies which make up that final outcome (for example, to have new doctors graduate who are competent in clinical skills); then the process is repeated to define the outcomes for each step of the process of learning. The concept has never been universally welcomed, with complaints that it is inherently reductionist, and that 'competency' implies a 'lowest common denominator' approach to training (62). However, there is value in defining what clinical education should aim for, and in naming the various components that are required to get there. Ten Cate and Schumacher describe competencies as 'by their nature, need[ing] a context to make them visible' (63). They use the example of a pianist – without a piano nearby, you have no way of knowing how competent they are at playing. Moreover, they may be fluent in Arabic, and a fast sprinter, but you would not know that even if they are playing the piano. The other criticism of the word 'competency' is the implication of a threshold which once reached is definitive – as with some current descriptions of 'cultural competency' (64). However, it seems likely that any alternative adopted (for example, ability, capability) could ultimately end up subject to the same drift in meaning and understanding. Consequently, we have in general retained the term 'competency' here.

Well-described competencies are (a) specific, (b) comprehensive (that is, include knowledge, attitude and skill), (c) durable, (d) trainable, (e) measurable, (f) related to professional activities and (g) connected to other competencies (61). We are observing a shift in how competencies are articulated and emphasised, moving from a previously quite mechanistic description of the tasks and roles of a doctor to emphasise a more generalist perspective, which must necessarily be followed with appropriate changes to assessment (9) (Figures 7.3 and 7.4). It should be noted, however, that these wider, more holistic competencies (or overarching meta-competencies) come in addition to the requirements to demonstrate codified knowledge. Thus clinical education continues to be codified and subdivided, with assessment required for each component, then integrated into a final decision about the learner's competence or otherwise (Table 7.2).

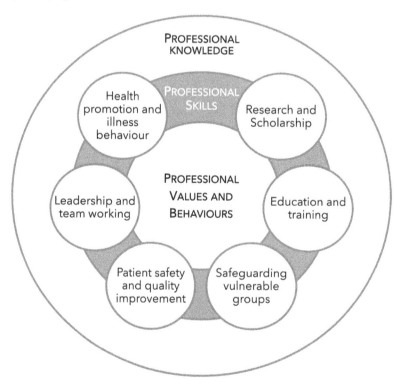

Figure 7.3 Clinical competencies, then and now: The UK General Medical Council's Generic Clinical Capabilities Framework 2017. © General Medical Council, reproduced with permission, not for adaptation and revision or for reproduction in condensed versions or excerpts of this book

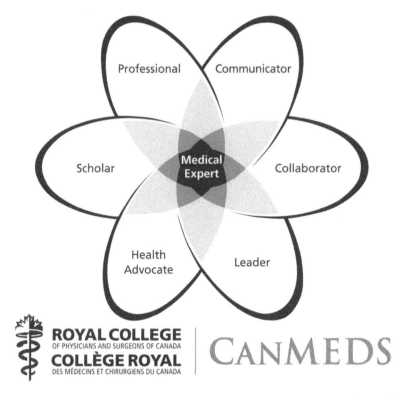

Figure 7.4 Clinical competencies, then and now: The Royal College of Physicians and Surgeons of Canada's CanMEDs framework 2015

Table 7.2 Clinical competencies, then and now: The Association of American Medical Colleges Medical School Objectives Project (AAMC MSOP) 1999 (72)

Altruistic	Knowledgeable	Skillful	Dutiful
• Ethical decision-making • Compassionate treatment of patients	• Knowledge of normal structure and function of the body and the organs • Knowledge of molecular, biomedical and cellular mechanisms of homeostasis	• Obtain accurate medical history • Carry out complete and organ-specific examinations including mental state	• Know the importance of non-biological determinants of health • Know epidemiology and prevent common maladies

(continued)

Table 7.2 (Cont.)

Altruistic	Knowledgeable	Skillful	Dutiful
• Honesty and integrity • Understand other healthcare professionals • Advocate for the patient • Understand the conflicts of interest • Recognise and accept own limitations	• Knowledge of causes of maladies, and pathogenesis • Knowledge of pathology and pathophysiology • Understand aetiology and treatment, including traditional / non-traditional • Understand need for lifelong learning	• Perform routine technical procedures • Interpret common diagnostic procedures • Knowledge of manifestations and common maladies • Reason deductively • Construct appropriate management strategy • Recognise and manage life-threatening conditions • Recognise and manage serious conditions • Relieve pain • Communicate effectively	• Identify individual risk factors • Retrieve and manage medical information • Know about organisation, management and financing of healthcare • Commit to provide healthcare for people and communities who are unable to pay

Redefining how we assess

We have demonstrated how the changing emphasis in clinical education has changed some of the competencies which should be assessed,
but have so far only seen ways in which current assessment modalities
are adjusted to attempt to accommodate some of these. This somewhat
tokenistic approach to changing emphasis reflects the as-yet unresolved tension between the needs of institutions to provide assessments
which are robust and defensible and generalism's experiential approach
(Figure 7.5).

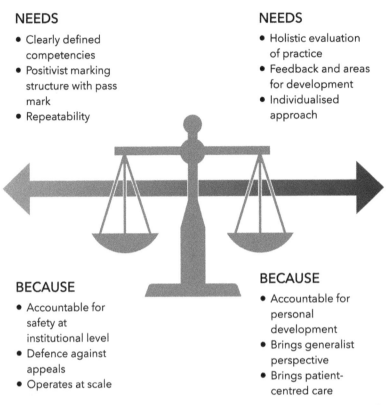

NEEDS
- Clearly defined competencies
- Positivist marking structure with pass mark
- Repeatability

NEEDS
- Holistic evaluation of practice
- Feedback and areas for development
- Individualised approach

BECAUSE
- Accountable for safety at institutional level
- Defence against appeals
- Operates at scale

BECAUSE
- Accountable for personal development
- Brings generalist perspective
- Brings patient-centred care

Figure 7.5 The fundamental conflict between traditional institutional approaches to assessment and generalism. © Eleanor Hothersall

Programmes of assessment (and their formal version, programmatic assessment), discussed above, offer one way of negotiating this conflict: accumulating enough data points of assessment that the sum demonstrates the achievements of the learner, while not needing any individual assessment to stand up to excessive positivist scrutiny (51). Another area currently under development is 'entrustable professional activities' (EPAs) (61,65). This is an intuitively appealing extension of competency-based learning, formalising the process whereby a trainer can decide when a learner may be trusted to bear responsibility to perform a professional activity, given the level of competence they have reached (61). The examples offered are often quite mechanistic (for example, venepuncture), but actually they can apply just as well to generalist approaches. As an example, one requirement of the GMC's General Professional Competencies Framework is 'sharing decision-making by informing the patient, prioritising the patient's wishes, and respecting the patient's concerns and expectations' (65, p.11). We can imagine a learner might be trusted to have discussions about decision-making under supervision, whereas around qualification they might be trusted to have the discussions and then share them with a supervisor. Then, once they were more experienced they could be trusted to have those conversations entirely unsupervised and simply relay or document the outcomes. The concept of 'trust' is key here: applied appropriately it changes the nature of the learner's relationship to their trainers, and may simultaneously reduce the risk of 'failing to fail' discussed earlier. Using an EPA structure may be one way to allow assessors to emphasise key values from generalism, such as integrating and co-constructing and decision-making in each individual patient's context.

The challenge for the future

As outlined above, the challenge for assessment of healthcare professionals is to achieve a programme of assessment that is at once authentic, holistic and achievable. Initial steps are to include patient and learner users alongside academic stakeholders in the production of assessment modalities. As outlined in Table 7.1, many assessments could increase their authenticity by increasing the input from patients or the public. There is a growing body of research outlining the ways that patients and patient groups can contribute to undergraduate (10,66) and postgraduate clinical education (11), including curriculum design and contributing to formative and summative assessment through clinical skills exams such as OSCEs, but there has been little reference to involvement in design of assessment (67). This is surely an important area for future development, reducing the risk of potential bias that is a concern when patients act as examiners (68,69). With learners, a critical discussion about the constraints of existing assessment approaches can begin by asking them to write a question (e.g. SBA) about a recent clinical experience. This makes visible to the learner the small subsection of knowledge possible to assess through this modality, in relation to the wider knowledge they have used to tackle complex decision-making in practice. Learners can then become partners in the production of alternative assessment approaches which make visible a broader range of generalist expertise and drive generalist learning.

While we have outlined many areas where improvements can already be made, some challenges remain unmet. Some of these are dimensions of a generalist approach which are not captured currently, such as curiosity, and moving more generally from an emphasis on 'knowing' to 'implementing knowledge'. Similarly, could we envisage an assessment of clinical reasoning in the future which evaluates a learner's 'inductive foraging' (70)? It is difficult to imagine an assessment which brings core values and beliefs of learners to light, but unless and until such an assessment is created, we will not be able to determine properly whether our learner 'gets it', or is just acting the role until they qualify.

We finish with a call to stakeholders (learners and educationalists) to focus their energies on moving to a system of assessment in which they are no longer focusing on a single form or set of knowledge, but balancing a range of interrelated knowledge forms (see Chapter 1). For as long as it remains true that assessment is the engine that drives learning (Cowan quoted in (71)), it remains vital to drive it in the right direction.

References

1. Fenton R. Performance assessment system development. *Alsk Educ Res J*. 1996;2(1):13–22.
2. Hafferty FW. Beyond curriculum reform: confronting medicine's hidden curriculum. *Acad Med*. 1998;73(4):403–7.
3. Norcini J, Anderson MB, Bollela V, Burch V, Costa MJ, Duvivier R, et al. 2018 Consensus framework for good assessment. *Med Teach*. 2018;40(11):1102–9.
4. Harden RM. Five myths and the case against a European or national licensing examination. *Med Teach*. 2009;31(3):217–20.
5. Jaye P, Thomas L, Reedy G. 'The Diamond': a structure for simulation debrief. *Clin Teach*. 2015;12(3):171–5.
6. Kurtz S, Draper J, Silverman J. *Teaching and Learning Communication Skills in Medicine*. CRC Press; 2017.
7. Ben-David MF. AMEE Guide No. 18: Standard setting in student assessment. *Med Teach*. 2000;22(2):120–30.
8. Yeates P, Cope N, Luksaite E, Hassell A, Dikomitis L. Exploring differences in individual and group judgements in standard setting. *Med Educ*. 2019;53(9):941–52.
9. Norcini J, Anderson B, Bollela V, Burch V, Costa MJ, Duvivier R, et al. Criteria for good assessment: Consensus statement and recommendations from the Ottawa 2010 Conference. *Med Teach*. 2011;33(3):206–14.
10. Dijk SW, Duijzer EJ, Wienold M. Role of active patient involvement in undergraduate medical education: a systematic review. *BMJ Open*. 2020;10(7):e037217.
11. Khalife R, Gupta M, Gonsalves C, Park YS, Riddle J, Tekian A, et al. Patient involvement in assessment of postgraduate medical learners: A scoping review. *Med Educ*. 2022;56(6):602–13.
12. Kane MT. Validation. In: Brennan RL, editor. *Educational Measurement*. 4th ed. Praeger; 2006. pp. 17–64.
13. Cook DA, Brydges R, Ginsburg S, Hatala R. A contemporary approach to validity arguments: a practical guide to Kane's framework. *Med Educ*. 2015;49(6):560–75.
14. Apple MW. *Ideology and Curriculum*. 2nd ed. Routledge; 1990.
15. Livingston SA, Zieky MJ. A comparative study of standard-setting methods. *ETS Res Rep Ser*. 1983;1983(2):i–48.
16. Medical Schools Council Selection Alliance. Indicators of Good Practice in Contextual Admissions. 2018. Available from: www.medschools.ac.uk/media/2413/good-practice-in-contextual-admissions.pdf (accessed 14 March 2024).

17. GMC. Outcomes for Graduates. 2018. Available from: www.gmc-uk.org/-/media/documents/dc11326-outcomes-for-graduates-2018_pdf-75040796.pdf (accessed 14 March 2024).
18. Hothersall E, Rodrigues V, Gordon M, Mclachlan JC, McAleer S. Making it fit: examining the assessment of contextual knowledge and understanding in the positivist assessment modality of medical education. In: *EDULEARN20 Proceedings*. IATED; 2020. pp. 2566–74.
19. Newble DI, Jaeger K. The effect of assessments and examinations on the learning of medical students. *Med Educ*. 1983;17(3):165–71.
20. Newble DI. Assessment. In: *Medical Education in the Millenium*. 1st ed. Oxford University Press; 1998. pp. 131–42.
21. Biggs J. Enhancing teaching through constructive alignment. *High Educ*. 1996;32(3):347–64.
22. Patricio M. A best evidence medical education (BEME) systematic review on the feasibility, reliability and validity of the objective structured clinical examination (OSCE) in undergraduate medical studies. Doctoral thesis, University of Lisbon. 2012.
23. Harrison CJ, Könings KD, Dannefer EF, Schuwirth LWT, Wass V, Van Der Vleuten CPM. Factors influencing students' receptivity to formative feedback emerging from different assessment cultures. *Perspect Med Educ*. 2016;5(5):276–84.
24. Miller GE. The assessment of clinical skills/competence/performance. *Acad Med*. 1990;65(9). Available from: https://journals.lww.com/academicmedicine/Fulltext/1990/09000/The_assessment_of_clinical.45.aspx (accessed 14 March 2024).
25. Devine OP, Harborne AC, McManus IC. Assessment at UK medical schools varies substantially in volume, type and intensity and correlates with postgraduate attainment. *BMC Med Educ*. 2015;15(1):146.
26. Paxton M. A linguistic perspective on multiple choice questioning. *Assess Eval High Educ*. 2000;25(2):109–19.
27. Millar KR, Reid MD, Rajalingam P, Canning CA, Halse O, Low-Beer N, et al. Exploring the feasibility of using very short answer questions (VSAQs) in team-based learning (TBL). *Clin Teach*. 2021;18(4):404–8.
28. Sam AH, Field SM, Collares CF, van der Vleuten CPM, Wass VJ, Melville C, et al. Very-short-answer questions: reliability, discrimination and acceptability. *Med Educ*. 2018;52(4):447–55.
29. Royal College of Physicians and Surgeons of Canada. CanMEDS: Better standards, better physicians, better care. 2015. Available from: www.royalcollege.ca/rcsite/canmeds/canmeds-framework-e (accessed 14 March 2024).
30. Ricker KL. Setting Cut-Scores: A Critical Review of the Angoff and Modified Angoff Methods. *Alta J Educ Res*. 2006;52(1):53–64.
31. Clauser JC, Hambleton RK, Baldwin P. The effect of rating unfamiliar items on Angoff passing scores. *Educ Psychol Meas*. 2017;77(6):901–16.
32. Lahner FM, Schauber S, Lörwald AC, Kropf R, Guttormsen S, Fischer MR, et al. Measurement precision at the cut score in medical multiple choice exams: theory matters. *Perspect Med Educ*. 2020;9(4):220–8.
33. Wass V, Van Der Vleuten C. The long case. *Med Educ*. 2004;38(11):1176–80.
34. Gleeson F. AMEE Medical Education Guide No. 9. Assessment of clinical competence using the Objective Structured Long Examination Record (OSLER). *Med Teach*. 1997;19(1):7–14.
35. Harden RM, Stevenson M, Downie WW, Wilson GM. Assessment of clinical competence using objective structured examination. *Br Med J*. 1975;1(5955):447.
36. Martin J, Regehr G, Reznick R, Macrae H, Murnaghan J, Hutchison C, et al. Objective structured assessment of technical skill (OSATS) for surgical residents. *Br J Surg*. 1997;84(2):273–8.
37. Hodges B. Validity and the OSCE. *Med Teach*. 2003;25(3):250–4.
38. Williamson M, Walker T, Egan T, Storr E, Ross J, Kenrick K. The Safe and Effective Clinical Outcomes (SECO) clinic: learning responsibility for patient care through simulation. *Teach Learn Med*. 2013;25(2):155–8.
39. Ten Cate O. Summative assessment of medical students in the affective domain. *Med Teach*. 2000;22(1):40–3.
40. Health Education England. Using Multisource feedback (MSF) as an assessment tool. 2022. Available from: https://nshcs.hee.nhs.uk/programmes/hsst/trainees/multi-source-feedback-msf/ (accessed 16 March 2023).
41. Mercer SW, Howie JGR. CQI-2 – a new measure of holistic interpersonal care in primary care consultations. *Br J Gen Pract*. 2006;56(525):262–8.

42. UK Foundation Programme. Practice SJT Paper1, with answers. Practice SJT Papers. Available from:https://foundationprogramme.nhs.uk/resources/situational-judgement-test-sjt/practice-sjt-papers/ (accessed 1 June 2023).
43. Olaru G, Burrus J, MacCann C, Zaromb FM, Wilhelm O, Roberts RD. Situational judgment tests as a method for measuring personality: development and validity evidence for a test of dependability. Gnambs T, editor. *PLoS One*. 2019;14(2):e0211884.
44. Sam AH, Bala L, Westacott RJ, Brown C. Is academic attainment or situational judgment test performance in medical school associated with the likelihood of disciplinary action? A national retrospective cohort study. *Acad Med*. 2021;96(10):1467–75.
45. De Leng WE, Stegers-Jager KM, Husbands A, Dowell JS, Born MPh, Themmen APN. Scoring method of a situational judgment test: influence on internal consistency reliability, adverse impact and correlation with personality? *Adv Health Sci Educ*. 2017;22(2):243–65.
46. ISFP Project. FP technical reports 2013–2020. Work Psychology Group; Improving Selection to the Foundation Programme. Available from: https://isfp.org.uk/fp-technical-reports/ (accessed 28 March 2023).
47. Nabavi N. How appropriate is the situational judgment test in assessing future foundation doctors? *BMJ*. 2023;p101.
48. Sam AH, Fung CY, Reed M, Hughes E, Meeran K. Time for preference-informed foundation allocation? *Clin Med Lond Engl*. 2022 Nov;22(6):590–3.
49. Health Education England. Annual Review of Competency Progression. Available from: www.hee.nhs.uk/our-work/annual-review-competency-progression (accessed 16 March 2023).
50. Cook DA, Kuper A, Hatala R, Ginsburg S. When assessment data are words: validity evidence for qualitative educational assessments. *Acad Med*. 2016;91(10):1359–69.
51. van der Vleuten CPM, Schuwirth LWT, Driessen EW, Dijkstra J, Tigelaar D, Baartman LKJ, et al. A model for programmatic assessment fit for purpose. *Med Teach*. 2012;34(3):205–14.
52. Wood DF. Formative assessment. In: Walsh K, editor. *Oxford Textbook of Medical Education*. Oxford University Press; 2013. pp. 478–88. Available from: https://academic.oup.com/book/25271/chapter/189859752 (accessed 28 March 2023).
53. Mak-van der Vossen M. 'Failure to fail': the teacher's dilemma revisited. *Med Educ*. 2019;53(2):108–10.
54. Adkins DA, Aucoin JW. Failure to fail – factors affecting faculty decisions to pass underperforming nursing students in the clinical setting: a quantitative study. *Nurse Educ Pract*. 2022;58:103259.
55. Bearman M, Nestel D, Andreatta P. Simulation-based medical education. In: Walsh K, editor. *Oxford Textbook of Medical Education*. Oxford University Press; 2013. pp. 186–97. Available from: https://academic.oup.com/book/25271/chapter/189849636 (accessed 28 March 2023).
56. Royal College of General Practitioners. MRCGP: Simulated Consultation Assessment (SCA). 2023. Available from: www.rcgp.org.uk/mrcgp-exams/simulated-consultation-assessment (accessed 28 April 2023).
57. Evans AW, McKenna C, Oliver M. Self-assessment in medical practice. *J R Soc Med*. 2002;95(10):511–3.
58. Johnson WR, Durning SJ, Allard RJ, Barelski AM, Artino Jr AR. A scoping review of self-monitoring in graduate medical education. *Med Educ*. 2023. Available from: https://doi.org/10.1111/medu.15023 (accessed 27 March 2023).
59. General Medical Council. MLA Content Map. 2021. Available from: www.gmc-uk.org/education/medical-licensing-assessment/mla-content-map (accessed 16 March 2023).
60. Harden RM. AMEE Guide No. 14: Outcome-based education: Part 1 – An introduction to outcome-based education. *Med Teach*. 1999;21(1):7–14.
61. Ten Cate O. Entrustability of professional activities and competency-based training. *Med Educ*. 2005;39(12):1176–7.
62. Ross S, Hauer KE, Van Melle E. Outcomes are what matter: competency-based medical education gets us to our goal. *MedEdPublish*. 2018;7:85.
63. Ten Cate O, Schumacher DJ. Entrustable professional activities versus competencies and skills: Exploring why different concepts are often conflated. *Adv Health Sci Educ*. 2022;27(2):491–9.
64. Lekas HM, Pahl K, Fuller Lewis C. Rethinking cultural competence: shifting to cultural humility. *Health Serv Insights*. 2020;13:117863292097058.

65. General Medical Council. Generic Professional Capabilities Framework. 2017. Available from:www.gmc-uk.org/education/standards-guidance-and-curricula/standards-and-outcomes/generic-professional-capabilities-framework (accessed 13 June 2023).
66. Ten Cate O. Nuts and bolts of Entrustable Professional Activities. *J Grad Med Educ*. 2013;5(1):157–8.
67. Jha V, Quinton ND, Bekker HL, Roberts TE. Strategies and interventions for the involvement of real patients in medical education: a systematic review. *Med Educ*. 2009;43(1):10–20.
68. Tew J, Gell C, Foster S. Learning from experience. Involving service users and carers in mental health education and training. UK Higher Education Academy/National Institute for Mental Health in England/Trent Workforce Development Confederation; 2004. Available from: www.swapbox.ac.uk/692/1/learning-from-experience-whole-guide.pdf (accessed 19 November 2022).
69. Moreau K, Eady K, Jabbour M. Patient involvement in resident assessment within the Competence by Design context: a mixed-methods study. *Can Med Educ J*. 2019;10(1):e84–102.
70. Donner-Banzhoff N. Solving the diagnostic challenge: a patient-centered approach. *Ann Fam Med*. 2018;16(4):353–8.
71. Quality Assurance Agency for Higher Education. *Reflections on Assessment: Volume 1*. QAA Scotland; 2005. Available from: www.enhancementthemes.ac.uk/docs/ethemes/assessment/reflections-on-assessment-volume-i.pdf (accessed 14 March 2024).
72. Medical School Objectives Writing Group. Learning objectives for medical student education. Guidelines for medical schools: Report I of the Medical School Objectives Project. *Academic Medicine* 1999;74(1):13–18.

Part III: Systems approaches

In Part I, we described the foundational principles and academic practices of generalism. In Part II, we explored generalist approaches to education. Part III looks at generalism at a systems level: how the structure of health and social care systems can enable or inhibit generalism, how and why generalism contributes to efficient, effective and sustainable healthcare, and generalist strategies for systems innovation and improvement.

8

Organisation and design of healthcare for generalism

Stewart Mercer, John Gillies and Clare MacRae

Introduction

This chapter examines how traditional, existing and future healthcare systems can support or undermine generalism in practice. We discuss current issues within UK general practice, although our reflections and suggestions on the crucial contribution of generalism to healthcare systems are by no means limited to this context. The relevance of generalism within all healthcare systems is emphasised. We provide historical examples from medicine with relevance to generalist clinical learning and practice today and beyond.

Drawing on Don Berwick's seminal paper published in 2016 'Era 3 for Medicine and Health Care' (1), we describe how the 'epic collision of two eras with incompatible beliefs' has undermined generalism, and emphasise the achievable changes required in the organisation and delivery of care to make 'Era 3' a reality with generalism at its core. We highlight the importance of generalism and Era 3 approaches now and in the future, as healthcare systems worldwide face the increasing challenges posed by mobile and ageing populations, isolation, multimorbidity and frailty. We describe how and why the organisation and design of healthcare systems, and their surrounding social, political and physical environments, are crucial to enabling effective and efficient generalist care.

Generalism is not a panacea for poverty, poor housing, unemployment, insecurity, abuse or injustice and will never fully mitigate health inequalities. However, generalism can help work towards ensuring health services work best where they are needed most. We highlight the key partnerships required – between health and social care providers and between care providers, care users and the general public – for generalism to flourish in the interests of the people that need it, now and in the future.

The value of generalism

> Man is the measure of all things.
>
> Protagoras the Sophist (c.490–c.420 BCE)

Protagoras's epigram suggests that, in much of what we ('man') do and decide to do, there are few truly objective truths. We have the freedom and the responsibility to decide what we measure and therefore what we regard as important. This is relevant because, for the organisation and design of healthcare to reflect generalist principles, it must embrace and balance different ways of seeing, knowing and understanding the world by integrating statistical evidence with a deep understanding of patient, community and population perspectives. For generalism to be valued, research should therefore reflect the science of qualities as well as the science of quantities. It should also include what has been described as the 'tacit knowledge' that experienced clinicians and patients acquire over years of engagement with individual patients, including their knowledge and understanding of what has worked well and less well in the organisation and delivery of healthcare (see Chapters 4 and 5).

Joanne Reeve has defined generalism as:

> a philosophy of practice which is person, not disease centred; continuous, not episodic; integrates biotechnical and biographical perspectives; and views health as a resource for living and not an end in itself.
>
> Reeve 2010 (2)

This 'way of looking at the world' is similarly reflected in what Launer describes as 'attentiveness' or paying close attention to every aspect of the patient's story (see Chapter 10). This attentiveness relies on the perceptual capacity of the clinician (3). Perceptual capacity is founded on *phronesis*: the ability to read or assess a situation correctly, in depth and breadth. Wiggins called this '*aisthesis*' or 'situational appreciation' (4), and Nussbaum 'some sort of complex responsiveness to the salient features of one's situation' (5). It is based on sound clinical knowledge, the exercise of empathy and compassion and the judicious use of imagination

and finely tuned emotional responses. To achieve this, health professionals should aim while consulting to become 'a person on whom nothing is
lost' (Henry James as paraphrased in 6,7).

This perceptual capacity or situational appreciation also applies to
the organisation, structure and delivery of healthcare. This must reflect a
broader understanding, contained within the above definitions, of individual health and ill health in the context of families, communities and
cultures, how these constrain or enhance physical and mental health
from both biographical and biotechnical perspectives.

An economic argument for generalism

All countries are eager to contain the costs of healthcare, and this has
become especially important with the growing costs associated with ageing, mobile and multimorbid societies. Indeed, the challenge of ageing
has been defined as one of the grand challenges facing modern society.
Secondary care consumes most healthcare costs, relating largely to hospital admission and length of stay. As specialists become increasingly
super-specialised, the complexity of care increases and costs escalate
further. Delivery of generalist care is a key method of mitigating these
spiralling costs, as well as reducing fragmentation of care which leads
to treatment burden for the patient as well as harmful effects from polypharmacy. Thus, developing generalism across healthcare systems will
be an important way to make care more rational and sustainable, to
reduce waste and duplication, and to reduce harm to the patient.

At the population level, a strong primary care system based on generalism is key to cost containment and the provision of high-quality care.
The groundbreaking work of Barbara Starfield (8) showed clearly that
countries with strong primary care systems deliver higher quality care
and are more cost-effective than countries without strong primary care
(Figure 8.1).

Generalism: past, present and future

Effective healthcare is one of the huge successes of the post-Enlightenment
age. The evolution of healthcare, however, has been a long journey with
periods of stasis punctuated by episodic rapid advances. Aseptic surgical
techniques, anaesthetics, immunisation against infectious disease, joint
replacements and antibiotics, are only some of these advances. However,
not all progress has been based on 'medical' advances. In addition, public

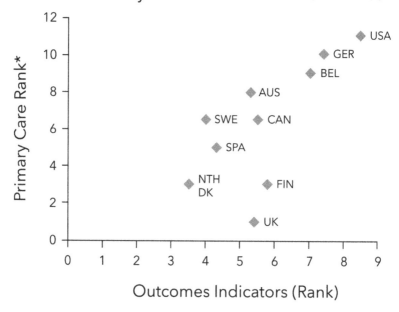

Relationship between Strength of Primary Care and Combined Outcomes

*1 = best : 11 = worst

Figure 8.1 Relationship between strength of primary care and outcomes. Barbara Starfield (8), reproduced under the Creative Commons licence CC BY-NC-ND 4.0

health measures, such as housing and sanitation, have arguably made a much greater contribution to people's health than any of the previous examples. Florence Nightingale's 'proper use of fresh air, light, warmth, cleanliness, quiet and proper diet' in 1854 dramatically reduced deaths among casualties during the Crimean War. Infectious diseases, such as tuberculosis, scarlet fever, diphtheria, pertussis and measles, were common and led to the building of hundreds of isolation hospitals usually with a focus on Nightingale's principles, as no specific treatments were generally available.

In the UK, the National Health Service (NHS) was established in 1948 on the principles that it should be comprehensive (meet the needs of everyone); that it should be universal (free to all at the point of delivery to access GP consultations or hospital treatment); and that it be based on clinical need, not ability to pay (9). The establishment and functioning of the NHS were dependent on medical cadres adopting a generalist approach. The surgical techniques and therapeutic advances that have subsequently led to increased specialisation and super-specialisation were not yet developed. So, most doctors had, by necessity, to be clinical generalists managing the widest range of clinical problems and presentations with a limited range of equipment and therapies. The founding of the Royal College of General Practitioners (RCGP) in the UK in 1952 included a commitment to an approach to generalism that embraced science and compassion as *'cum scientia caritas'*. That broad approach to the care of patients is at heart a generalist one and necessitates a way of looking at the organisation and delivery of care that goes far beyond the immediate clinical problem. Although central to the philosophy of good general practice, it is not necessarily unique to general practice (2,10).

Berwick describes Era 1 as the establishment and ascendancy of the power of the medical profession (dating back to the time of Hippocrates) in which the doctor is regarded as noble, beneficent, with knowledge that is inaccessible to everyday people (and patients), and thus all-powerful. Many of the advances described above occurred during this Era 1, an era of professional autonomy. The 'doctor as God' construct led to the profession being exempt from external scrutiny, and able to judge the quality of its own work and to self-regulate. This model of medicine, based on prerogative and blind trust, continued well after the establishment of the NHS in 1948, and only began to be challenged when researchers studying healthcare systems uncovered issues such as enormous unexplained variation in practices, high rates of clinical errors, and inequities in care relating to sex, race and social class, together with evidence that the soaring costs of healthcare were not always related to better patient outcomes.

This heralded the birth of Era 2 medicine, characterised by accountability, governance, scrutiny, measurement, targets, incentives and (in many countries) marketisation. In the UK, the evolution of Era 2 can be traced back to the rising influence and power of managerialism within the NHS, including the separation of health and social care, and the introduction of the provider–purchaser split by the UK's Thatcher government in 1998. Berwick contends that the inherent tensions between these two eras continue to play out. In his own words, 'this conflict impedes the pursuit of the social goals of fundamentally better care, better health, and lower cost' (1).

One of the developments of Era 2 healthcare has been the enormous growth of specialist and super-specialist care and the single-disease paradigm that has come to dominate clinical care and evidence-based medicine (discussed also in Chapters 2 and 5). However, recent concerns around the wastes and harms of overdiagnosis and overtreatment have led to an increased focus on a generalist approach which uses a much wider view of the patient and their life as part of a community to complement a disease-focused approach (11). A related development has been a vision of clinical care in the future being delivered through 'realistic medicine'. Championed by the Chief Medical Officer (CMO) in Scotland in 2015, this concept aims to reduce the burdens of overdiagnosis and overtreatment, reduce waste and harm, increase patient involvement in decision-making, and encourage innovation (12). Arguably this is only possible by adopting a generalist approach to the organisation and delivery of care (11) and can be seen as part of a broader move to Era 3 medicine.

> Era 3 medicine is guided by reduced measurement, improvement science, transparency, and co-production with patients. Achieving this requires a paradigm shift to an approach to medicine that has realistic and proportionate, high-quality, high-value care as its aim and collaboration at its core.
>
> Smith et al. 2017 (13) referencing Berwick 2016 (1)

Both the philosophy of generalism described in Chapter 1, and the day-to-day practices of health professionals, support a shift from Era 2 to Era 3: reduced mandatory measurement and incentivisation; complete transparency; shifting the business model from forefronting revenue to quality; embracing improvement science; replacing individual professional prerogative with a team identity; working collaboratively in the interests of patients and populations through co-production, co-design and person-centred approaches; protecting civility; and rejecting greed.

A common question, given that an Era 3 approach is inherently responsive to local needs, is how the success or otherwise of local approaches should be assessed or assured; and given reduced incentivisation, how healthcare systems can be organised to encourage excellence. Letting go of Era 2 thinking and embracing Era 3 requires moving from a culture of measurement and incentivised targets (that are often poorly, or at best crudely, aligned to people's needs) towards a culture of transparency and collaborative engagement in continuous improvement. We argue that Era 3 approaches are necessary to realise the key advantages of generalism as outlined by the Essence of General Practice group (14):

- **Trust** in both professional intentions and competence.
- **Coordination** between people, community and hospital services.
- **Continuity** of care with attention to both current and future needs.
- **Flexibility** of thinking and approach.
- **Coverage** for all, including disadvantaged and marginalised people.
- **Leadership** based on situated and multidisciplinary knowledge.

General practice and generalism

Generalism, as explored in Chapters 1 and 2, is applicable in all aspects of healthcare. General practice, however, is where the philosophy of generalism, its practical application and evolution are currently most clearly reflected. General practice is underpinned by a holistic, biopsychosocial approach to care that combines the biomedical with the biographical. This is one of the reasons why the consultation between clinician and patient is such a key feature of general practice training and research. The rise of specialism and super-specialism has to some extent endangered generalist learning by focusing on narrowly biomedical rather than more holistic approaches, a trend that must be reversed if the needs of patients and populations are to be met in ways that are both person-centred and future-proof. The role of general practice in the delivery of generalism remains central to the functioning of universal healthcare systems. The WHO estimates that effective public health and primary care could prevent up to 70 per cent of the disease burden through primary prevention, supported self-care, and health in all policies (15).

General practice plays a key role in the enactment of generalism within healthcare systems for the reasons set out in Figure 8.2. General practice is the central hub of effective healthcare systems, providing people with contact (the average person in the UK consults a GP approximately six times a year), coverage (almost the entire population is registered with a single GP practice in the UK), continuity (both informational and relational), comprehensive (there is no condition or population group that GPs will not consult with or manage as an initial presentation), coordinated care (GPs are the gatekeepers of the NHS, and refer fewer than 10 per cent of the patients who consult them to secondary care services) built on historically good relationships and high levels of trust.

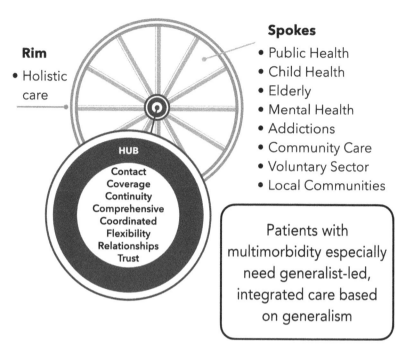

Rim

• Holistic care

HUB

Contact
Coverage
Continuity
Comprehensive
Coordinated
Flexibility
Relationships
Trust

Spokes

• Public Health
• Child Health
• Elderly
• Mental Health
• Addictions
• Community Care
• Voluntary Sector
• Local Communities

Patients with multimorbidity especially need generalist-led, integrated care based on generalism

Figure 8.2 General practice as the hub of generalist healthcare. Reproduced with permission from Graham Watt

Example 8.1: Current threats to UK general practice

In 2008, Don Berwick described UK general practice as the 'jewel in the crown' of the NHS (16). However, there is, at the time of writing, a crippling workforce crisis in UK general practice. This is driven by rising patient demand and complexity, insufficient numbers of general practitioners, unsustainable workloads, insufficient resources, political scapegoating and outdated infrastructure (17). A focus on Era 2 approaches has increased the compartmentalisation and commodification of general practice work, reducing opportunities for relational expertise and continuity (18). General practice delivers approximately 90 per cent of healthcare activity in the UK, using only approximately 10 per cent of NHS funding – which has only returned to this level recently after falling as low as 8 per cent in 2013 (19,20). Between 2008 and 2018, there was a rapid rise in new hospital NHS consultants compared with either

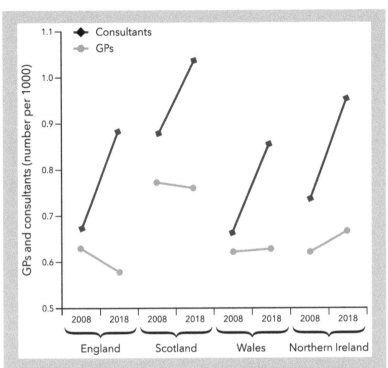

Figure 8.3 Rise in hospital consultants versus GPs in the UK. Data Source: Anderson et al. (26)

very small increases, or actual decreases, in GP numbers across the four nations of the UK (Figure 8.3).

The delivery of generalist care to the population is only possible through a strong general practice foundation that provides continuous cradle-to-grave care for all citizens. Precisely the opposite has been encouraged under successive UK governments. An ideological belief in market forces has neither improved efficiency nor increased capacity. Instead, it has created a fragmented, supply-driven system that has catastrophically failed to address the demand side of healthcare (21). Resource allocation towards hospitals rather than primary care has increased costs without reducing demand (22) and financial cuts to public health and social care may actually be increasing demand (23). Accompanying this is the influence of industry and pharmaceutical companies, and the 'industrialisation' of medicine – which thrives on demand and treats advanced healthcare as a commodity to be bought and sold, irrespective of the detrimental implications for patients and populations (24).

Secondary care, with its focus on super-specialism and biomedicine, thus continues to dominate the UK's healthcare system, and, largely, clinical education. Unfortunately, part of this culture is to denigrate general practice as a career ('just a GP') – the so-called 'hidden agenda' or 'hidden curriculum', which, for many young doctors in training, is not so hidden. So, although generalism is still present in UK general practice, it is clearly under threat (25,26).

Improving access to generalist healthcare

Ensuring that people who need care have access to it is one of the foundational principles of an equitable healthcare system. Generalism is central to universal health coverage and equitable access to healthcare internationally. As part of the United Nations' Sustainable Development Goals, member states have agreed to work toward worldwide universal health coverage by 2030, and the WHO has specified that good primary care is fundamental to universal health coverage (15,27). 'Healthcare as a universal human right' is also an important aspect of Era 3 medicine. Universal health coverage is defined by the World Health Organization (WHO) as follows:

> Universal health coverage is defined as ensuring that all people have access to needed health services (including prevention, promotion, treatment, rehabilitation, and palliation) of sufficient quality to be effective while also ensuring that the use of these services does not expose the user to financial hardship. Universal health coverage has therefore become a major goal for health reform in many countries and a priority objective of WHO.
>
> World Health Organization 2022 (28)

Gulliford and colleagues conceptualise improving access to healthcare across four domains (29): increasing supply (building capacity), removing barriers (personal, financial and systems-based), optimising utility (the right service at the right time and place) and ensuring equity (priority access for those with the greatest need). Each domain will have different impacts on health service availability, utilisation and outcomes, and each domain indirectly impacts the others. For example, reducing barriers through online booking systems may reduce equitable access for those without online access, and increasing supply without attention to quality might reduce utility. No single strategy is likely to be effective, rather a judicious combination of all four.

Attention to authenticity when building capacity

The role of generalism internationally varies widely due to variations in the structure of healthcare systems. The World Health Organization (WHO) describes how, in developed countries, future emphasis is likely to be on quality and sustainability, whereas in developing countries, priorities include building capacity and improving access (15). The WHO warns against fragmentation, unregulated commercialisation and hospital centrism, and argues instead for systems that are based on health equity, that put the care of people first, that secure the health of both communities and individuals, that invite participation and that provide reliable, responsive care.

The WHO also warns against oversimplification of generalism when building capacity in developing countries. Generalism is not one-way delivery of a small range of priority health interventions, nor is it isolated community health workers, nor community clinics for common ailments, nor cheap, low-tech, non-professional care for the rural poor who cannot afford any better. Instead, they argue for attention to the core attributes of generalism: comprehensive care for all people and all health problems; collaborative care, referring and guiding people through a range of services; relationship-based care that involves people, families and communities in the decisions that affect them; care that opens opportunities for health promotion, disease prevention and early detection of disease; and care that combines sophisticated biomedical and social skills through adequate resources and investment in education and training. Countries with developed general practice have generalism as a core tenet within postgraduate training, and qualifications that are specific to this role.

Many developed countries are also seeking to extend existing models of working with allied healthcare professionals and creating additional roles to address challenges with primary care capacity. Such expansion may well be warranted, given the key role of primary care in healthcare systems, and the global shortage of GPs. It is not, however, clear to what extent allied health professionals are trained in, or indeed practise, generalism. If the expansion of allied health professionals into the primary care team is to be effective, then all practitioners need to understand the vital role of generalism, their role in it, and how to best put it into practice. The implications for generalism of expanding capacity in this way are not yet clear. Simply co-locating healthcare professionals who are specialists in a specific area of healthcare, such as physiotherapists, pharmacists, mental health nurses and so on, will not in itself lead to the integration of care (see Chapters 2 and 9) and may indeed simply replicate the fragmentation of care that is seen in specialist services in secondary care.

Good primary care requires GPs and other healthcare staff to be trained to a high standard in the core aspects of holistic care, and hence generalism (30). True integration of the multidisciplinary team into primary care will therefore require training and education in generalist approaches. This is likely to require mentorship and leadership from experienced generalists, potentially adding to the workload of already overstretched general practitioners (31). In Scotland, the new GP contract aims to engage generalists in training allied health professions, but recent evaluation suggests problems exist with its implementation (32) most of which were predicted (33) but not acted upon. Internationally, barriers to effective transformation of primary care identified poor leadership, resistance to change, inadequate resources, and a lack of clear targets or outcomes as key themes (32). Challenges integrating multidisciplinary health workers into primary care are likely to be similar to those encountered when integrating teams across health and social care (see below).

Influences on the quality of generalism

Funding models

Funding and payment mechanisms have important impacts on both patients and clinicians. Relying on out-of-pocket payments at the point of service can lead to catastrophic expenditure that pushes people into poverty or bankruptcy (34). Point-of-care payments are also a barrier for people on low to medium incomes where they do not qualify for free care, further exacerbating health inequalities (35). These inequalities can also be driven at a national level, for example the affordability of cancer treatments in low- to middle-income countries driving global health inequalities (36). Incentivisation systems have consistent impacts on physician behaviour, but mixed or limited impacts on patient outcomes (37). Incentives can subvert the intrinsic motivations of clinicians to provide personalised holistic care and influence decision-making through micro-incentives to over- or under-treat people (38). They can also cause a focus on the incentive (for example, waiting time) to the detriment of overall quality (39). Fee-for-service, for example, incentivises clinicians to provide as many (short) consultations as possible and may disadvantage people with more complex problems requiring longer consultations compared to capitation-based funding systems (40). A US study comparing fee-for-service to managed care found preventive screening was lower, hospital admission rates higher, and health outcomes virtually identical (41).

Consultation length

Studies have shown wide variations in consultation length in general practice (where longer consultation times are assumed to correlate to a more generalist approach), ranging from a mean of under one minute in Bangladesh to 23 minutes in Sweden (42). It is inconceivable that a generalist approach, that combines the biomedical with the biographical, and includes shared decision-making, collaborative planning and opportunistic health promotion, can take place in a very short consultation. Indeed, a study in a general outpatient clinic in the public healthcare sector in Hong Kong, in which three-quarters of consultations were shorter than five minutes in duration, found that 99 per cent of patients were consulting about physical problems, mostly about one problem (despite being a largely elderly multimorbid population), with reported low rates of continuity of care, GP empathy, and patient enablement (43,44). As discussed in Chapter 11, using interactional knowledge well, may make for a more efficient use of time within consultations and thus the 'ideal' consultation length will depend on multiple factors including continuity of care and the therapeutic relationship (45). There is some evidence that longer consultations result in more patient enablement, lower GP stress and better patient outcomes, as well as being highly cost-effective (46). Increasing the duration of generalist consultations might also reduce the use of unnecessary investigations and downstream referrals, thereby improving care, avoiding iatrogenic harm and improving the patient experience.

Continuity of care

Continuity of care has been threatened by incentives to operate in larger practices, increases in remote healthcare, and systems that do not give people the choice of a named doctor. Other threats include mobile populations, multidisciplinary working, part-time working, portfolio careers, shift-working and the commoditisation of patient needs into discrete components. Many people, however, still prefer to see a known, regular GP, and evidence suggests that older people, those with multimorbidity and those with mental health conditions are most likely to benefit from continuity of care (18). Continuity of care could be prioritised for people most likely to benefit (18); however, identifying those most likely to benefit in advance of an appointment is challenging, and patients may prefer to prioritise speed over continuity for different problems. Patient-led strategies include giving people clear information about how and when to get an appointment with their chosen doctor, how to request a longer appointment, and how and when to contact their chosen doctor between face-to-face appointments (47).

Empathy and compassion

Regardless of financial resource constraints, care providers must be able to interact with compassion and empathy alongside technical clinical expertise, because a care provider must first understand the situation from the person's perspective to effectively propose suitable solutions (48). Empathy is the ability to understand and share someone else's feelings or experiences by imagining what it would be like to be them, and includes three domains: emotional; cognitive; and behavioural (49). Empathy in the consultation is beneficial for both the care user, in terms of improved satisfaction and treatment adherence, and for the care provider, where empathy can protect against stress (48). Nevertheless, it is challenging for individual care providers to engage cognitively and emotionally or to behave with empathy when they are not supported by the systems in which they work. Policymakers need to be aware of structural aspects such as relational continuity that affect how clinicians empathise with patients' needs (48).

Integrated care

Fragmented healthcare systems tend to focus clinicians' attention on small and local 'savings', rather than focusing on the bigger ecosystem and ultimate cost-effective strategies for patients across the health and social care system. People with complex problems can find themselves pushed from service to service. Strengthening the delivery of generalist care needs to combine integrative approaches (where there is effective coordination both between primary and secondary care, and across multidisciplinary teams) and interpretive approaches (where clinical decision-making involves careful consideration of the needs of the individual in addition to guidelines) (50). The United Model of Generalism, devised by Reeve et al. in 2017 (Figure 8.4), describes types of care

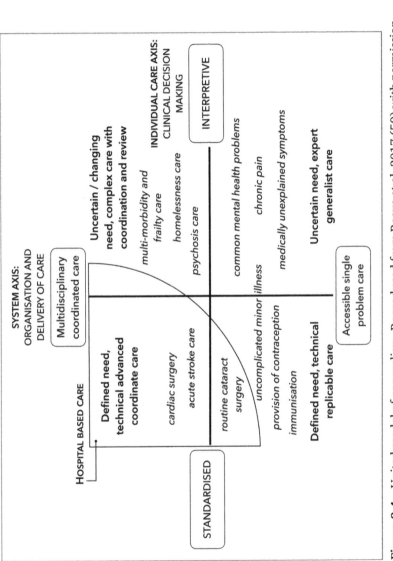

Figure 8.4 United model of generalism. Reproduced from Reeve et al. 2017 (50) with permission

provision suitable for meeting the needs of the whole person (50). The goals of integrating health and social care include the reduction of this fragmentation and the improvement of health and wellbeing of the people who require these services (51). Another driver for integrating across sectors is to reduce cost and improve efficiencies. Although integration in the UK does not appear to have reduced emergency hospital use, there is some evidence that it has improved user outcomes and experience (51).

Commodification and marketisation

Julian Tudor Hart, in his essay on the inverse care law (52) over half a century ago, warned of the negative impacts of market forces on disadvantaged groups:

> This inverse care law operates more completely where medical care is most exposed to market forces, and less so where such exposure is reduced. The market distribution of medical care is a primitive and historically outdated social form, and any return to it would further exaggerate the maldistribution of medical resources.
>
> Hart 1971 (52)

Since then, there has been a steady move towards privatisation of the NHS, especially in England, under consecutive governments. One way in which this has been done is to 'commodify' care by cutting comprehensive generalist services into individual bits that can be delivered by the private sector. Such segmentation of care damages possibilities for generalism and often increases rather than decreases costs. Furthermore, it often allows 'cherry-picking' by the private sector of 'easier' patients and problems, leaving public services to support people with complex needs (53).

Where generalism is needed most

Ageing populations

People are living longer, and the world's population is ageing. It is anticipated that one in six people globally will be aged 60 years or over by the year 2030 (54). There will be a substantial increase in people with complex care needs, including higher levels of dementia, multimorbidity and frailty, with associated dependence on health and social care services (55). When the process of ageing and the experience of longevity are accompanied by good health this brings opportunities for people to contribute to their families and communities. However, multimorbidity increases with age and brings many health and care challenges, and this stage of life can also be associated with social life transitions such as the death of a partner, with associated loss of support (54). Application of generalism to clinical practice, using approaches such as more widespread training in geriatric medicine for hospital-based clinicians, could improve generalist care for such patients within secondary care (56). However, if future healthcare needs of ageing populations with complex needs are to be met holistically and cost-effectively, countries must invest in growing general practice as well as supporting generalism in hospital specialties.

Complex needs

As discussed in Chapter 1, the term 'complex' can be used to mean 'atypical' or 'technically difficult'. Here, however, we use the term to mean multiple and potentially interrelated factors where the outcome can be unclear and/or the process continuous or ongoing. People with complex needs, such as those with learning disabilities and long-term health problems, or people with complex childhood trauma combined with substance misuse, have additional health- and social-care requirements while also experiencing illness and treatment burden (57). They also have additional challenges negotiating the complexities of a fragmented health- and social care system (58). Inadequate social support and poverty further contribute to ill health (see Chapter 10). The co-existence of mental and physical multimorbidity is more common and occurs up to 40–45 years younger in people living in areas of high deprivation compared with those living in affluent areas in the UK (57). This adds to the existing challenges facing both the people living in, and the clinicians working in, areas of deprivation (59,60). Generalism is of crucial importance in the delivery of integrated health and social care, particularly for a population with rising needs and where inequalities are marked (51). Multimorbidity and personalised approaches to care are discussed further in Chapter 18.

Marginalised communities

Special attention to marginalised groups is central to Era 3 medicine. With generalism at the core of organisational structures and culture, healthcare systems can maximise their inclusivity and adaptability to meet the needs of people in need. There are many marginalised communities requiring expert generalist care. Perhaps the largest and most pressing relates to people affected by conflict, famine, trafficking, persecution and environmental threats. The United Nations estimates that 1 in 74 people on earth has been forced to flee (61). The UK's Equality and Human Rights Commission points out that forced migrants may have fled traumatic circumstances, had traumatic journeys, and arrived with little or no resources or support, leaving them at risk of further exploitation (62). Dispersal on arrival may further disrupt supportive social networks, and people often fall outside formal asylum systems. These traumas are compounded by barriers to accessing health and social care. These include language barriers, discrimination, being unaware of their rights or entitlements, fear of arrest or detainment, as well as structural barriers such as the need to provide an address, or pay for services and medicines. Rights-based interventions are discussed in Chapter 10.

Health and social inequalities

Inequalities exist in the organisation and quality of care for people living in areas of high deprivation. These groups are less likely, for example, to receive good quality end-of-life care where they are less commonly consulted about advance care planning and decisions about their care (56). Patients living in areas of higher deprivation often have more problems to address during a single consultation, and these problems are often more complex (mental, physical and social) than for those people living in more affluent areas. However, due to the inequitable distribution of GPs relating to the allocation of funding, the consultations they receive are often shorter and less patient-centred than in affluent areas, and result in higher stress levels in the GPs, less patient enablement and poorer outcomes following clinical encounters (59,62). Patients in deprived areas have lower patient satisfaction and GPs have lower job satisfaction compared with affluent areas (63). Structural approaches to address social inequalities (housing, education, employment, social security) are also needed in parallel to approaches that address health inequalities (64).

Addressing the 'inverse care law'

Throughout this book it is argued that generalism is central to high quality, person-centred care. This is particularly important for patients with the largest burden of health and social care needs, who in practice often have the least access to good quality generalist care. Such inequity in care provision stems from the organisation of healthcare. Over 50 years ago, this mismatch between need and supply was coined the 'inverse care law' by GP and epidemiologist, Julian Tudor Hart, in a seminal essay in the Lancet (52). Tudor Hart explained the inverse care law as follows: 'The

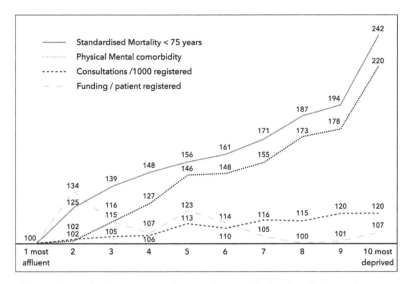

Figure 8.5 The inverse care law at the population level. Reproduced from McLean et al. 2015 (65) with permission

availability of good medical care tends to vary inversely with the need for it in the population served.' A series of papers from Scotland over the last 20 years have shown how the inverse care law still operates within the NHS. The fundamental problem is a historical mismatch of need and supply – as Figure 8.5 shows, increasing levels of need in more deprived areas of Scotland (as reflected by higher levels of premature mortality, multimorbidity, and poor general health compared with more affluent areas) are not matched by the funding or distribution of GPs (65).

Recent research by the Health Foundation has confirmed the ongoing existence of the inverse care law in the English NHS (66). Ongoing research in Scotland on the new GP contract, which outlines how GP services are funded, also suggests that there has been little emphasis on the needs of older patients or those exposed to health inequalities (32).

The effect of the inverse care law is most apparent in patients with multimorbidity. In affluent areas, multimorbid patients get substantially longer consultations than non-multimorbid patients (on average 40 per cent longer), perceive their GPs as more empathic, and the GPs deliver more patient-centred care when measured objectively using video recorded consultations. In deprived areas, no such differences between multimorbid and non-multimorbid patients exist (67) (Table 8.1).

Table 8.1 Issues affecting communities and consultations in deprived areas. Based on data from Mercer and Watt 2007 (59) and Mercer et al. 2012 (68), reproduced with permission from Graham Watt

Issues affecting communities	Issues affecting clinical encounters
Unemployment	Multiple morbidity
Benefits sanctions	Social complexity
Cuts to services	Shortage of time
Drugs and alcohol	Reduced expectations
Child protection	Lower enablement
Migrant health	Health literacy
Vulnerable adults	Practitioner stress
Bereavement	Weak interfaces

Future policy must address the inverse care law. Generalism must be at the centre of care systems that support all patients, particularly for vulnerable groups such as those with multimorbidity who live in deprived areas. A holistic approach is needed, with continuity, integration of services and a patient-centred balance of approaches and priorities. Providing services for people with complex clinical and care needs requires them to be designed around people and populations rather than single diseases, and for there to be intelligent and adequate funding for health and social care that is targeted towards the most vulnerable so that care is responsive and personalised. High-quality generalist care for such patients requires several components: time, continuity, an empathic patient-centred approach, and (at least initially) support for practitioners in managing such complexity. The feasibility, effectiveness, and cost-effectiveness of such an approach has been demonstrated through the CARE Plus Study (69,70) meaning in the future it could be implemented at scale. However, this will require re-investment in primary care in deprived areas with sufficient staff, training and funding to make it a reality, together with a shift in how generalist work is understood and valued by society and populations.

Major opportunities exist to effectively harness scientific and technological advances while maintaining the basic principles of generalism, and such innovations need to be rapidly developed, evaluated and implemented equitably and at scale within primary care. Future strategies in the UK include enhancing the use of digital infrastructure, integrated care records and responsive data tools such as risk-based screening, digital health checks, access to online peer support, virtual consultations, and at-home diagnostics to deliver 'flexible, tailored services that promote people's health, wellbeing, and independence' (71).

To meet these increasing needs, systems and processes must become responsive to the needs of individuals and populations. Additionally, systemic participatory approaches such as engendering a culture that invites and welcomes feedback from people using services, involvement of people and carers in service design, and providing appropriate training for people who provide health and social care, could be used to make real-time changes to services and improve the generalist approach (56).

For changes of this nature to occur, the organisers of a healthcare system and the individuals working within it must share a common holistic view of healthcare provision (69). For people with complex care needs, effective provision of generalist care requires that clinicians working in all disciplines understand the specific needs of individuals, promote shared decision-making, and collaborate skilfully across teams of professions (50). For this to occur, healthcare systems at the population level must enable generalist systems to thrive.

A vision for the future: making generalism a reality

Quoting from the Health Foundation document on modern medical generalism: 'the essential quality is that the generalist sees health and ill health in the context of people's wider lives, recognising and accepting wide variation in the way those lives are lived, and in the context of the whole person' (10). Implementing generalism at scale throughout the healthcare system must therefore overcome current barriers.

The well-known saying 'culture eats strategy for breakfast' has been attributed to the management expert Peter Drucker but is often quoted in healthcare management circles in relation to quality improvement. Thus, in the ambition to expand and enhance generalism, as argued for in this book, we must be mindful that any strategies will need to understand and address issues of culture within healthcare. Healthcare systems around the world remain dominated by the biomedical, reductionist model of disease and treatment, and the supremacy of secondary care specialties. It is also reflected in the single-disease paradigm that still dominates healthcare practice, education and systems. Implementing generalism, especially in secondary care, will require a change in culture amongst specialists, so that generalism is seen as everyone's job and not just that of the geriatrician and the GP (see also Chapter 2). Delivering expert generalism at scale, as discussed earlier, will undoubtedly require a substantial investment in general practice, since hospital care is episodic and most care for most patients (especially those with multimorbidity) is, across their life course, delivered in general practice (72). This is a political and practical challenge as there is a global shortage of trained GPs. Bold actions are required by governments to boost GP numbers by encouraging more trainee doctors to become GPs, help retain experienced GPs, and, above all, ensure the work of GPs is meaningful and sustainable for both professionals and patients.

The WHO suggests focusing on the following drivers of reform to ensure the future of generalism (15):

- **Mobilising the production of knowledge**: ensuring policy reviews stimulate organisational imagination, intelligence and ingenuity; address the technical and political obstacles to the advancement of generalist knowledge; and ensure that new knowledge is effectively shared and implemented.
- **Mobilising the commitment of the workforce**: ensuring generalist careers are more stimulating and gratifying, and more socially and economically rewarding than past models, and that generalist clinicians are attracted to the areas that need them most.
- **Mobilising the participation of people**: harnessing the dynamics of civil society so that the perspectives of people are included within policy debate; so that all people have reliable protection against health threats and equitable access to quality healthcare without fear of financial exploitation.

The facilitators to integrating generalism into the organisation and design of healthcare systems are summarised in Table 8.2. Because the quality of care is a combination of technical and interpersonal effectiveness, generalism – with its integration of the biomedical and the biographical – is important in all aspects of healthcare. Yet, as clinical care has become more specialised and super-specialised, the balance has inexorably shifted towards the biomedical. Generalism is the key to delivery of effective, sustainable and compassionate care. However, generalist services, especially UK general practice, currently suffer from financial under-investment, chronic workforce shortages and compartmentalisation. Healthcare challenges, including an ageing population, rising complexity, marginalised groups and health inequalities, mean that adoption of generalist approaches will become even more necessary. Organisational structures must support and encourage generalist ways of working, generalism must be a key theme in clinical and postgraduate training, together with a culture change within the clinical professions that challenges the dominant reductionist, overtly biomedical model to one that

Table 8.2 Facilitators of generalism in healthcare systems

• Universal coverage: a healthcare system free at the point of care, with a strong general practice-led primary care base • A healthcare system that adequately responds to the needs of all patients, including those suffering health inequalities • Widespread training in generalism for all medical students and doctors in training • Putting generalism at the heart of the integration of health and social care • Organisational support for the factors that enable generalism to flourish such as appropriate leadership training, supporting effective communication within and between teams and system interfaces, flexibility, continuity of care, relationship-centred care.

prioritises and rewards generalism. Politically, there is an urgent imperative to halt commodification and profit-based approaches to organising clinical care systems, in order to deliver the most cost-effective and clinically appropriate care to all members of society.

From the seminal publication on generalism by the Health Foundation in 2011 (10) to Berwick's moral prescription in 2016 (1) and since, the philosophical and empirical case for situating generalism at the heart of healthcare systems and their organisation and delivery has grown and developed. Urgent action is now required.

References

1. Berwick DM. Era 3 for medicine and health care. *JAMA*. 2016;315(13):1329–30.
2. Reeve J. Protecting generalism: moving on from evidence-based medicine? *Br J Gen Pract*. 2010;60(576):521.
3. Kortum RD. Review of *Mind, Value, and Reality*, by John McDowell. *Essays Philos*. 2004;5(2): 521–30.
4. Wiggins D. *Needs, Values, Truth: Essays in the Philosophy of Value*. 2nd edn. Oxford: Blackwell; 1991.
5. Nussbaum M. The discernment of perception: an Aristotelian conception of private and public rationality. P. 145, in Sherman N. (ed.) *Aristotle's Ethics: Critical Essays*. New York: Rowman & Littlefield; 1999.
6. Gillies JCM. Getting it right in the consultation: Hippocrates' problem; Aristotle's answer. *Occas Pap R Coll Gen Pract*. 2005;(86):5–35.
7. Gillies J. Ethics and the professional identity of a general practitioner in twenty-first century Britain. In: *Handbook of Primary Care Ethics*. 1st edn. CRC Press; 2018. p. 213–24.
8. Starfield B. Is primary care essential? *Lancet*. 1994;344(8930):1129–33.
9. Rivett G. From Cradle to Grave: The history of the NHS. Nuffield Trust; 2023. Available from: www.nuffieldtrust.org.uk/health-and-social-care-explained/the-history-of-the-nhs (accessed 15 March 2024).
10. The Health Foundation. Guiding patients through complexity – Modern medical generalism. 2011. Available from: www.health.org.uk/publications/guiding-patients-through-complexity-modern-medical-generalism (accessed 2 May 2023).

11. Treadwell J, McCartney M. Overdiagnosis and overtreatment: generalists – it's time for a grass-roots revolution. *Br J Gen Pract*. 2016;66(644):116–7.

12. NHS Scotland. Chief Medical Officer's Annual Report 2014–15. Available at www.gov.scot/binaries/content/documents/govscot/publications/progress-report/2016/01/chief-medical-officers-annual-report-2014-15/documents/chief-medical-officers-annual-report-2014-15/chief-medical-officers-annual-report-2014-15/govscot%3Adocument/00492520.pdf (accessed 24 March 2023).

13. Smith GI, Mercer SW, Gillies JC, McDevitt A. Improving together: a new quality framework for GP clusters in Scotland. *Br J Gen Pract*. 2017;67(660):294–5.

14. Gillies JCM, Mercer SW, Lyon A, Scott M, Watt GCM. Distilling the essence of general practice: a learning journey in progress. *Br J Gen Pract*. 2009;59(562):e167–76.

15. World Health Organization. *The World Health Report 2008: Primary health care now more than ever*. WHO Press; 2008.

16. Berwick DM. A transatlantic review of the NHS at 60. *BMJ*. 2008;337:a838.

17. Spooner S, van Marwijk H, Mcdermott I. GP crisis: how did things go so wrong, and what needs to change? The Conversation. 2023. Available from: https://theconversation.com/gp-crisis-how-did-things-go-so-wrong-and-what-needs-to-change-208197 (accessed 15 March 2024).

18. Jeffers H, Baker M. Continuity of care: still important in modern-day general practice. *Br J Gen Pract*. 2016;66(649):396–7.

19. House of Commons Health Committee. Primary Care. Fourth Report of Session 2015–16. 2016. Available from: https://publications.parliament.uk/pa/cm201516/cmselect/cmhealth/408/408.pdf (accessed 15 March 2024).

20. NHS Digital. Investment in General Practice, 2013/14 to 2017/18, England, Wales, Northern Ireland and Scotland. Available from: https://digital.nhs.uk/data-and-information/publications/statistical/investment-in-general-practice (accessed 1 January 2023).

21. Cameron G, Alderwick H, Bowers A, Dixon J. *Shaping Health Futures*. Health Foundation; 2019.

22. Donaldson M. The value of primary care. In: Donaldson M, Yordy K, Lohr K, Vaneslow N, eds. *Primary Care: America's Health in a New Era*. National Academies Press; 1996. Available from: www.ncbi.nlm.nih.gov/books/NBK232636/ (accessed 15 March 2024).

23. Appleby J, Galea A, Murray R. *The NHS Productivity Challenge: Experience from the front line*. The King's Fund; 2014.

24. Montori VM. Turning away from industrial health care toward careful and kind care. *Acad Med*. 2019;94(6):768–70.

25. Heath I, Montori VM. Responding to the crisis of care. *BMJ Online*. 2023;380:464–464.

26. Anderson M, O'Neill C, Macleod Clark J, Street A, Woods M, Johnston-Webber C, et al. Securing a sustainable and fit-for-purpose UK health and care workforce. *The Lancet*. 2021;397(10288):1992–2011.

27. World Health Organization. *Declaration of Alma-Ata*. Regional Office for Europe; 1978.

28. World Health Organization. Universal Health Coverage (UHC). 2022. Available from: www.who.int/news-room/fact-sheets/detail/universal-health-coverage-(uhc) (accessed 24 March 2023).

29. Gulliford M, Figueroa-Munoz J, Morgan M, Hughes D, Gibson B, Beech R, et al. What does 'access to health care' mean? *J Health Serv Res Policy*. 2002;7(3):186–8.

30. Gunn JM, Palmer VJ, Naccarella L, Kokanovic R, Pope CJ, Lathlean J, et al. The promise and pitfalls of generalism in achieving the Alma-Ata vision of health for all. *Med J Aust*. 2008;189(2):110–2.

31. Pope L, Dubras L. Delivering medical education for future healthcare needs: a community-focused challenge. *Educ Prim Care*. 2020;31(5):266–9.

32. Donaghy E, Huang H, Henderson D, Wang HH, Guthrie B, Thompson A, et al. Primary care transformation in Scotland: qualitative evaluation of the views of national senior stakeholders and cluster quality leads. *Br J Gen Pract*. 2023;73(728):e231–41.

33. Kidd C, Donaghy E, Huang H, Noble-Jones R, Ogilvie S, McGregor J, et al. Challenges in implementing GP clusters in Scotland: A comparison of the views of senior primary care stakeholders in 2016 and 2021. *BJGP Open*. 2023;7(2).

34. Xu K, Evans DB, Carrin G, Aguilar-Rivera AM, Musgrove P, Evans T. Protecting households from catastrophic health spending. *Health Aff (Millwood)*. 2007;26(4):972–83.

35. Schokkaert E, Steel J, Van de Voorde C. Out-of-pocket payments and subjective unmet need of healthcare. *Appl Health Econ Health Policy*. 2017;15(5):545–55.

36. Ocran Mattila P, Ahmad R, Hasan SS, Babar ZUD. Availability, affordability, access, and pricing of anti-cancer medicines in low- and middle-income countries: a systematic review of literature. *Front Public Health*. 2021;9:462.

37. Heider AK, Mang H. Effects of monetary incentives in physician groups: A systematic review of reviews. *Appl Health Econ Health Policy*. 2020;18(5):655–67.

38. Roland M, Campbell S, Bailey N, Whalley D, Sibbald B. Financial incentives to improve the quality of primary care in the UK: predicting the consequences of change. *Prim Health Care Res Dev*. 2006;7(1):18–26.

39. Propper C, Burgess S, Gossage D. Competition and quality: evidence from the NHS internal market 1991–9. *Econ J*. 2008;118(525):138–70.

40. Gosden T, Forland F, Kristiansen I, Sutton M, Leese B, Giuffrida A, et al. Capitation, salary, fee-for-service and mixed systems of payment: effects on the behaviour of primary care physicians. *Cochrane Database Syst Rev*. 2000;3. Available from: https://doi.org//10.1002/14651858.CD002215

41. Steiner A, Robinson R. Managed care: US research evidence and its lessons for the NHS. *J Health Serv Res Policy*. 1998;3(3):173–84.

42. Irving G, Neves AL, Dambha-Miller H, Oishi A, Tagashira H, Verho A, et al. International variations in primary care physician consultation time: a systematic review of 67 countries. *BMJ Open*. 2017;7(10):e017902–e017902.

43. Fung CSC, Hua A, Tam L, Mercer SW. Reliability and validity of the Chinese version of the CARE measure in a primary care setting in Hong Kong. *Fam Pract*. 2009;26(5):398–406.

44. Mercer SW, Fung CSC, Chan FWK, Wong FYY, Wong SYS, Murphy D. The Chinese-version of the CARE measure reliably differentiates between doctors in primary care: a cross-sectional study in Hong Kong. *BMC Fam Pract*. 2011;12(1):43–43.

45. Elmore N, Burt J, Abel G, Maratos FA, Montague J, Campbell J, et al. Investigating the relationship between consultation length and patient experience: a cross-sectional study in primary care. *Br J Gen Pract*. 2016;66(653):e896–903.

46. Mercer SW, Fitzpatrick B, Gourlay G, Vojt G, McConnachie A, Watt GCM. More time for complex consultations in a high-deprivation practice is associated with increased patient enablement. *Br J Gen Pract*. 2007;57(545):960–6.

47. Hill AP, Freeman GK. Promoting continuity of care in general practice. Royal College of General Practitoners; 2011.

48. Kerasidou A, Bærøe K, Berger Z, Caruso Brown AE. The need for empathetic healthcare systems. *J Med Ethics*. 2020;47(12):e27–e27.

49. Moudatsou M, Stavropoulou A, Philalithis A, Koukouli S. The role of empathy in health and social care professionals. *Healthc Basel*. 2020;8(1):26.

50. Reeve J, Byng R. Realising the full potential of primary care: uniting the 'two faces' of generalism. *Br J Gen Pract*. 2017;67(660):292–3.

51. Reed S, Oung C, Davies J, Dayan M, Scobie S. Integrating health and social care: A comparison of policy and progress across the four countries of the UK. The Nuffield Trust; 2021. Available from: www.nuffieldtrust.org.uk/files/2021-12/integrated-care-web.pdf (accessed 24 March 2023).

52. Hart JT. The inverse care law. *The Lancet*. 1971;297(7696):405–12.

53. Guthrie B, Mercer SW. Divided we fall: the commodification of primary medical care. *BMJ Online*. 2018;360:k787–k787.

54. World Health Organization. Ageing and Health. 2022. Available from: www.who.int/news-room/fact-sheets/detail/ageing-and-health (accessed 24 March 2023).

55. Kingston A, Comas-Herrera A, Jagger C. Forecasting the care needs of the older population in England over the next 20 years: estimates from the Population Ageing and Care Simulation (PACSim) modelling study. *The Lancet Public Health*. 2018;3(9):e447–55.

56. Oliver D, Foot C, Humphries R. Making our health and care systems fit for an ageing population. The King's Fund; 2014. Available from: www.kingsfund.org.uk/sites/default/files/field/field_publication_file/making-health-care-systems-fit-ageing-population-oliver-foot-humphries-mar14.pdf (accessed 24 March 2023).

57. MacRae C, Mercer SW, Henderson D, McMinn M, Morales DR, Jefferson E, et al. Age, sex, and socioeconomic differences in multimorbidity measured in four ways: UK primary care cross-sectional analysis. *Br J Gen Pract*. 2023;73(729):e249–56.

58. Moffat K, Mercer SW. Challenges of managing people with multimorbidity in today's healthcare systems. *BMC Fam Pract*. 2015;16(129).

59. Mercer SW, Watt GCM. The inverse care law: clinical primary care encounters in deprived and affluent areas of Scotland. *Ann Fam Med*. 2007;5(6):503–10.

60. Mercer SW, John P, Robson JP, Smith S, Walton E, Watt G. The inverse care law and the potential of primary care in deprived areas. *The Lancet*. 2021;397(10276):775–6.

61. Global Trends: Forced displacement in 2022. United Nations High Commissioner for Refugees (UNHCR); 2023. Available from: www.unhcr.org/global-trends-report-2022 (accessed 15 March 2024).

62. Mercer SWP, Higgins MMs, Bikker AMMs, Fitzpatrick BP, McConnachie AP, Lloyd SMBs, et al. General practitioners' empathy and health outcomes: a prospective observational study of consultations in areas of high and low deprivation. *Ann Fam Med*. 2016;14(2):117–24.

63. Mercer SW, Lunan CJ, MacRae C, Henderson DAG, Fitzpatrick B, Gillies J, et al. Half a century of the inverse care law: A comparison of general practitioner job satisfaction and patient satisfaction in deprived and affluent areas of Scotland. *Scott Med J*. 2023;68(1):14–20.

64. Marmot M. Society and the slow burn of inequality. *The Lancet*. 2020;395(10234):1413–4.

65. McLean G, Guthrie B, Mercer SW, Watt GCM. General practice funding underpins the persistence of the inverse care law: cross-sectional study in Scotland. *Br J Gen Pract*. 2015;65(641):e799–805.

66. Gopfert A, Deeny S, Fisher R, Stafford M. Primary care consultation length by deprivation and multimorbidity in England: an observational study using electronic patient records. *Br J Gen Pract*. 2021;71(704):e185–92.

67. Mercer SW, Zhou YP, Humphris GMP, McConnachie AP, Bakhshi AP, Bikker AMs, et al. Multimorbidity and socioeconomic deprivation in primary care consultations. *Ann Fam Med*. 2018;16(2):127–31.

68. Mercer SW, Jani BD, Maxwell M, Wong SY, Watt GC. Patient enablement requires physician empathy: a cross-sectional study of general practice consultations in areas of high and low socioeconomic deprivation in Scotland. *BMC Fam Pr*. 2012;13(6).

69. Mercer SW, Fitzpatrick B, Guthrie B, Fenwick E, Grieve E, Lawson K, et al. The CARE Plus study – a whole-system intervention to improve quality of life of primary care patients with multimorbidity in areas of high socioeconomic deprivation: exploratory cluster randomised controlled trial and cost-utility analysis. *BMC Med*. 2016;14(1):88–88.

70. Mercer SW, O'Brien R, Fitzpatrick B, Higgins M, Guthrie B, et al. The development and optimisation of a primary care-based whole system complex intervention (CARE Plus) for patients with multimorbidity living in areas of high socioeconomic deprivation. *Chronic Illn*. 2016;12(3):165–81.

71. NHS England. A plan for digital health and social care. 2022. Available from: www.gov.uk/government/publications/a-plan-for-digital-health-and-social-care/a-plan-for-digital-health-and-social-care (accessed 24 March 2023).

72. The King's Fund. Improving the quality of care in general practice. 2011. Available from: www.kingsfund.org.uk/sites/default/files/improving-quality-of-care-general-practice-independent-inquiry-report-kings-fund-march-2011_0.pdf (accessed 24 March 2023).

9
Collaborative and integrated working

Emily Owen, Charles Coombs and Sophie Park

Introduction

There have been significant changes in recent years that aim to promote collaborative and integrated working across clinical systems, disciplines and institutional organisations. These strategies have often evolved as organisations, including their workforce and client base, become larger in size. Effective collaborative and integrated working may facilitate co-creative learning communities, the cross-pollination of knowledge and ideas, increase accessibility to services, and reduce costs in the healthcare system (1,2,3). Healthcare professionals have also described how collaborative and integrated working practices may foster greater job satisfaction, self-awareness and professional growth, through providing opportunities to develop mutual respect and appreciation for one another's competencies and contributions (3,4,5). Despite the many benefits, there remains limited evidence on how collaboration and integration can be achieved in practice and how specific regulatory, organisational and systemic barriers may be overcome. For instance, existing research has found that limited time and financial remuneration models, geographical separation, concerns about patient confidentiality, imbalances of authority, turbulent political and organisational contexts, and incompatible information systems are challenges that should be considered when designing collaborative and integrated working practices (5,6).

Collaboration and integration can happen at multiple levels – from the individual patient consultation, through to how care is organised within a clinical institution, through to coordination of care across different organisations and disciplinary boundaries. Many of the principles, opportunities and challenges are comparable across these levels. As you progress through this chapter; we invite you to reflect upon your own experiences of collaborative and integrated working. For instance, what are the opportunities and challenges you have personally encountered? Think about who you collaborate with routinely in your practice, what works well about this? What do you (or they) find challenging? And how does (or might) this impact on patient care?

Throughout this chapter, we will explore how collaboration and integration may support a generalist philosophy of care through combining and capitalising on the perspectives, knowledge and skills of diverse professionals to provide comprehensive, whole-person care that is responsive to the needs of individuals, families and communities (7) (see also Chapter 2). We argue that the intention to work collaboratively and in integrated ways needs to be made explicit, and related strategies and policies developed to support this. We will present examples within primary healthcare settings, across community organisations and at the interfaces between primary, secondary and social care. We recognise that not all readers are based within the UK, but we believe the key concepts, ideas and examples shared can be generalised or transferred to other geographical settings and countries.

We begin our chapter by first defining the concepts of collaboration and integration within the context of healthcare. An overview and critique of practices that support or undermine collaborative and integrated working is then presented. Finally, interventions, strategies and recommendations will be provided for overcoming barriers to collaborative and integrated working despite challenging sociopolitical structures and organisational contexts.

The concepts of collaboration and integration

Collaboration and integration are both complex phenomena, with various definitions and meanings attached to them (8,9). Some of the definitions within the literature indicate that collaboration is the synergistic combination of skills, knowledge, and resources from different sectors and organisational contexts (10). It has been frequently equated with shared goals and responsibility, mutual respect and understanding, open communication and dialogue (11). Integration has been described as subsuming healthcare professionals under a shared identity, common policy and regulatory framework, and organisation (for example, joint commissioning initiatives, common information systems, defined referral mechanisms, and formal contractual arrangements) (9,12). Specifically, there are two main types of integration described within the literature: horizontal and vertical. Horizontal integration takes place between organisations that provide similar services (at the same hierarchical level), and might comprise, for instance, collaboration between primary care, social care and community sectors (13). Vertical integration takes place between organisations offering different services or functions (at different levels of the hierarchical structure), and might involve, for example, primary care, secondary and tertiary services (10,13). Successful integration may require collaboration between different professionals as a precondition to achieve high-quality healthcare (9,10). As such, collaboration has been recognised as a key element for improving integration of care (9).

The focus and aims of collaborative and integrated working are to improve alignment and continuity of care for patients as they access, engage with, and navigate different parts of the healthcare system (14). Although many definitions of continuity exist, it may be characterised as care delivered over time that is consistent, person-centred and holistic (15,16). Importantly, continuity consists of multiple dimensions (14,15). Examples of these dimensions include:

- **Informational continuity**
  This arises when there is an awareness of the patient's clinical and psychosocial history and use of previous services.
- **Longitudinal continuity**
  This occurs when patients receive most of their care from a team of healthcare professionals who work together and share collective responsibility for coordinating services.
- **Relational continuity**
  This refers to an ongoing personal relationship characterised by trust, care and a sense of responsibility.

What factors support or undermine collaboration and integration between healthcare professionals?

In the face of an increasingly changing healthcare environment, collaborative and integrated ways of working inherently require professionals to respond to complexity and uncertainty, while acting collectively as one unit maintaining the best interests of the patient. In healthcare, this can take abundant forms. For instance, in day-to-day practice, clinicians will often collaborate with patients, across specialties, and beyond their own practices to hospital and community services. Importantly, collaboration and integration refer not only to the interrelations between healthcare professionals but also involve the interactions and relationships between professionals and patients. Collaborative and integrated working have become essential to the way healthcare is delivered. While this often means that expertise is outsourced and shared across specialties, a generalist philosophy of care (see Chapter 1) may help to maintain a holistic, integrative and comprehensive picture (17). To enhance this fundamental pillar of modern clinical practice, the challenges involved in collaboration and integration need to be recognised and addressed. Drawing upon the findings of two reviews (18,19), and knowledge and information in the existing literature, we discuss the factors which can support or undermine collaborative and integrated ways of working. These factors range from macro-level (structure), meso-level (institution) and micro-level (practice). We highlight some of these challenges through empirical examples and consider ways in which they may be either overcome or mitigated. As you read, consider how they may relate to your own practice and working environment. Are there specific changes you can make to how you work with others, encourage others (for example, in your role modelling and leadership), or questions you can ask of those who coordinate particular elements of the organisation? How may this shape opportunities for patient care?

Macro-level challenges

At the macro level, economic, systemic and regulatory factors support or undermine collaborative and integrated working. While collaboration and integration may seem 'common sense', there are often significant tensions between these ambitions and other structural, organisational 'rules', and governance frameworks. As one example, policy might encourage 'competition' between organisations to bid for the same or similar work. Consequently, this might not only affect the potential income of employers and employees and related possible investment in services, but also the range and location of patient services and resources. This, in turn, might impact on how patients navigate access to care. For example, by offering the same services or functions in different settings, or by expecting patients to be able to self-select or navigate 'appropriate' access to each service, depending on how they may perceive their problems.

Limited structural funding and financial remuneration models for healthcare professionals may also limit their contributions and involvement in collaborative and integrated ways of working (20). For instance, because collaboration and integration require establishing, developing, and maintaining trusting and mutually respectful relationships, professionals have described the process as exceedingly time consuming, resource-intensive and emotionally exhausting (5,21,22). As such, optimal financial arrangements including remuneration for healthcare professionals' time and effort may be needed to promote collaboration and ensure effective and sustainable integration of services (5,22,23).

Alongside financial reimbursement models, government and managerial support has been shown to act as both facilitators and barriers to collaborative and integrated ways of working (23). Despite varied healthcare settings, previous studies have shown that when government and management are in favour of collaborative and integrated working, they are more likely to establish an organisational context and culture where collaboration and integration is supported and encouraged for all healthcare professionals (21,23). This support may be demonstrated through creating and rewarding spaces for dialogue, encouraging exploration of differences, diversity of opinion, possibilities for mutual gain, and organising multidisciplinary training initiatives and professional development opportunities (21). In contrast, when an organisational culture is established where collaboration and integration is not valued or promoted, this may result in professionals feeling discouraged and reluctant to work with others on collaborative tasks (23). Interestingly, government and managerial support may be influenced by the perceived benefits of collaboration and subsequent costs in relation to human resources, institutional and technological infrastructure (23). The perception that the National Health Service does not contract or incentivise professionals to create and maintain well-functioning collaborative relationships has also been identified as a barrier (23,24). Macro-level factors can have a direct or indirect influence on meso-level factors and may be inextricably linked with one another. Think about an organisation you learn or work within. How is it structured? How does competition, financial remuneration, government/managerial support, and the issue of contracting and incentivising impact how you learn, work and communicate with others, and the opportunities for patient interaction?

Meso-level challenges

Meso-level challenges comprise organisational, technical, ethical and cultural barriers. One example is the organisational challenges facing general practice and the potential implications for continuity of care. For instance, in the UK, Australia and many other countries, the number of general practices continues to decline steadily, while the population is expanding exponentially (25,26). As such, there is an international trend towards rising patient numbers and an increasing list size of patients registered at general practices (27,28). In such contexts, this has resulted in many general practices merging to form larger group practices. It is argued that, through exposure to a diverse interdisciplinary team of professionals, access to more resources and comprehensive care options, larger practices may result in more equitable service access, improved patient safety, and the delivery of more cost-effective healthcare (29). Yet, the benefits of larger practice sizes are ambiguous given the lack of strong scientific evidence that patient experience or clinical outcomes can improve (30,31,32). Preliminary evidence has in fact identified an association between larger practice sizes and decreased patient perceptions of access and satisfaction with care (27). Shifting expectations from individual to team, or organisational rather than personal continuity, has many important implications for patient relationships, trust and experience of healthcare. There is concern that the continuity of care traditionally experienced in primary care may be compromised if larger teams result in patients engaging with a greater number of unfamiliar professionals (30,33).

The rationale behind continuity is that healthcare professionals can accumulate knowledge of a patient's values, clinical and personal circumstances over time and tailor healthcare provision based on their individualised needs (34,35). This relational continuity may be established through repeated consultations and interactions between the same care provider or team of providers and patient (35). Through an ongoing therapeutic and collaborative relationship, patients may develop and maintain trust, perceptions of psychological safety, and interpersonal ties with a small number of healthcare providers (36). Relational continuity implies mutual commitment and association between patient and clinicians. This commitment, in turn, may reduce a 'collusion of anonymity', whereby decisions regarding a patient's care are passed from one clinician to another (that is, passing the buck) (37). Patients with multimorbidities and complex healthcare needs often benefit from continuity most (see Chapter 18); especially when their care needs can be addressed early and comprehensively (38).

A fundamental requirement for effective collaborative and integrated working is the sharing of information between healthcare professionals. The implementation of electronic information systems and tools may facilitate informational continuity by ensuring patient records and previous encounters can be preserved among professionals. Healthcare professionals may rely upon informational continuity to reduce medical errors, improve decision-making, and efficiency when managing or assuming care for patients they are unfamiliar with (39,40,41). Unfortunately, different disciplines and professions may use incompatible systems, making it increasingly difficult to communicate, access, and interpret information (42). Simple as it may seem to address this, many of these systems individually reflect the focus and attention of that disciplinary approach to patient care – the knowledge a particular professional might find most important to record, and the way in which they do this, might therefore differ across professional groups in different organisational settings. The narrative elements of the patient story being 'heard' subsequently differ. As such, attempts to standardise IT systems across disciplines need to be mindful of these distinctions to ensure that the records remain useful and feasible to use within busy clinical situations. Additionally, concerns about the logistics and suitability of sharing information through electronic systems as well as limited computer literacy skills may act as barriers to collaborative and integrated ways of working (43,44,45,46). Consequently, improving electronic information systems and tools at the group and organisational levels, by making them easier to navigate, more secure and interoperable may be critical to facilitate informational continuity. Although the benefits of informational continuity are not tantamount to relational continuity. There is a further risk that substituting relational with informational continuity may lose associated benefits to patient experience and outcomes. As practices expand and patients see increasing numbers of different healthcare professionals patients see increases, practices may come to depend more heavily on informational rather than relational continuity.

Micro-level challenges

Micro-level factors include the skills, capacity and previous experiences of healthcare professionals. The ability to effectively communicate with a wide range of healthcare workers and a diversity of patients is considered a generalist skill. These types of skills include knowing how to speak well and listen well, how to display compassion and empathy, and how to work together as a team to prevent and solve problems (47). Unfortunately, many healthcare professionals have described limited confidence in their ability to collaborate with other professional disciplines and organisations. One possible explanation for this is that education, training and development opportunities have occurred largely within discipline-specific 'silos' (48). Consequently, the introduction of more collaborative and integrated ways of working has contributed to role confusion and ambiguity among professionals. A lack of definition, awareness, and understanding of other professionals' roles and responsibilities have been shown to contribute to role overlap, protectionism, accountability confusion, and the blurring of professional boundaries (5,45,46,49,50). This can be particularly challenging within the context of unselected comprehensive, universal care (although readers working in other disciplines may feel the same), where healthcare professionals may require flexibility and adaptation in roles to respond to identified patient needs and problems. Once the problem has been 'set', then it may be easier to refer on to different disciplinary roles and areas (51). As one example, in a specialist clinic, a patient may bring symptoms relevant to that specialist but might also mention other symptoms which may or may not be relevant to the structural boundaries of that clinic appointment. Chapter 2 presents an additional discussion of these types of challenges.

Before you continue reading, take a few minutes to reflect upon your experience learning or working within a group of multidisciplinary professionals. This may, for example, have been in a workplace-based setting, or a formal institutional-based session, or you may have been expected to learn with and from another disciplinary expert. How did such experiences feel? What supported or challenged learning opportunities?

To enhance role clarity, the provision of, and opportunities for, interprofessional education and multidisciplinary training have been identified as strategies to create opportunities for dialogue and enable professionals to interactively learn with, from and about each other to build mutual trust, facilitate collaboration, and the delivery of safe and efficient care (52,53). Over the past few decades, initiatives designed to enhance interprofessional education have included: case-based interprofessional discussions; shared seminars and lectures; community-based projects; simulation training; online learning and reflective activities; interprofessional student teamwork in clinical placements; and interprofessional living-learning accommodations (54,55). In line with adult learning theory and contact hypothesis (56), such opportunities may affect cultural change, by enabling learners to develop an understanding of the roles of other professions, promote shared values, reconcile any differences, and reduce prejudice (54). Empirical evidence supports the efficacy of early exposure to interprofessional education as negative attitudes towards other professionals may become more entrenched with time and can act as a powerful barrier to effective collaboration (57,58). Although progress has been made to promote interprofessional education at the undergraduate level, it is critical that professionals consider interprofessional learning to be an ongoing, lifelong process. As such, qualified professionals should have opportunities available to engage in regular multidisciplinary training and learning activities (53).

Example 9.1: Multidisciplinary training

One example of a multidisciplinary training scheme is 'Walk in my Shoes'. In 2015, Lewisham Clinical Commissioning Group (CCG) commissioned an interprofessional exchange project between general practices and community pharmacies in South London, UK. In total, 93 exchange visits took place comprising 42 general practitioners and 45 community pharmacists. Throughout the exchange visits, general practitioners and community pharmacists were provided the opportunity to 'experience life in primary care from a different perspective', to learn from each other, to enhance feelings of trust, improve health systems, and work together to solve local problems (59).

Interventions/strategies to improve collaborative and integrated working

There are many factors that may act as either facilitators or barriers to effective collaborative and integrated working between healthcare professionals. There is no single, one-size-fits-all solution to addressing such barriers; multi-pronged, multifactorial and multidisciplinary solutions may need to be designed that consider barriers which operate at the macro, meso and micro levels. Here we discuss potential interventions and strategies that may overcome these barriers across all three levels to help improve collaborative and integrated working practices and the quality of patient care. You may already be implementing some of the strategies we discuss, or as a learner, you may have already experienced these during placements. Some strategies may be more suitable for you than others. We hope you can use the information in this section to reflect on your own practice and how you may develop and nurture more effective collaborative relationships with those around you.

Micro teams

To overcome the barriers at the meso level, micro teams have been proposed. They are a structural intervention to organise the workforce of a practice. In particular, micro teams may address challenges initiated by practice expansion, including maintaining continuity of care. Micro teams are mini multidisciplinary teams embedded within the wider practice workforce. They aim to establish continuity with the flexibility of part-time staff and absences. In conjunction with a named general practitioner, patients can establish long-term relationships with several members of a multidisciplinary team (60). As such, micro teams are thought to address a loss of continuity, by providing continuity through teams, not just an individual practitioner. When a patient is unable to book a consultation with their preferred doctor or clinician, they can be seen by a member of the micro team responsible for their care. By employing the continuity that several individuals can offer by operating collectively, micro teams aim to address the documented loss of continuity in the UK.

The novelty of micro teams has meant flexibility in how they are defined, and which roles are incorporated into the team. In addition to established roles such as nursing and pharmacy, the team may comprise emerging roles including, but not limited to, physician associates, physiotherapists, dietitians, and health coaches (61,62). The Royal College of General Practitioners (RCGP) has advocated building well-established trusting relationships between patients and their named general practitioner, a requirement set out in the UK General Medical Services contract within 20 days of registration (60). The importance of responsibility and accountability for patient care is also raised. In addition to a named general practitioner, patients can establish long-term relationships with other members of the team whom they might see more regularly or who deliver augmented continuity.

Collaborative and integrated ways of working raise the question of who is responsible and ultimately accountable for a patient's care. There is a potential risk with micro teams that patients slip through the net and are not cared for by an allocated team. To address this, micro teams should have clearly defined expectations in roles and responsibilities. Frequent communication and discussion of care plans may help to develop collective responsibility, but also act as a safety net to ensure care plans for all patients are optimised (63). Additionally, there must be a straightforward pathway to allocate patients to teams on a recurring basis.

Micro teams can be resource-intensive and may require an increased number of staff for each consultation. This implies potential fiscal consequences; yet no research has directly addressed these outcomes to date. The resources required can be considerable and a potential barrier to successful implementation (64). Prior planning and preparation for the application of resources are required to mitigate challenges which might arise following implementation. In the long term, it is hoped a micro-team approach may decrease the overall number of consultations a patient requires, thus, making a positive step towards sustainable healthcare goals and systems. Fewer consultations may be achieved by dealing with a wider range of issues more effectively within a single visit. In practice, this could mean spending longer with a member of the team or incorporating multiple members into a single visit (65). This may involve, for example, a health coach enabling patients' engagement in self-management, thereby addressing a micro-level factor of healthcare professional–patient interaction.

The organisation of primary care has the potential to impact the nature and quality of patient care. Primary care today builds its foundations upon collaborative and integrated systems to deliver efficient and effective care to patients and their families. Micro teams are a structural intervention at the meso level of practice. They are established from a team of healthcare professionals who promote generalist care by responding to patients' needs holistically to address the biological, social, relational and psychological aspects of an individual's life.

Huddles

Huddles are structured, brief, routine, face-to-face communication of the team's full membership (63,66). As practices expand in the range of roles and numbers employed, huddles aim to address the complexities that arise as communication becomes more and more difficult. Huddles may be used as an adjunct or independently to a micro-team structure. They provide a structured opportunity for team members to communicate and collectively strategise daily practice. This may, for instance, include managing workflow, addressing patients' needs and preferences, and improving the provision of preventive services through pre-consultation planning. Huddles address micro-level factors of primary care (63,66). They can facilitate social interaction across disciplinary and organisational boundaries to promote collaborative and integrated ways of working.

Huddles can help align continuity which might be offered in micro teams (63). Through discussion of a team's full membership, patient-specific issues can be clarified, and care plans scrutinised. Regular discussion of patients under the team's care increases familiarity and knowledge of each patient by all members of the team (62). Using huddles enables an additional level of safety netting to be applied, drawing on distributed expertise to cross-check and minimise important aspects being neglected or missed.

Huddles may facilitate timely communication and ensure consensus is promptly established. Information can then be shared directly with patients. They are designed to be brief (lasting approximately 10 minutes), to enable a team to develop a care plan for patients and anticipate potential needs and/or special circumstances so that team members can support each other throughout the day. Importantly, protected time slots should be adopted to ensure all members can attend and participate in huddles, limiting their flexibility (67). Over time, huddles may promote job satisfaction and once routinely embedded in daily practice, should become more efficient, curbing the impact on time limitations. A predetermined template or framework to standardise the structure of discussions may further streamline huddles.

Huddles have been adapted to secondary care to improve patient safety and set expectations for daily practice. An example of this includes surgical teams embracing huddles to start their day (68,69). The teams follow a pre-operative huddle template which comprises discussing each planned case (69). Huddles provide the surgical team with the opportunity to scrutinise the day's operation list, pre-identify risk factors and address foreseen demands for each operation. In addition, the World Health Organization (WHO) Surgical Safety Checklist is then completed before and after each operation (70). A limitation of the surgical component of the WHO Surgical Safety Checklist is that it is typically completed once the patient has been anaesthetised. This is often too late to identify and correct critical demands to proceed with the operation due to inadequate time. For example, routine safety items on the checklist include the availability of specialist equipment. The pre-operative huddle can anticipate the need for missing equipment. That day's surgical procedures can then be restructured to allow time to obtain equipment, thereby optimising workflow through the list. The WHO Surgical Safety Checklist's improvement in mortality and operation-related complications should not be underestimated (71). Huddles can, however, complement the use of the checklist to address foreseen requirements at the start of the day before these demands delay workflow. The use of huddles to supplement current surgical work systems highlights opportunities for their implementation in secondary care.

Huddles provide an opportunity to promote team debate, cohesion and communication transparency (63,66). They have been reported to raise awareness of the interdependence of team members and individual responsibilities. Those who have applied huddles (72) to daily practice have reported improved overall work satisfaction, team cohesion and practice climate. Importantly, team members have become more attuned to other members' troubles and seek solutions and knowledge as a team. Huddles provide a structure to support and encourage collaboration and integration at the micro level of practice. Before you continue reading, consider whether you think huddles could influence your practice. If so, how?

Example 9.2: Show me your meds, please

Shared by Dr Deborah Gompertz (GP and Complex Care / Frailty Clinical Lead in South Somerset).

A new model of care asking a simple screening question, during routine home visits, by community staff, provides the potential for reduction in medicines waste with subsequent environmental and cost saving benefits, along with improved individualised patient care (72).

The problem

The role of the complex care general practitioner in South Somerset is to perform holistic assessments of patients' needs within their homes. These patients may have recently been discharged from hospital, had frequent admissions to hospital, and/or may be involved with multiple services. During assessments, patients were identified who were not adhering to their medication as prescribed and subsequent wastage of large amounts of medication. This was only apparent from asking to see a patient's medication and would not have been identified otherwise. Viewing medication is not part of a normal medication review (in Chapter 16, medication reviews are discussed in more detail), yet, if this simple task is performed, we can identify a cohort of the population that are at increased risk from adverse events from erratically taking medication, poor optimisation of long-term conditions, and missed diagnosis (for example, dementia).

The solution

The solution was a simple screening question asked on routine visits by community staff:

'Show me your meds, please'

The staff reported after viewing the patient's medications, if they had any concerns that the medications were not being taken properly. This included the complex care team, health coaches, district nurses, community physiotherapists and adult social care. The information was then fed back to primary care and the patients were discussed in huddles to decide which staff member was most appropriate to follow up with the patient. Follow-up could range from a phone call to a comprehensive assessment aligned with patient needs and goals. The Primary Care Network (PCN) pharmacist, pharmacy technician, complex care team (which includes general practitioner, nurse and support worker), and primary care team all played a vital role.

The challenges

There needs to be sensitivity to the psychological impact of removing or stopping medication in case patients feel their medical care is being withdrawn. There is a potential challenge of increased clinical workload, which was addressed through the involvement of the PCN pharmacist and pharmacy technician who were invaluable in helping with assessments and liaising with community pharmacists around communication and altering medication regimes.

Two potential methods of addressing the workload involved in this intervention are to:

1. Fund extra pharmacy support required through financial savings (initial impact assessment has suggested this would significantly exceed the costs).
2. Reallocation of resources away from an emphasis on routine, high volume but low impact medication reviews.

The results

The first pilot over a 3-month period identified 40 patients not adhering to their medication as prescribed:

- 1,049 individual months of unused prescription items were identified.

- Wasted medication was valued at £10,866 (see Chapter 13 for a discussion on sustainable healthcare).
- It is estimated that every pound spent on pharmaceuticals generates greenhouse gas emissions of 0.1558 kg CO_2 per pound (£), representing avoidable CO_2 emissions of 1,693 kg.
- 39 medications were stopped providing predicted cost saving over the next 12 months of £3,529 and 549 kg CO_2 emissions prevented.
- Medication regimes were simplified in more than 50 per cent of cases.
- Social prescribing was initiated in 30 per cent of cases.
- New cognitive impairment was identified in 35 per cent of cases.

Co-location

A powerful facilitator of collaborative and integrated working is co-location. By co-locating healthcare professionals within the same or adjacent physical space, opportunities are created for informal social interaction, knowledge dissemination, and the sharing of ideas and information within and across different disciplines and professional boundaries (24,73,74). Realistic patient access and travel arrangements are, however, paramount to consider. In primary care, the co-location of multiple disciplines, including general practitioners, clinical pharmacists, dieticians, dentists, opticians, social workers, physiotherapists, and paramedics in a 'one-stop-shop' format, has been shown to facilitate access and communication, reduce fragmentation of services as well as provide more equipment, resources and financial capital (46,75,76). Yet, although there are benefits to be gained from sharing a common space, co-location may not be enough on its own to foster collaborative and integrated working between healthcare professionals. For instance, differences in relation to status, authority, culture, ideological values and working practices may serve as barriers to effective collaboration (46,74). Within some contexts, co-location could also translate into unrealistic expectations and greater informality, which may undermine professional practice and preparedness (46). Interestingly, there is some evidence to suggest that the benefits of co-location may also be achieved through frequent and regular face-to-face interaction and planned multidisciplinary meetings (24).

Example 9.3: General Practitioner & Consultant Forum evenings

Shared by Dr Hannah Cowling (GP at Bridgewater Surgeries and Education Committee member for Watford and West Herts Medical Society).

The problem

Significant changes in the day-to-day working patterns of general practitioners and hospital-based consultants have led to limited opportunities to listen and learn from one another. Previously, there had been regular lunchtime meetings involving general practitioners and consultants along with other team members. These meetings provided meaningful opportunities to discuss patient cases and new guidelines.

The solution

A local consultant and general practitioner met through the Medical Society – which has a well-established history having been in existence for 160 years as a forum for local doctors to meet with an educational and social purpose. They decided to restart these opportunities for learning and networking between consultants and general practitioners. To do this, they began by inviting new consultants who had recently joined the trust to speak on their area of specialty, while focusing this for a general practitioner audience. This then moved on to inviting a range of speakers (for example, general practitioners and consultants to talk about relevant topics such as respiratory and cardiology evenings, or sessions focused on managing the 'dizzy patient').

The challenges

A main challenge was ensuring the whole general practitioner and consultant / hospital doctor community were cognisant of the meetings. They used the Medical Society mailing list, but this did not cover all general practitioners. As such, general practitioner trainers' networks and word of mouth were helpful to reach out to trainees. Challenges were experienced when inviting consultants from other trusts to talk as they had different expertise. This led to some discussion around local and trust politics.

The results

The meetings have stimulated critical reflection and dialogue between the clinical interface of the hospital trust and primary care, increasing understanding and awareness of a range of general practitioner and consultant priorities. These are interactive evenings with lively debates and opportunities to ask open questions. A recent 'Women's Health' evening was a great success, covering the hotly debated topic of hormone replacement therapy (HRT) in addition to cardiovascular health and inequalities in research and treatment.

Conclusion

Collaboration and integration have become increasingly important for healthcare professionals as they strive to provide the highest quality care to their patients. Collaborative and integrated ways of working can take abundant forms, but many potential barriers exist due to different and incompatible systems, competition between professionals, limited structural funding, role overlap and accountability confusion. This chapter has provided an overview and critique of practices that may support or undermine collaborative and integrated working. We hope that the contents of our chapter can stimulate critical reflection and discussion, and that the recommendations suggested can be considered by healthcare professionals and decision-makers when designing and implementing collaborative and integrated working practices within their own organisation.

Acknowledgements

The authors would like to thank Dr Deborah Gompertz and Dr Hannah Cowling for kindly providing their in-depth examples and for the outstanding work they are doing to promote collaborative and integrated ways of working.

Emily Owen is a research fellow funded by an NIHR School of Primary Care Research (SPCR) project (567988) led by Sophie Park. This 'Companion Study' examined collaboration and integration between Community Pharmacies and GPs (see https://ora.ox.ac.uk/objects/uuid:2a2c0cde-1ec9-4a05-9cdf-3c60fbbdb0b8/files/s7h149r801). Charles Coombs received an NIHR School of Primary Care Research medical student internship in 2022 to support work on a project about primary care micro-teams.

References

1. Stanley P, Peterson CQ. Interprofessional collaboration: issues for practice and research. *Occup Ther Health Care*. 2001;15(3–4):1–12.
2. Morley L, Cashell A. Collaboration in health care. *J Med Imaging Radiat Sci*. 2017;48(2): 207–16.
3. Jove AM, Fernandez A, Hughes C, Guillen-Sola M, Rovira M, Rubio-Valera M. Perceptions of collaboration between general practitioners and community pharmacists: findings from a qualitative study based in Spain. *J Interprof Care*. 2014;28(4):352–7.
4. Howard M, Trim K, Woodward C, Dolovich L, Sellors C, Kaczorowski J, et al. Collaboration between community pharmacists and family physicians: lessons learned from the Seniors Medication Assessment Research Trial. *J Am Pharm Assoc*. 2003;43(5):566–72.
5. Bollen A, Harrison R, Aslani P, van Haastregt JCM. Factors influencing interprofessional collaboration between community pharmacists and general practitioners – a systematic review. *Health Soc Care Community*. 2019;27(4):e189–e212.
6. Cvetkovski B, Cheong L, Tan R, Kritikos V, Rimmer J, Bousquet J, et al. Qualitative exploration of pharmacists' feedback following the implementation of an 'allergic rhinitis clinical management pathway (AR-CMaP)' in Australian Community Pharmacies. *Pharmacy (Basel)*. 2020;8(2).
7. Royal College of Physicians and Surgeons of Canada. Report of the Generalism and Generalist Task Force. 2013. Available from: https://srpc.ca/resources/ESS/Library/Rural%20 Generalist%20Medicine%20and%20Surgery/Report-by-the-Royal-College-on-Generalism-2013.pdf (accessed 16 March 2024).
8. Henneman EA, Lee JL, Cohen JI. Collaboration: a concept analysis. *J Adv Nurs*. 1995;21(1):103–9.
9. Boon HS, Mior SA, Barnsley J, Ashbury FD, Haig R. The difference between integration and collaboration in patient care: results from key informant interviews working in multiprofessional health care teams. *J Manipulative Physiol Ther*. 2009;32(9):715–22.
10. Axelsson R, Axelsson SB. Integration and collaboration in public health – a conceptual framework. *Int J Health Plann Manage*. 2006;21(1):75–88.
11. Way D, Jones L, Busing N. Implementation Strategies: 'Collaboration in Primary Care – Family Doctors & Nurse Practitioners Delivering Shared Care': Discussion Paper Written for The Ontario College of Family Physicians. 2000. Available from: https://citeseerx.ist.psu.edu/document?repid=rep1&type=pdf&doi=9178e66dbd2e917215bab9c04824f59146914dea (accessed 16 March 2024).
12. Leutz WN. Five laws for integrating medical and social services: lessons from the United States and the United Kingdom. *Milbank Q*. 1999;77(1):77–110, iv–v.
13. Bywood P, Brown L, Raven M. Improving the integration of mental health services in primary health care at the macro level. Primary Health Care Research & Information Service (PHCRIS); 2015. Available at: https://core.ac.uk/download/pdf/43335677.pdf (accessed 16 March 2024).
14. Schmied V, Mills A, Kruske S, Kemp L, Fowler C, Homer C. The nature and impact of collaboration and integrated service delivery for pregnant women, children and families. *J Clin Nurs*. 2010;19(23–24):3516–26.

15. Haggerty JL, Reid RJ, Freeman GK, Starfield BH, Adair CE, McKendry R. Continuity of care: a multidisciplinary review. *BMJ*. 2003;327(7425):1219–21.
16. Rogers J, Curtis P. The concept and measurement of continuity in primary care. *Am J Public Health*. 1980;70(2):122–7.
17. Kelly MA, Wicklum S, Hubinette M, Power L. The praxis of generalism in family medicine: six concepts (6 Cs) to inform teaching. *Can Fam Physician*. 2021;67(10):786–8.
18. Coombs C, Cohen T, Duddy C, Mahtani KR, Owen E, Roberts NW, et al. Opportunities, challenges and implications of primary care micro-teams for patients and healthcare professionals: an international systematic review. *Br J Gen Pract*. 2023;73(734):e651–8.
19. Owen EC, Abrams R, Cai Z, Duddy C, Fudge N, Hamer-Hunt J, et al. Community pharmacy and general practice collaborative and integrated working: a realist review protocol. *BMJ Open*. 2022;12(12):e067034.
20. Vassbotn AD, Sjovik H, Tjerbo T, Frich J, Spehar I. General practitioners' perspectives on care coordination in primary health care: a qualitative study. *Int J Care Coord*. 2018;21(4):153–9.
21. Lasker RD, Weiss ES, Miller R. Partnership synergy: a practical framework for studying and strengthening the collaborative advantage. *Milbank Q*. 2001;79(2):179–205, III-IV.
22. Cheadle A, Beery W, Wagner E, Fawcett S, Green L, Moss D, et al. Conference report: community-based health promotion – state of the art and recommendations for the future. *Am J Prev Med*. 1997;13(4):240–3.
23. Rubio-Valera M, Jove AM, Hughes CM, Guillen-Sola M, Rovira M, Fernandez A. Factors affecting collaboration between general practitioners and community pharmacists: a qualitative study. *BMC Health Serv Res*. 2012;12:188.
24. Bradley F, Elvey R, Ashcroft DM, Hassell K, Kendall J, Sibbald B, et al. The challenge of integrating community pharmacists into the primary health care team: a case study of local pharmaceutical services (LPS) pilots and interprofessional collaboration. *J Interprof Care*. 2008;22(4):387–98.
25. BMA. Pressures in general practice data analysis. 2024. Available from: www.bma.org.uk/advice-and-support/nhs-delivery-and-workforce/pressures/pressures-in-general-practice-data-analysis (accessed 16 March 2024).
26. Manski-Nankervis JE, Sturgiss EA, Liaw ST, Spurling GK, Mazza D. General practice research: an investment to improve the health of all Australians. *Med J Aust*. 2020;212(9):398–400 e1.
27. Edwards P. Bigger practices are associated with decreased patient satisfaction and perceptions of access. *Br J Gen Pract*. 2022;72(722):420–1.
28. Forbes L, Forbes, H, Sutton, M, Checkland, K, Peckham, S. Changes in patient experience associated with growth and collaboration in general practice: observational study using data from the UK GP Patient Survey. *Br J Gen Pract*. 2020;70(701).
29. Jansen L. Collaborative and interdisciplinary health care teams: ready or not? *J Prof Nurs*. 2008;24(4):218–27.
30. Pineault R, Provost, S, Silva, R, Breton, M, Levesque, J. Why is bigger not always better in primary health care practices? The role of mediating organizational factors. *Inquiry*. 2016;53:1–9.
31. Pettigrew LM, Kumpunen S, Mays N, Rosen R, Posaner R. The impact of new forms of large-scale general practice provider collaborations on England's NHS: a systematic review. *Br J Gen Pract*. 2018;68(668):e168–e77.
32. Pettigrew LM, Kumpunen S, Rosen R, Posaner R, Mays N. Lessons for 'large-scale' general practice provider organisations in England from other inter-organisational healthcare collaborations. *Health Policy*. 2019;123(1):51–61.
33. Devlin RA, Hogg W, Zhong J, Shortt M, Dahrouge S, Russell G. Practice size, financial sharing and quality of care. *BMC Health Serv Res*. 2013;13:446.
34. Freeman G, Hughes, J. Continuity of care and the patient experience. The King's Fund; 2010. Available from: https://archive.kingsfund.org.uk/concern/published_works/000094996?locale=zh#?cv=0 (accessed 16 March 2024).
35. Pereira Gray DJ, Sidaway-Lee K, White E, Thorne A, Evans PH. Continuity of care with doctors – a matter of life and death? A systematic review of continuity of care and mortality. *BMJ Open*. 2018;8(6):e021161.
36. Green CA, Polen MR, Janoff SL, Castleton DK, Wisdom JP, Vuckovic N, et al. Understanding how clinician–patient relationships and relational continuity of care affect recovery from serious mental illness: STARS study results. *Psychiatr Rehabil J*. 2008;32(1):9–22.
37. Balint M. The doctor, his patient, and the illness. *Lancet*. 1955;268(6866):683–8.

38. Engamba SA, Steel N, Howe A, Bachman M. Tackling multimorbidity in primary care: is relational continuity the missing ingredient? *Br J Gen Pract*. 2019;69(679):92–3.

39. McMurray J, Hicks E, Johnson H, Elliott J, Byrne K, Stolee P. 'Trying to find information is like hating yourself every day': the collision of electronic information systems in transition with patients in transition. *Health Informatics J*. 2013;19(3):218–32.

40. Wright DJ, Twigg MJ. Community pharmacy: an untapped patient data resource. *Integr Pharm Res Pract*. 2016;5:19–25.

41. Menachemi N, Collum TH. Benefits and drawbacks of electronic health record systems. *Risk Manag Healthc Policy*. 2011;4:47–55.

42. Weller J, Boyd M, Cumin D. Teams, tribes and patient safety: overcoming barriers to effective teamwork in healthcare. *Postgrad Med J*. 2014;90(1061):149–54.

43. Ben-Assuli O. Electronic health records, adoption, quality of care, legal and privacy issues and their implementation in emergency departments. *Health Policy*. 2015;119(3):287–97.

44. Gagnon MP, Ghandour el K, Talla PK, Simonyan D, Godin G, Labrecque M, et al. Electronic health record acceptance by physicians: testing an integrated theoretical model. *J Biomed Inform*. 2014;48:17–27.

45. Cameron A, Lart R, Bostock L, Coomber C. Factors that promote and hinder joint and integrated working between health and social care services: a review of research literature. *Health and Social Care in the Community*. 2014;22(3).

46. Kharicha K, Iliffe S, Levin E, Davey B, Fleming C. Tearing down the Berlin Wall: social workers' perspectives on joint working with general practice. *Fam Pract*. 2005;22(4):399–405.

47. Abrams TE , Lloyd AA, Held ML, Skeesick JD. Social workers as members of burn care teams: A qualitative thematic analysis. *Burns*. 2022;48(1):191–200.

48. Gilligan C, Outram S, Levett-Jones T. Recommendations from recent graduates in medicine, nursing and pharmacy on improving interprofessional education in university programs: a qualitative study. *BMC Med Educ*. 2014;14:52.

49. Gardiner C, Gott, M, Ingleton, C. Factors supporting good partnership working between generalist and specialist palliative care services: a systematic review. *Br J Gen Pract*. 2012.

50. Kraft M, Blomberg K, Hedman AM. The health care professionals' perspectives of collaboration in rehabilitation – an interview study. *Int J Older People Nurs*. 2014;9(3):209–16.

51. Park S, Abrams R, Wong G, Feder G, Mahtani KR, Barber J, et al. Reorganisation of general practice: be careful what you wish for. *Br J Gen Pract*. 2019;69(687):517–8.

52. Hopkins D. Framework for action on interprofessional education and collaborative practice. World Health Organization; 2010.

53. Bidwell S, Copeland A. A model of multidisciplinary professional development for health professionals in rural Canterbury, New Zealand. *J Prim Health Care*. 2017;9(4):292–6.

54. Abu-Rish E, Kim S, Choe L, Varpio L, Malik E, White AA, et al. Current trends in interprofessional education of health sciences students: a literature review. *J Interprof Care*. 2012;26(6):444–51.

55. Frenk J, Chen L, Bhutta ZA, Cohen J, Crisp N, Evans T, et al. Health professionals for a new century: transforming education to strengthen health systems in an interdependent world. *Lancet*. 2010;376(9756):1923–58.

56. Barr H. Toward a theoretical framework for interprofessional education. *J Interprof Care*. 2013;27(1):4–9.

57. Cooper H, Carlisle C, Gibbs T, Watkins C. Developing an evidence base for interdisciplinary learning: a systematic review. *J Adv Nurs*. 2001;35(2):228–37.

58. Barrington D, Rodger M, Gray L, Jones B, Langridge M, Marriott R. Student evaluation of an interactive, multidisciplinary clinical learning model. *Medical Teacher*. 1998;20(6):530–5.

59. PSNC. PSNC Briefing 041/17: 'Walk in my Shoes' toolkit. 2017. Available from: https://psnc.org.uk/wp-content/uploads/2017/06/PSNC-Briefing-041.17-Walk-in-my-Shoes-toolkit.pdf (accessed 16 March 2024).

60. BMA. Requirement for all patients to have a named GP. 2020. Available from: www.bma.org.uk/advice-and-support/gp-practices/managing-your-practice-list/requirement-for-all-patients-to-have-a-named-gp (accessed 16 March 2024).

61. Risi L, Bhatti N, Cockman P, Hall J, Ovink E, Macklin S, et al. Micro-teams for better continuity in Tower Hamlets: we have a problem but we're working on a promising solution! *Br J Gen Pract*. 2015;65(639):536.

62. Baird B, Chauhan K, Boyle T, Heller A, Price C. How to build effective teams in general practice. The King's Fund; 2020. Available from: www.kingsfund.org.uk/publications/effective-teams-general-practice#space (accessed 16 March 2024).

63. Rodriguez HP, Meredith LS, Hamilton AB, Yano EM, Rubenstein LV. Huddle up! The adoption and use of structured team communication for VA medical home implementation. *Health Care Manage Rev*. 2015;40(4):286–99.

64. Forman J, Harrod M, Robinson C, Annis-Emeott A, Ott J, Saffar D, et al. First things first: foundational requirements for a medical home in an academic medical center. *J Gen Intern Med*. 2014;29(Suppl 2):S640–8.

65. Hofer A, McDonald M. Continuity of care: why it matters and what we can do. *Aust J Prim Health*. 2019.

66. Gale RC , Asch SM, Taylor T, Nelson KM, Luck J, Meredith LS, Helfrich CD. The most used and most helpful facilitators for patient-centered medical home implementation. *Implementation Science*. 2015;10(1):1–11.

67. Panayiotou H, Higgs C, Foy R. Exploring the feasibility of patient safety huddles in general practice. *Prim Health Care Res Dev*. 2020;21:e24.

68. Chan AY, Vadera S. Implementation of interdisciplinary neurosurgery morning huddle: cost-effectiveness and increased patient satisfaction. *J Neurosurg*. 2018;128(1):258–61.

69. Jain AL, Jones KC, Simon J, Patterson MD. The impact of a daily pre-operative surgical huddle on interruptions, delays, and surgeon satisfaction in an orthopedic operating room: a prospective study. *Patient Saf Surg*. 2015;9:8.

70. World Health Organization. Implementation manual: WHO Surgical Safety Checklist. 1st edn. 2008. Available from: https://policycommons.net/artifacts/483645/implementation-manual/1458044/ (accessed 16 March 2024).

71. Treadwell JR, Lucas S, Tsou AY. Surgical checklists: a systematic review of impacts and implementation. *BMJ Qual Saf*. 2014;23(4):299–318.

72. Gompertz D. BGS Green Issues: Show me your meds, please. British Geriatrics Society; 2022. Available from: www.bgs.org.uk/bgs-green-issues-show-me-your-meds-please (accessed 16 March 2024).

73. Lalani M, Marshall M. Co-location, an enabler for service integration? Lessons from an evaluation of integrated community care teams in East London. *Health Soc Care Community*. 2022;30(2):e388–e96.

74. Barsanti S, Bonciani M. General practitioners: between integration and co-location. The case of primary care centers in Tuscany, Italy. *Health Serv Manage Res*. 2019;32(1):2–15.

75. Rumball-Smith J, Wodchis WP, Kone A, Kenealy T, Barnsley J, Ashton T. Under the same roof: co-location of practitioners within primary care is associated with specialized chronic care management. *BMC Fam Pract*. 2014;15:149.

76. Eaton G, Wong G, Tierney S, Roberts N, Williams V, Mahtani KR. Understanding the role of the paramedic in primary care: a realist review. *BMC Med*. 2021;19(1):145.

10
Supporting generalism through health justice partnerships
Hazel Genn and Sophie Park

Introduction

This chapter explains the positive opportunities presented by partnership between health services and social welfare rights services in promoting health and wellbeing. It provides a practical guide to incorporating a health justice approach in generalism, particularly providing effective support for challenges. Rooted in an understanding of the impact of social determinants on health, health justice partnerships (HJPs) are practitioner-led collaborations that integrate free social welfare rights services and healthcare services to address the health-harming social needs of patients. They address social and economic drivers of poor health such as debt, income, housing and employment issues. Such partnerships have been in existence around the world for at least three decades. While the examples in this chapter are drawn from experience in England, the development of HJPs is an international phenomenon. In Scotland, integrating advice services into general practice has become well-established over the last two decades (1) and there has been growth in what are called 'welfare advice and health partnerships' (WAHPs) across Scotland, supported by funding from the Scottish government, in which advice workers, with consensual access to medical records, are embedded within health settings (2). In the USA, medical legal partnerships, which frequently involve lawyers fully integrated into healthcare teams, have been developing for over 40 years and have a national representative body, the National Center for Medical-Legal Partnership (3). There is also a rapidly developing network of HJPs in Australia. Their growth has been accelerated by the activities of the Australian national centre of excellence for HJPs, Health Justice Australia (4).

Social determinants of health and social welfare legal issues

Historically, the conceptualisation of illness and health and the organisation of healthcare has been based on a biomedical model that focuses on physical and biological aspects of specific diseases and conditions (5). Since at least the middle of the twentieth century, however, there has been an increasing appreciation and understanding that health and wellbeing are affected by a broad range of factors besides individual biology, genetic endowment and access to good quality healthcare services. Social and environmental factors such as income and social status, living conditions, education and literacy, employment and working conditions are now understood to exert a powerful influence over health and wellbeing. The impact of social determinants on health is well-researched and documented (6). Estimates of the impact of social and environmental determinants on health status range between around 45 to 60 per cent (7) and in health discourse, the connection between social disadvantage and health, leading to significant health inequalities, has become widely accepted. The Health Foundation has put a great deal of effort into promoting greater emphasis on the social determinants of health. They have commented that the UK health system has focused disproportionately on treating disease and that more emphasis should be placed on action that promotes the conditions for good health (8).

While the links between poverty and health are complex, it is clear that unmet basic needs are strongly associated with poor health outcomes and that people with fewer resources are likely to experience complex health challenges (9). The legal system, through social welfare law, provides a basic level of protective and 'safety net' rights and entitlements to shield low income and vulnerable groups from many of the social factors ('social pathogens') known to harm health and wellbeing. These rights and entitlements to critical services and support run across a wide range of social determinants of health. Essentially the law 'prescribes' measures to ameliorate inequality and social exclusion (10). Social welfare law provides people with rights in relation to matters such as state benefits and social housing, fair treatment in employment, access to education and community care. But these legal protections often fail to benefit the most disadvantaged groups experiencing the greatest burden of ill health because people do not receive or access the benefits, goods and services to which they are entitled (11,12). Many of the health issues experienced by patients result from unenforced laws or incorrect denial of critical services, leading to preventable poor health outcomes. For these individuals and families, the provision of advice and support by free social welfare rights services can have preventive and remedial impact in crisis situations such as potential eviction, loss of income, or threatened termination of employment (13). The inability to access critical services and benefits to which people are legally entitled is often referred to as 'unmet legal need' or 'lack of access to justice'. Research on the health impact of health-harming unmet legal needs highlights the very clear overlap between underserved groups experiencing health challenges and those needing the support of free social welfare advice services (14).

There is a bidirectional link between health and social welfare law. Social issues with a legal dimension can create or exacerbate ill health and, conversely, ill health can create legal problems (15). We know from two decades of research (12,16) that social welfare legal problems are not evenly distributed in the population, but occur more commonly among certain groups and tend to occur in 'clusters' creating complex challenges for individuals and families. People experiencing poor mental or physical health, those on low incomes and those with other vulnerabilities disproportionately experience difficulties relating to obtaining appropriate welfare benefits (17), long-term indebtedness, and adverse housing circumstances (18). They are also more likely to have difficulty accessing professional support and advice for such issues giving rise to 'health harming legal needs'. Without resolution, such problems can lead to a cascade of consequences that may push people into poverty or other challenges. They are also accompanied by stressful living and working conditions that are associated with high blood pressure, development of diabetes, and heart disease (19). People in lower socioeconomic groups experience greater chronic stress exposure than more materially advantaged groups and these differences in stress exposure may result in differing biologic risk for diseases. In simple terms, being 'stressed' makes people ill through direct impact on health and ageing as well as telomere shortening, plus indirectly through influencing health behaviour such as smoking, diet and exercise (20,21).

This relationship highlights how legal problems contribute to cycles of deprivation and poor health, adding to the entrenchment of health inequalities (15). Legal problems can also increase health service workloads (22) through people seeking help from healthcare professionals in the absence of knowing where else to go for help (16). Social welfare advice services, providing support for basic needs, can improve the socioeconomic circumstances of patients, address underlying problems that are causing or exacerbating ill health, and mitigate the financial and social costs of illness (23).

Patients frequently bring a complex mix of health and social challenges into generalist healthcare encounters. In this respect generalist clinicians are in the position of *'critical noticers'* of situations that require a broad approach to improving the health and wellbeing of their patients. They are in a unique position to identify, possibly at an early stage, problems affecting health that would benefit from non-clinical services or interventions. Biomedical training and mindset naturally focus attention on addressing a patient's medical symptoms, even though the underlying cause of presenting complaints may be susceptible – and indeed require – an additional or alternative approach. Healthcare professionals, recognising the need for non-clinical intervention and support with social welfare issues, often struggle to know how best to assist patients having been trained in disease mechanisms rather than health mechanisms (24,25). They cannot be expected to resolve such underlying problems, but the opportunity for them to identify problems and connect patients with assistance such as welfare advice services can make a crucial difference.

A case in point is that of an infant death in England caused by long-term exposure to mould in social housing, which created something of a media storm following the Coroner's public comments at the conclusion of the inquest. The case illustrated the vital role that health professionals sometimes occupy in navigating patients experiencing health-harming legal needs toward positive outcomes. In 2020, toddler Awaab Ishak died eight days after his second birthday, following 'chronic exposure' to mould in the flat in which he lived (26). Despite concerns expressed repeatedly by his parents in the two years leading up to Awaab's death, the landlord failed to fix the mould or improve ventilation. At the inquest into Awaab's death in November 2022 the Coroner described this as a 'defining moment'. Awaab's parents said: 'We cannot tell you how many health professionals we have cried in front of and Rochdale borough housing staff we have pleaded to expressing concern ... We shouted out as loudly as we could.'

For individuals and families facing multiple health, social and economic challenges, the provision of social welfare advice services through what are known as health justice partnerships (HJPs) can offer preventive and remedial impact in challenging situations. In HJPs, patients are linked in with welfare rights advice services via their healthcare provider so that welfare rights advice is integrated with patient care. The aim is to support health and maximise recovery by tackling social and economic circumstances that are harmful to health and wellbeing. There is a significant overlap between patients with the greatest need for legal services and those dealing with complex health challenges – and in both cases often dealing with significant social disadvantage. 'Because the same low-income and marginalised populations experiencing poor health also experience poor access to justice, formal partnerships among service providers working with these populations can facilitate both justice and better health equity' (27). The logic seems plain and is supported by research evidence, to better integrate health services with those that secure rights and entitlements that would alleviate health-harming social needs.

Health justice partnerships as an integrated health intervention

Health justice partnerships are practitioner-led collaborations between free social welfare legal services and healthcare services to better address the health-harming unmet legal needs of patients. The provision of free legal advice has long been understood, within the legal sector at least, to have value for the health and wellbeing of low income and vulnerable groups where legal support can make the difference between stable housing, money, and employment or crisis (10). Poverty, substandard living conditions, insecure employment and debt all directly impact health and wellbeing and have indirect impacts in denying citizens the capacity to make healthy lifestyle choices.

Protecting housing security, improving living conditions, or increasing benefit income can reduce anxiety and stress and result in longer-term improvements in mental and physical health and health behaviours (28). This can diminish the impact of adverse events that are harming health and support the work of health services. Put simply, legal practitioners have the knowledge, training and skills to address legal needs that arise from or are caused by the social determinants of health. Welfare rights advice can be seen as a critical tool in supporting health and wellbeing, tackling the underlying causes of illness that predominantly affect people living on low incomes or underserved communities. Left unresolved, welfare rights issues can perpetuate or exacerbate poor living conditions, poverty and other stressful life situations. This directly impacts on mental health through anxiety and distress but can also influence physical health through lack of adequate food and warmth.

Integration of health and social welfare advice services is not a novel proposition. In the UK, social welfare legal services have been working in partnership with healthcare providers through different models since the late 1980s to better serve the needs of patients (29,30). Historically, such partnerships have developed as a result of local initiatives between healthcare practitioners and providers of free legal services. Grassroots practitioner experience, together with research, including the Marmot Review into health inequalities, noting the value of providing free legal advice services in primary care (6) have supported the development of HJPs in the UK, USA, Australia and Canada (27). The spread internationally of HJPs is evidence in itself of their effectiveness, as service innovations are more likely to spread if they work (31). Their value lies in reaching vulnerable patient groups – who might not otherwise obtain help – at a time and place of need (32). This is because health settings are accessible and the professionals with whom patients interact are trusted. This creates the conditions in which patients may discuss difficult matters about which they feel anxious or embarrassed, although as discussed below, such interactions require skilful handling. In the short and medium term, ensuring that low income and vulnerable groups benefit from existing legal safety net entitlements, such as income maintenance, secure employment and healthy housing, is important for mitigating the worst effects of deprivation and disadvantage for individuals and populations more broadly.

In the UK there is a wide spectrum of health justice collaborations ranging from welfare rights advisers embedded in multidisciplinary teams, to co-located services, 'pop-up' services, clinician direct referrals, and navigation referrals via social prescribing link workers (30). There is no single model for HJPs and multiple examples exist in a wide range of health settings, both in the UK and abroad, delivering dedicated and specialist advice services in GP practices, hospitals, maternity services, mental health services and so on (27,30,33).

Examples of partnerships include those defined by a particular health condition (such as cancer, mental health, HIV) or in particular circumstances (such as pregnancy or life limiting conditions); those targeted at particular demographic characteristics (such as age, gender, ethnicity); or people living in a particular geographical region. Other partnerships might target particular types of legal need (such as housing, benefits, education, employment, domestic abuse, immigration status).

Example 10.1: A health justice partnership in primary care

In 2016, UCL Centre for Access to Justice established an HJP (Integrated Legal Advice Clinic [iLAC]) with a GP surgery at a Health and Wellbeing Centre in an area of East London with historically high levels of deprivation (Newham). The Guttmann Health Centre, intended to be a model for healthcare delivery in the local area, offered a range of healthcare services under one roof. iLAC operated within the health centre for two years, providing assistance for practice patients and local residents. Patients would be referred by the practice clinicians or self-refer to the service. The service provided free face-to-face social welfare advice, casework and representation by qualified lawyers and specialist welfare advisers supported by students from UCL Faculty of Laws. During the two years of co-location, services were provided to ethnically diverse clients on low or very low incomes. The most common issues dealt with were welfare benefits and housing. Consistent with legal needs research, many clients were experiencing clusters of social welfare legal problems. Research evaluation of the HJP, tracking clients' health and wellbeing scores over time, revealed statistically significant improvements in mobility, self-care, usual activities, pain/discomfort, and anxiety/depression (EQ5D) as well as global assessment of health. Mental wellbeing scores also showed an upward trend over time (34). 'I have improved mentally due to having some peace after help to deal with my claims. I had nowhere to turn to and felt very vulnerable and afraid.' [Respondent, Female, 50–64 years]

Example 10.2: A hospital-based health justice partnership

Camden Citizens Advice Bureau in partnership with Great Ormond Street Hospital (GOSH) provides a specialist welfare rights service on site. The service is situated within GOSH in recognition of the overwhelming evidence linking poverty and inequality to poorer health. The service specialises in social security law and welfare rights and advises families at GOSH on a range of issues, including welfare benefits; employment; housing and homelessness; landlord and tenant problems; debt and money management; community care, including Children Act assessments; immigration and asylum. The service provides advice face-to-face, by telephone and by email as well as carrying out casework. The work of the service is free, impartial, independent and confidential. The service is delivered by a group of paid staff and volunteer advisers.

Interest in HJPs has been growing steadily in recent years and has accelerated since the COVID-19 pandemic. This reflects concern about the specific association between deprivation and mortality and the broader issue of tenacious social and geographical health inequalities (35,36). The emphasis on addressing health inequalities within the UK Health and Care Act 2022 via greater integration of health with non-medical services, has accelerated thinking around the potential and practicalities of developing HJPs. The 42 English integrated care systems (ICSs) that have been established bring together a variety of medical and non-medical organisations and services to provide more joined-up health and care for patients. There is now, apparently, a more determined focus on prevention and early intervention, especially among high risk groups, to reduce ill health and care needs. At the same time, the UK's Ministry of Justice is concentrating more closely on the value of early intervention in preventing the downstream costs to both the health and justice systems of unmet legal needs, and is currently supporting the development and evaluation of welfare rights services co-located in health settings (37).

The health justice approach offers important opportunities for legal and health services to work together to ameliorate health inequalities and HJPs can be a vehicle through which social welfare law becomes part and parcel of the approach to improving the health of citizens. Research evaluations of HJPs show strong evidence of effectiveness in improving the socioeconomic circumstances of individuals; reaching patient groups most likely to be affected by health-harming legal needs who would otherwise not seek help for social welfare issues; and improvements in stress, depression, anxiety and wellbeing, occurring as a direct result of the legal interventions. There is also good research evidence for improvements in social determinants, including access to food, heating and healthcare, and increased social participation, self-care and self-confidence. Studies of the impact of HJPs on health services show benefits in freeing up beds in hospitals, support for healthcare professionals to manage patients' non-medical needs and improving both practitioner and patient experience (38).

Incorporating an integrated partnership approach in generalism

The [HJP] approach focuses on prevention by addressing upstream structural and systemic social and legal problems that affect population health. It leverages medical and legal resources through an interprofessional model of care delivery.

Elizabeth Tobin-Tyler 2017 (39)

Chapter 1 outlined how generalist clinical practice and education requires multiple lenses and points of engagement with patients. Sometimes, this might require clinicians to address a range of discrete and different problems shared by a patient. At other times, problems may be enmeshed and interwoven. In these situations, while clinicians are not able to solve underlying health-harming unmet legal needs, they are nonetheless in the position of 'critical noticers' who may have significant impact on health through providing a gateway to non-medical services and interventions. Part of the task is working out together the key issues that need to be addressed and for the clinician to make a judgement about the most effective approach. This requires a clinician to elicit, through careful and sensitive questioning, what matters most to the patient at that point in time, and to determine what is most likely to make a meaningful difference to the patient's health and wellbeing. Very often this is not simply about looking for the presence or absence of disease, but rather requires an exploration of the broader context in which the patient functions or survives, and identification of ongoing health-harming events or problems. Whether a problem is framed as 'clinical', 'social', 'legal', or a combination of all, depends on the patient, clinician and the resources available to them. Problem identification and framing is complicated not merely by the particular lens through which it is viewed, but also by the lack of common understanding and vocabulary. A threat of eviction causing anxiety and/or depression may be seen by the patient simply as a nightmare from which they want to escape, but feel helpless. They may have no idea of the existence of any legal rights or remedies or how to pursue them if available. The clinician may see this as a medical problem requiring medication and understandably focus on dealing with the presenting mental health issue without further exploring the underlying cause. However, a social welfare lawyer will see this as a legal need that requires rapid protective action via available justice system remedies.

A generalist, integrated health justice partnership approach therefore requires a number of steps. These steps may not occur in a linear fashion and could happen over a relatively brief or longer period, involving a series of appointments or conversations.

- Step 1 requires the professional's mindset to have an appreciation of the interconnectedness between a patient's health and disease, with additional factors such as stress; the impact of material wellbeing on how a patient can experience and / or manage their illness; the support a patient might need or expect (and whether this is available and / or feasible to achieve).

- Step 2 involves an exchange between patient and professional that leads to some shared understanding of the range of factors shaping the patient's current experiences or problems and their priorities. This is likely to be led initially by professional, patient or both and could possibly include another individual (such as a social prescribing link worker).
- Step 3 involves patient and professional agreeing a problem-set (for example, depression which needs treating, but also identifying factors contributing to this such as relationship breakdown, financial struggles, housing difficulties, employment problems).
- Step 4 involves an honest and realistic discussion about the feasibility and likely scope and timelines to expect if accessing or approaching other organisations for support.
- Step 5 involves a cross-disciplinary connection – enabling a patient to benefit directly from welfare rights advice and support that would ideally lead to an improvement in the patient's situation, reducing stress and leading to an overall improvement in health and wellbeing (38) as well as an increase in confidence about how to manage ongoing and future challenges.
- Step 6 ideally involves continuity and a sustained relationship between patient and professional – to ensure that a plan (as it evolves) can be reviewed and assessed by both patient and clinician.
- Step 7 involves an ongoing and critical discussion about how service provision and systems can evolve and learn from each collaborative case. Ideally, this includes space to reflect on and address any ways involvement in a case has impacted on professionals, before they move on to attend to another patient.

Tables 10.1 and 10.2 illustrate the different approaches and outcomes for example clinical conditions. This compares the traditional biomedical model with a service model that integrates social welfare legal advice and support in order to address underlying 'social pathogens' in a way that may more effectively alleviate poor health for the longer term (Tables 10.1 and 10.2).

The health justice approach in practice

> Both medical and legal professionals are trained to obtain and rely on information provided by the patient or client to define, clarify and craft a solution to a problem ... both professions rely on questioning and listening skills to obtain accurate, relevant and complete stories from patients and clients.
>
> Bliss and colleagues 2011 (40)

Table 10.1 Traditional biomedical model of health

Clinical condition	Clinical intervention
Chronic asthma	Increase asthma medication dose and frequency, refer to specialist clinic, advise stop smoking
Insomnia in pregnant woman	Sleep hygiene advice, hypnotic medications, investigate for medical causes of sleeplessness e.g. thyroid function, breathing, pain, referral to psychological therapies
Suicidal ideation or deliberate self-harm	Mental health support or referral, safeguarding, emergency assessment, psychotropic medications
Lower back pain	Analgesia, imaging investigations, physiotherapy, surgical referral
Malnutrition, anaemia, iron deficiency	Investigation of bowel health, supplemental nutrition milkshakes, iron supplements, vitamin B12 and folate, alcohol history

Table 10.2 Integrating interrelated (upstream) social pathogens and using legal interventions to achieve long-term solutions

Social pathogen	Clinical condition	Clinical intervention	Legal remedy
Poor quality damp housing	Chronic asthma	Increase asthma medication dose and frequency. Support smoking cessation. Refer to specialist clinic if needed	Compel landlord to comply with legal duty to provide healthy safe housing. Check income entitlements. Increase income to enable move to better accommodation
Employer illegally threatening with redundancy	Insomnia in pregnant woman	Sleep hygiene advice, hypnotic medications, referral to psychological therapies	Compel employer to comply with legal duty to protect employment of pregnant employees

(continued)

Table 10.2 (Cont.)

Social pathogen	Clinical condition	Clinical intervention	Legal remedy
Landlord threatening eviction	Suicidal ideation or deliberate self-harm	Mental health referral, safeguarding, emergency assessment, psychotropic medications	Prevent eviction and or compel local authority to provide housing assistance
Unsafe working conditions	Lower back pain	Analgesia, imaging investigations, surgical referral	Compel employer to modify working conditions or provide reasonable adjustments to accommodate
Insufficient income for healthy diet	Malnutrition, anaemia, iron deficiency	Supplemental nutrition milkshakes, iron supplements, vitamin B12 and folate. Food vouchers	Check income entitlements. Increase income by applying for unclaimed benefit. Appeal decision to deny or withdraw benefits

If we acknowledge that health is considerably more than the absence of disease, then the boundaries and overlaps between stress, illness and disease become vital to acknowledge and explore. As discussed in Chapter 1, generalists are not a 'catch all' for dealing with issues that others decline to touch, nor are generalists looking after the 'basics' while others focus on specialist problems. Generalists' expertise lies in the application of dynamic and agile capabilities required to examine the potential range, breadth and depth of issues experienced by patients affecting their health and wellbeing. They must then skilfully navigate a variety of options in order to direct attention in a way that most effectively achieves the outcomes that matter most to a patient. This requires exploration of long- and short-term preferences and needs within the boundaries of service possibilities and the constraints imposed by the patient's other conditions and context. In some cases this could be relatively straightforward, for example a patient expressing extreme anxiety and possibly suicidal thoughts as a result of pending eviction and potential homelessness. In other, more complex cases, there is a 'risk' that the generalist will identify such a broad range of challenges to tackle, that both patient and professional feel overwhelmed and unable to cope or act.

The generalist needs to mitigate this risk by focusing on the problem-set, enabling each participant to review and discuss what is named and recognised within the problem-set at that moment in time, and review how this is framed in relation to possible trajectories or outcomes. The value of integrating the expertise and understanding of the generalist clinician with the specialist knowledge and skills of the welfare adviser is the ability to address interlocked social welfare issues as a set rather than attempting to 'unbundle' and address issues individually. Building a sustained relationship between patient and clinician can help to identify priorities, triggers and possibilities for interventions that would deliver effective improvement in the patient's health and broader wellbeing in the longer term.

A generalist cannot always be inclusive, comprehensively attending to all identified problems. They may, however, be one of the only professionals a member of the public has ready access to, bringing a range of distress, suffering and potential needs. While their suffering or distress may initially therefore appear difficult to unpack, we have noted earlier that while the generalist cannot deal with everything, their role as critical noticer is crucial in signposting to additional services where needed (for example, a link worker). It is necessary to be able and willing to shift perspective and perhaps let go of some issues as a patient's story evolves. Hearing, for example, how a patient's experience has changed through a set of interactions with another (for example, carer, family member, professional) is key to ensuring that healthcare remains responsive to a patient's needs and relevant to the priorities of that time. This might involve both tackling short-term challenges, as well as periodically revisiting longer-term threads about more entrenched difficulties. This critical noticing approach therefore requires a balance of active planning with the patient, connecting to and with colleagues, and agreement to hold or monitor some problems, where no immediate solution or activity is possible.

How can we implement a health justice partnership approach into clinical care?

The health justice partnership approach offers the possibility of effective holistic care that addresses health issues and ameliorates underlying social and economic circumstances that are causing or exacerbating ill health. In this approach to healthcare, the clinician plays a catalytic role, mobilising other services and resources that will impact health in a way that medicine alone cannot.

Implementing a health justice approach in generalism requires the professional to be ready to adopt a broad approach in dealing with the issues brought by the patient. It requires insightful questioning, listening and discussion skills to disentangle the issues that are most important to the patient and most likely to achieve a positive impact on health and wellbeing. A health justice approach also requires the generalist to have knowledge of the range of relevant non-clinical services that might be mobilised to assist the patient and preferably to establish strong links between the practice and those services. Local service provision is highly diverse and fluid depending on resources. Effective learning systems within organisations are both an essential precursor to developing a health justice approach and an important method of remaining updated on developments in the health justice field and the provision of welfare rights services local to a practice. This includes learning with and along-side patients as they move through and navigate a particular system or process. Learning might range from very practical elements (for example, knowledge about a single point of contact for referral via a link worker, or changes to service arrangements over time), through to more detailed knowledge about the approaches or limits of available service provision.

The overlap and integrated nature of legal and health problems is messy and often blurred. A generalist clinician who delves into 'causal' level discussions for every attending patient might encounter challenges in terms of time, energy and ability to complete other competing tasks. However, part of the skill and expertise of a generalist will be to listen with curiosity and select with the patient how and when to pick up on particular cues and clues. These may help to invite a conversation about issues beyond (but in addition to) a traditional disease-focused discussion. This more inclusive approach is a key part of generalist clinical practice. Key elements include:

- **Active listening** to note 'cues' and 'clues' which hint at additional elements of a patient's stories or contributory factors needing to be explored.
- **Curiosity** to probe and explore where gaps or ambiguities arise (for example, about causal contributors or triggers).
- **Decision-making in partnership with patients**, to recognise the limitations of time and resources at particular moments; acknowledging there is more to discuss; and selecting whether to focus on this now or

at another time; once a problem is clarified, considering whether to own the problem and its exploration together, whether to delegate, or move a discussion to another setting or set of individuals.

- **Familiarity with what others can achieve.** Clinical encounters need to be able to address both what is explicitly expressed as a problem within the clinical encounter or directly possible to address, and beyond. Each professional (and patient) needs not only to have an awareness of what each other can readily achieve, but also know how other services or individuals might relate to or support identified needs. For example, co-working within a building (if enabling regular informal discussions) might support professionals to share stories about how and what they do in work, helping generalists to identify relevant elements of a patient interaction which might be relevant to share or distribute with others.

- **System-level 'health checks'** about how healthcare professionals and patients work together. This process and the ability to act on broader, shared information requires regular attention and calibration to the system in which healthcare professionals work. So, for example, is a generalist able to share, distribute or shift identified problems with colleagues to explore and address 'gaps'? This might be within a healthcare organisation (for example, a lawyer situated for a certain number of hours per week, within a clinical setting), or through movement or communication with another organisation (for example, signposting a patient to contact a Women's Centre for support following domestic violence).

- **Advocacy.** Politics can feel overwhelming and dissonant with the identified needs of patients (for example, hunger, homelessness, conflict). However, there are many levels at which healthcare professionals can interact and work with the public (as a collective) and patients (as individuals) to tackle such challenges – and regain a sense of control to either or both. An example from the UK is the commissioning of services through integrated care boards (ICBs).

- **Recognition and response to social determinants of health.** No healthcare system is sustainable if it does not attend to social determinants of health. Moving from a focus on equal provision of care (providing the same for all), to equity (providing what each individual needs to enable fair access and opportunity) enables a system to adapt to the individual identified needs of patients, maximising their ability to meet particular outcomes. Often these do not involve getting rid of disease, but living well with it, or enabling its impact to be minimised.

What is needed to develop and implement a health justice approach?

A partnership is an alliance between organisations, brought together around common goals, shared values and commitments. By joining forces, the partners can tackle complex issues they could not address alone. Genuine collaboration and good working relationships can be a major strength of Health Justice Partnerships and ideally this interdisciplinary teamwork becomes a part of everyday practice that is routine, accepted and widely utilised. As well as working together to assist individual patients/clients, partnerships can be strengthened by mutual training, support and consultation between professionals (32).

Ways to support learning

Education and training are essential for clinicians and legal providers to work effectively in partnership. As with any innovative or reformist approach, learners may encounter teaching about certain priorities or services, before or alongside their being developed in practice. Learners may therefore need support to make sense of potential dissonance or tensions encountered (between teaching and service experience). Learners can, however, still feel empowered within boundaries, to shape their own clinical practice to meet particular moral imperatives and accountabilities. An understanding of how determinants of health may manifest as 'legal needs' is fundamental if clinicians are to be effective partners in addressing health-harming unmet legal needs. The lack of a well-developed shared vocabulary between clinicians and social welfare lawyers can lead to a limited interpretation of the issues patients bring to the clinical conversations and a consequent failure to see the 'legal' in what may appear to be merely 'social' or 'economic'.

This presents a challenge for clinical and legal education. Breaking down disciplinary silos in education can reveal shared professional values, such as respect for the individual, professional judgement and experience, as well as mutual concern for patient/client safety (27). Interprofessional learning, dialogue and contact during training also offers the opportunity to develop the interests, skills and cultural awareness referred to earlier that are necessary for taking a HJP approach in generalism.

Clinical example: Mother and baby

A mother repeatedly takes her baby to the GP with concerns about breathing, asthma and skin problems. They live in social housing with mould, insect infestations and rodents. The mother had tried to contact her local authority by telephone and email to discuss conditions in her home and the possibility of remedial works or rehousing but without success. On one visit to the surgery, the GP advised her to visit the free legal advice clinic, located in the health centre on the floor above the surgery. She did so. The adviser discussed her situation with her and then wrote to the local authority requesting a review of her situation for which they had a legal obligation. The local authority responded, undertook the review as required, assessed the housing to be inappropriate to the family's needs and provided alternative more suitable housing. The critical steps in this process are shown in Figure 10.1.

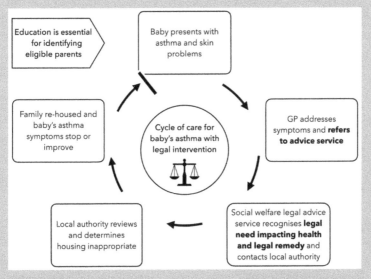

Figure 10.1 A health justice approach to the social determinants of health. © Hazel Genn

Educational example: Embedding health-justice learning into the core undergraduate medical curriculum at UCL

At UCL, all medical students learn about health justice in their penultimate year of study. This is positioned within the students' general practice clinical placement. The session is co-designed and co-delivered by the Faculty of Laws and Medical School team. Each contributes their insights and experience drawing on each other's disciplinary expertise, and building knowledge about the interface between the two. Students are encouraged to bring some anonymised examples of patient encounters from their placement relevant to the session. These discussions are supplemented with case vignettes and videos of clinical encounters. Following the session, students are encouraged to use the frameworks and questions from the session to inform their subsequent patient discussions, in addition to seeking out additional community resources local to their clinical placement. The teaching is assessed in written and OSCE end-of-year exams. Some students also use learning from the session to inform their patient with multimorbidity and carer essay assignment.

Key messages and discussion points

Key messages and discussion points are highlighted in this next section. The first is to explain that laws, regulations and policies are established to protect low-income families to reduce the negative impacts of poverty and health on wellbeing. The policies are designed to address the adverse social conditions that negatively impact health and livelihood and improve quality of life for those in need. However, rights and protections do not automatically happen. The process of identifying, communicating and claiming 'need' is complex. Social needs become framed as legal needs in order to access benefits, entitlements and rights protection prescribed by law. Health may be undermined at individual and population level, when people do not receive the benefits or protections that law provides (Figure 10.2).

Social welfare legal rights and potentially health-harming unmet legal needs can be diverse and/or multiple. So, for example, an individual might be eligible for benefits (for example, disability, income security or housing benefit); housing support (for example, tenant's rights, safe housing, or support if homeless); employment (for example, dismissal/redundancy, equal pay, bullying/harassment, discrimination); mental

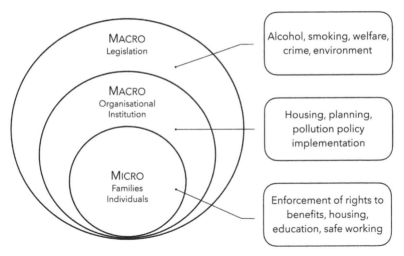

Figure 10.2 Three levels at which law influences health.
© Hazel Genn

capacity (for example, lasting power of attorney); family (for example, breakdown, residence/contact with children, child safety); immigration (for example, right to remain/work/benefits/asylum, deportation); violence (partner, relative); community care (right to support/services); education (exclusion, special needs); and discrimination (for example, protected characteristics such as age, sex, race, religion, sexual preference). At least in the UK, criminal and civil law are separate. The latter focuses on everyday life, often providing safety net protections for people on the lowest incomes prone to experiencing difficulties and less able to manage (Figure 10.3).

Some people with unmet social welfare legal needs experience considerable impact on their health and wellbeing. This is likely to result in recurrent health service use (for example, repeated Accident and Emergency or general practice visits). These presentations may appear (through a solely biomedical lens) as seemingly minor or irremediable health problems. Rather than framing their attendance as 'inappropriate', a health justice approach can potentially release people from this 'revolving door' of unmet needs (Figure 10.4).

Working together, it is possible to address problems and their severity through earlier action. Rather than a lawyer meeting with a person after a crisis has emerged, they can work with them earlier in the process, to avoid problems from arising or minimise the impact of difficulties faced. This can be achieved through HJPs that embed welfare advisers within multidisciplinary teams; combining health and legal tools to

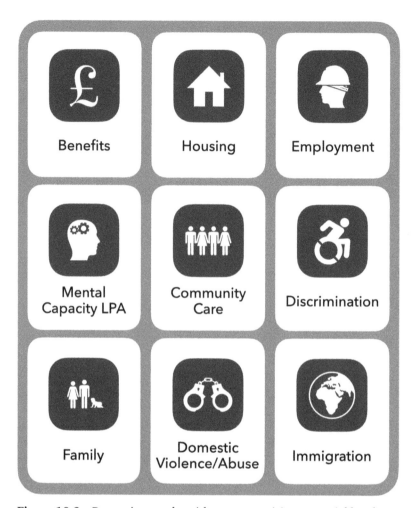

Figure 10.3   Protections and entitlements requiring potential legal assistance. © Hazel Genn

support outcomes; integrating health-justice learning into clinical curricula; maximising opportunities to reach people early, to improve material, mental and physical wellbeing; alongside support and transformation of community health services. In England, the latest integrated care systems (ICS) model offers a range of opportunities for potential collaboration, including at system level, to support provider collaboratives. Next, place-based partnerships or health and wellbeing boards. And finally, locally at neighbourhood level through primary care networks (or PCNs) (see The King's Fund (41) for more details). Potential changes for patients resulting from these services are highlighted in Figure 10.5.

Common Social Problems	Impact on Health and Healthcare	Potential Legal Intervention

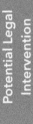

Unstable, unsafe or chaotic living conditions

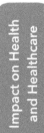

Unemployment due to physical or mental disability

 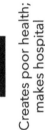

Creates poor health; makes hospital discharge difficult

Limits income, threatens housing, nutrition, health, child welfare

Eviction protection; rehousing; benefit review; enforcement of regulations; child protection

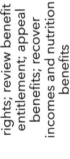

Review employment rights; review benefit entitlement; appeal benefits; recover incomes and nutrition benefits

Figure 10.4 Heavy health service use as an indicator of unmet social welfare needs. Adapted from E. Tobyn Tiler's presentation 'Addressing the social determinants of health through Medical-Legal Partnership', 15 July 2016

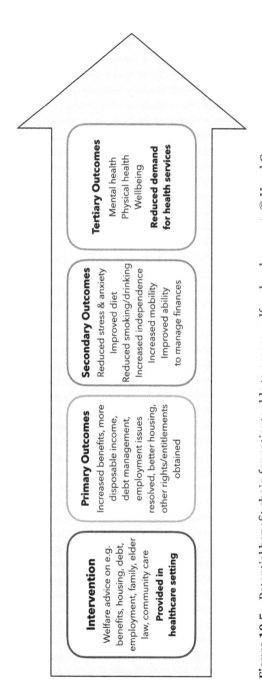

Figure 10.5 Potential benefit chain for patients able to access welfare legal support. © Hazel Genn

Intervention

Welfare advice on e.g. benefits, housing, debt, employment, family, elder law, community care

Provided in healthcare setting

Primary Outcomes

Increased benefits, more disposable income, debt management, employment issues resolved, better housing, other rights/entitlements obtained

Secondary Outcomes

Reduced stress & anxiety
Improved diet
Reduced smoking/drinking
Increased independence
Increased mobility
Improved ability
to manage finances

Tertiary Outcomes

Mental health
Physical health
Wellbeing

Reduced demand for health services

Pause and reflect

Consider your own 'advocacy barometer'. What influences the scope and limitations of how and when you feel able to a) notice and b) support others with the broader challenges related to a patient's health and social care needs? Many clinicians report a sense of disempowerment or lack of confidence to know how to act on problems beyond the biomedical lens. Have you found ways to enable or legitimise attention to a patient's broader social context (for example their housing or employment problems) when a patient or carer attends for help? Can you see the value of noticing and making explicit factors which might help a patient to improve? For example, not only attending to their low mood, but also signposting to social welfare advice services which could help with housing change. If these do not feel possible or valuable, why not? Do you feel a lack of know-how about who and how to access resources? Or maybe hopelessness that even if you do reach out, resources or timelines may not make a difference in practice? Or have you, in fact, seen positive change and impact through supporting patients in this multifaceted way? (see Table 10.3).

Table 10.3   Key learning action points

Learning challenge	How to do this
Knowledge and confidence	Find out about your local range of services (e.g. welfare legal support) and / or 'connectors' (e.g. link workers or social prescribers)
Maximise familiarity, trust and collaboration between you and local services	Consider informal and formal connections e.g. co-location, regular dialogue or learning systems, feedback.
Consider how you might identify social and legal unmet need in your clinical practice	Might this be informal curiosity in patient interactions, or a more formal questionnaire approach?
Patient advocacy	Clinicians' capacity and ability to advocate for patients will of course vary. But at the very least, become a critical noticer: model legitimising social and legal needs as a relevant dimension of patient care, and know who to approach where these needs are shared.

Overcoming challenges

> We see a high proportion of social problems … I'd say there's a social element to at least a third of the consultations that I deal with … It's a lot easier to medicalise problems than to address social determinants … We have 10 minutes. We often have multiple problems to deal with … and sometimes it's easier to ignore a problem than to try to take it on.
>
> GP in practice in HJP

A common criticism against clinicians noticing and supporting elements of social determinants of health, is workload. This broader range of focus with patients becomes positioned as overwhelming and just another addition to the list of jobs to do each day. Most clinicians who are working with patients who experience this broad range of challenges (impacting on both their health and social wellbeing) do notice these elements of allostatic load; they see how social stressors or challenges impact on patients' health and their ability to engage with and access healthcare. The key distinction is this: clinicians cannot be expected to include or achieve solutions to all the social determinant and legal challenges a patient might experience. However, they can notice *with* the patient, and ensure that a negotiated problem-set includes not only the biomedical elements in their management plan, but also acceptance that other factors are important to attend to. That process of acknowledgement in itself can be enough to help reframe and shift a patient's action plan for help-seeking approaches. But it might also include a clinician signposting or encouraging a patient to contact local relevant services who have more specialist expertise and knowledge of resources (for example, social prescribing or social welfare advice services) which offer a possibility of hope and / or change.

In the short term, 'noticing' might take another few minutes of a clinician's time, extending the intended scope of an appointment about pain, insomnia or low mood. Longer term, however, this noticing is likely to represent an overall time-saving and can make a significant difference to both patient and clinician. A burgeoning field of research around clinician burnout, particularly in areas of social deprivation (see deep end movements in Chapter 8), shows how permission to notice is key. It is not that clinicians would not otherwise notice patient suffering due to social deprivation. They might, however, develop ways to ignore this, position it as irrelevant, or accept a sense of disempowerment to effect change. Rather, if clinicians are given permission to notice and attend to these issues with patients, and make connections with others who do the same, patterns, systems and collective solutions become possible. Individuals can feel part of a broader collective movement as a social advocate, increasing their knowledge about how and when to signpost and access help for patients who need help.

It is important to nurture a sense of hope and agency, to sustain the energies and commitment many patients and carers require. Many of the challenges described in this chapter are directly related to broad national and international aspects of policy and economic challenge. For example, allocation of funds to social care systems; conflict necessitating populations to move (and therefore become 'migrants' in need of help and support); economic milieu impacting on the range and availability of possibilities for suitable employment. Clinicians, however motivated, cannot change all of this. However, in recognising these broader societal challenges, and how they impact on particular patients and local populations, clinicians work with patients and carers to help formulate and make explicit connections between elements of suffering and open up access to and ways of problematising issues in different ways, that might enable new ways of supporting and helping others. There will always be limits to a clinician's remit or scope for facilitating change: there will always be a limit to resources. However, without a sense of curiosity and ability to imagine things differently, these conversations might never happen.

Might this do more harm than good? Some prefer to think of clinical work as apolitical, but most will recognise that patient advocacy is inherently political. Clinicians might worry that reframing a problem as legal might in fact harm their patient. Might it raise their hopes and not in fact result in long-term change? Of course, this is a risk. But if we are honest with our patients, and prepared to advocate where we can, this partnership can improve capability to support patients with social challenges (42). A biomedical dominance to clinical practice has tended to draw clinicians' attention to problematise things which have an obvious solution. Thus 'medically unexplained symptoms' or 'social determinants of health' become irrelevant or unimportant, as no obvious or direct solution is visible to the patient or clinician. Communication, shared practice of examples where action has effected change, or feedback through local or national learning systems can, therefore, be really important in helping clinicians to recognise the value and potential benefit for patients of noticing and acknowledging broader elements of distress. Acknowledging this distress with patients can be a powerful act in itself, and possibilities exist for effecting change for some, if not all.

Conclusion

In conclusion, social determinants of health have long been recognised as impacting on health and wellbeing. However, clinicians often feel disempowered at local level to notice, name and act upon broader social and potentially legal and welfare unmet need. Health justice partnerships are one example of collaborative ways in which clinicians and lawyers can exchange knowledge and expertise locally, maximising the opportunities for patients to access support at the earliest possible opportunity. Modelling cross-faculty collaborations within clinical education curricula and workplaces is one way to enable clinicians to feel able and equipped to support patients: helping clinicians to see these aspects of patients' suffering and distress as relevant to notice, alongside familiarity with available services to signpost. So, can you be a curious and critical noticer? Can you observe when you are able to advocate for a patient? What will enable you to feel more empowered to support a patient with these challenges? And how can this empowerment become shared (or not) with your patient and shift their sense of possibility, agency or hope?

References

1. Scottish Public Health Network, NHS Health Scotland and the Improvement Service. Primary Care Improvement Plans: Specialist Link Workers (Welfare Rights Advice) in General Practice. 2018. Available from: www.improvementservice.org.uk/__data/assets/pdf_file/0017/9710/hscp-briefing-welfare-advisors-general-practice-mar18.pdf (accessed 25 June 2023).
2. Egan J, Robison O. Integrating money advice workers into primary care settings: an evaluation. Glasgow Centre for Population Health; 2019. Available from: www.gcph.co.uk/assets/0000/7293/Advice_workers_in_deep_end_GP_primary_care_setting.pdf (accessed 25 June 2023).
3. National Center for Medical-Legal Partnership. Available from: https://medical-legalpartnership.org/ (accessed 25 June 2023).
4. Health Justice Australia. Partnerships for better health and justice outcomes. Available from: www.healthjustice.org.au/ (accessed 25 June 2023).
5. Wade DT, Halligan PW. Do biomedical models of illness make for good healthcare systems? *BMJ*. 2004;329(7479):1398–401.
6. Institute of Health Equity. Fair Society, Healthy Lives – The Marmot Review. 2010. Available from: https://policycommons.net/artifacts/2297843/fair-society-healthy-lives/ (accessed 18 March 2024).
7. The King's Fund. Determinants of Health. Time to Think Differently. 2014. Available from: www.kingsfund.org.uk/projects/time-think-differently/trends-broader-determinants-health (accessed 25 June 2023).
8. The Health Foundation. Healthy lives for people in the UK. 2017. Available from: www.health.org.uk/publications/healthy-lives-for-people-in-the-uk (accessed 25 June 2023).
9. Tobin-Tyler E, Teitelbaum JB. *Essentials of Health Justice: Law, policy, and structural change*. Jones & Bartlett Learning; 2022.
10. Genn H. When law is good for your health: mitigating the social determinants of health through access to justice. *Curr Leg Probl*. 2019;72(1):159–202.

11. OECD/Open Society Foundations. *Legal Needs Surveys and Access to Justice*. OECD Publishing; 2019. Available from: www.oecd-ilibrary.org/content/publication/g2g9a36c-en (accessed 18 March 2024).

12. Genn H. *Paths to Justice: What people do and think about going to law*. Bloomsbury Publishing; 1999.

13. Sandefur RL. What we know and need to know about the legal needs of the public. *S C Law Rev*. 2016;67(2):16.

14. Forell S, Boyd-Caine T. Service models on the health justice landscape: a closer look at partnership. Discussion paper. Health Justice Australia; 2018.

15. Coumarelos C, Pleasence P, Wei Z. Law and disorders: illness/disability and the experience of everyday problems involving the law. *Justice Issues*. 2013;(17):1–23.

16. Pleasence P, Balmer NJ, Buck A. The health cost of civil-law problems: further evidence of links between civil-law problems and morbidity, and the consequential use of health services. *J Empir Leg Stud*. 2008;5(2):351–73.

17. Clegg A, Ghelani D, Charlesworth Z, Johnson T-M. Missing out: £19 billion of support goes unclaimed each year. Policy in Practice; 2023. Available from: https://policyinpractice.co.uk/wp-content/uploads/Missing-out-19-billion-of-support.pdf (accessed 26 June 2023).

18. Tunstall R, Bevan M, Bradshaw J, Croucher K, Duffy S, Hunter C, et al. The links between housing and poverty: an evidence review. Joseph Rowntree Foundation; 2013.

19. Siegrist J, Marmot M. Health inequalities and the psychosocial environment – two scientific challenges. *Health Inequalities Psychosoc Environ*. 2004;58(8):1463–73.

20. Tobin-Tyler E, Teitelbaum JB. Socioeconomic status, unmet social needs, and health. In: *Essentials of Health Justice: Law, Policy, and Structural Change*. Jones & Bartlett Learning; 2022.

21. Epel ES, Lin J, Wilhelm FH, Wolkowitz OM, Cawthon R, Adler NE, et al. Cell aging in relation to stress arousal and cardiovascular disease risk factors. *Psychoneuroendocrinology*. 2006;31(3):277–87.

22. Popay J, Kowarzik U, Mallinson S, Mackian S, Barker J. Social problems, primary care and pathways to help and support: addressing health inequalities at the individual level. Part I: the GP perspective. *J Epidemiol Community Health*. 2007;61(11):966–71.

23. Beardon S, Woodhead C, Cooper S, Genn H, Raine R. A comparative case study of health-justice partnerships in England: service models and implementation success. *J Epidemiol Community Health*. 2021;75:A80. Available from: https://jech.bmj.com/content/75/Suppl_1/A80.1 (accessed 12 April 2024).

24. Citizens' Advice, Royal College of General Practitioners. Advice in practice: Understanding the effects of integrating advice in primary care settings. 2018. Available from: https://assets.ctfassets.net/mfz4nbgura3g/7fstM4TyWfdqEhlN839GDl/8463eac58d3642ad44a410044b8a5cb9/_Global_Public_Impact_Understanding_the_effects_of_advice_in_primary_care_settings_research_report__final_.pdf (accessed 18 March 2024).

25. Antonovsky A. The salutogenic model as a theory to guide health promotion. *Health Promot Int*. 1996;11(1):11–8.

26. Box L. Awaab Ishak: another avoidable tragedy. Race Equality Foundation. 2022. Available from: https://raceequalityfoundation.org.uk/housing/awaab-ishak-anotvoidable-tragedy/ (accessed 5 November 2023).

27. Tobin-Tyler E, Genn H, Boyd-Caine T, Reis N. Health justice partnerships: an international comparison of approaches to employing law to promote prevention and health equity. *J Law Med Ethics*. 2023;51(2):332–43.

28. Marmot M, Allen J, Boyce T, Goldblatt P, Morrison J. Health Equity in England: The Marmot Review 10 Years On. 2020. Available from: www.health.org.uk/publications/reports/the-marmot-review-10-years-on (accessed 18 March 2024).

29. Jarman B. Giving advice about welfare benefits in general practice. *BMJ*. 1985;16(290):522–4.

30. Beardon S, Genn H. The health justice landscape in England and Wales: Social welfare legal services in health settings. UCL Centre for Access to Justice; 2018.

31. Leedham-Green K, Knight A, Reedy GB. Success and limiting factors in health service innovation: a theory-generating mixed methods evaluation of UK projects. *BMJ Open*. 2021;11(5):e047943.

32. Beardon S, Woodhead C, Cooper S, Genn H, Raine R. Health-Justice Partnerships in England: An implementation study. NIHR School for Public Health Research; 2022. Available

from:www.fph.org.uk/media/3487/research-briefing-health-justice-partnerships-in-england_implementation-study.pdf (accessed 18 March 2024).

33. Improvement Service. Welfare Advice and Health Partnerships. 2020. Available from:www.improvementservice.org.uk/products-and-services/consultancy-and-support/welfare-advice-and-health-partnerships (accessed 26 June 2023).

34. Genn DH, Beardon S. Health Justice Partnerships: Integrating welfare rights advice with patient care. The Legal Education Foundation; 2021. Available from: www.ucl.ac.uk/health-of-public/sites/health_of_public/files/health_justice_partnerships_integrating_welfare_rights_advice_with_patient_care.pdf (accessed 18 March 2024).

35. Marmot M. Society and the slow burn of inequality. *The Lancet*. 2020;395(10234):1413–4.

36. Barros AJD, Wehrmeister FC, Ferreira LZ, Vidaletti LP, Hosseinpoor AR, Victora CG. Are the poorest poor being left behind? Estimating global inequalities in reproductive, maternal, new-born and child health. *BMJ Glob Health*. 2020;5(1):e002229.

37. Ministry of Justice. Early Legal Advice Pilot. 2022. Available from: www.gov.uk/guidance/early-legal-advice-pilot (accessed 26 June 2023).

38. Beardon S, Woodhead C, Cooper S, Ingram E, Genn H, Raine R. International evidence on the impact of health-justice partnerships: a systematic scoping review. *Public Health Rev*. 2021;42.

39. Tobin-Tyler E. Medical-legal partnership in primary care: moving upstream in the clinic. *Am J Lifestyle Med*. 2019;13(3):282–91.

40. Bliss L, Caley S, Pettignano R. Client and patient relationships: understanding cultural and social context. In: Tobin-Tyler E, Lawton E, editors. *Poverty, Health and Law: Readings and cases for medical-legal partnership*. Carolina Academic Press; 2011. pp. 125–46.

41. The King's Fund. Primary care networks. Available from: www.kingsfund.org.uk/topics/general-practice/primary-care-networks (accessed 3 November 2023).

42. Pleasence P, Balmer NJ, Denvir C. How People Understand and Interact with the Law. The Legal Aid Foundation; 2015. Available from: www.thelegaleducationfoundation.org/wp-content/uploads/2015/12/HPUIL_report.pdf (accessed 18 March 2024).

11
Generalist approaches to community health needs

Jane Myat, Jane Riddiford, Sadie Lawes-Wickwar and Henry Aughterson

Introduction

Clinical practice is often only thought about only in relation to an individual one-to-one interaction between patient and clinician. There are, however, many forms of generalism which engage more broadly with aspects of the community and the health of local populations. This might require clinicians to assess and monitor local health needs as well as advocate for services to meet those needs. There is a growing shift towards patient support that aims not only to focus on direct disease management, but also to address underlying causes of poor health and/or wellbeing. The referral by generalist practitioners to these community-based interventions has come to be known by some as 'social prescribing' or 'health creation'. These initiatives have benefits in enabling clinicians to support patients in making changes to their lifestyle or health-related behaviours. There are competing and different definitions of social prescribing, but one important and common aspect is mutually respectful relationships. By patients and healthcare practitioners working in partnership this in turn can nurture social connectedness. This chapter focuses on a broad movement of social prescribing or health creation which is a key example of generalist principles. Recent developments in this area highlight the importance of the clinician knowing the community, the community knowing the clinician (continuity), and clinicians working with the community to promote opportunities for health and wellbeing. This community engagement work as a form of social prescribing is now well-established in some areas, and has been implemented using a range of important principles including flattening of hierarchies between clinician and patient; utilising community spaces for interactions outside of the clinical consulting room; and enabling public and patients to become local advocates and leaders of community groups (for example, sewing and textile groups, practice green spaces or gardens, connection cafes, story exchanges, cooking groups). Through these groups, a sense of belonging and engagement can be generated, enabling both patients and practitioners to develop insight, engage in dialogue and gain confidence to recognise their strengths, share dilemmas, problem-solve and listen to others.

This chapter reflects on the process of generalists supporting individual and community health needs, which can in turn support clinical practice to flourish. Chapters 3 and 15 explore how the generalist can work to understand and prioritise patient and carer needs during clinical encounters. Building on this, we focus in this chapter on the process of generalists and patients working together to uncover individual needs, and then to identify local community activities that might be appropriate to support physical health and/or wellbeing. The example of social prescribing is used in this chapter to highlight many of the principles, potential challenges and facilitators, for supporting community health and health creation within generalist clinical practice. We may think about social prescribing as an activity, intervention or service to which a clinician might refer – that is, a separate entity or resource. In this chapter, however, we share how clinicians can work together with their patients in close collaboration, and how the process of socially connecting patients and practitioners with new or existing community initiatives can inform and complement clinical care. For this to happen, we need to attend to the importance of relationships – not as something separate to clinical care – but as integral to its practice. Through this attention to relational expertise we can begin to understand how the often sporadic, intermittent or episodic nature of clinical interactions forms part of a connected continuum. In the context of generalism, public health and community care are not necessarily distinct from what is achieved through clinical encounters, but part of the same endeavour to support clinical practice, and maximise the appropriate use of interventions and treatments as and when they are needed.

Social prescribing: current evidence and practice

Social prescribing has fast evolved in the UK as an interface or conduit between clinical care and community activities to support health and wellbeing. While there is no universally agreed definition of social prescribing (1), it is generally understood to involve healthcare staff making referrals to non-medical interventions by linking individuals with activities and/or support services based in the community (2). Social prescribing happens within clinical contexts (for example, in the UK social prescribing generally sits within primary care), and aims to address social, emotional and/or practical challenges such as social isolation, financial issues, poor housing, low mood, and health behaviour change (3). Consistent with these aims, there is growing evidence about the efficacy of social prescribing activities for promoting biological and psychosocial benefits (4). For example, recent research reported that social prescribing can lead to improvements in anxiety, depression and social isolation (5–8). One recent ethnographic study (9) described some of the 'active ingredients' facilitating social prescribing which included interpersonal facilitator expertise, high regularity of activities, creation of a safe space, high affordability and accessibility and shared lived experiences. Ways in which this provided benefit (or 'mechanisms of action') included increased purpose and meaning, experience of pleasure or joy, increased social support, increased structure and routine, formation of friendships and reduced loneliness and an enhanced sense of community and belonging (9). The degree to which individuals benefit from this combination of active ingredients and engage with such spaces will be mediated through someone's ethnicity, age, socioeconomic status, geography, and other characteristics (4). These all make up the 'complex system' of social prescribing engagement (10). The practice of social prescribing, should, arguably, take this complexity into account.

One key aspect supporting the success of social prescribing efforts is the relationship between the individual and their practitioner, distinguishing the practice of 'prescribing' from simply picking up a flyer or leaflet about a local activity. A good relationship or rapport involves meaningful shared decision-making that identifies a need, empowers patients and assesses any barriers that may hinder the uptake of onward support. Recent research aligns with this, indicating that patients are more likely to accept a referral to a support service if the referral is presented in an acceptable way, is tailored to their individual needs, and they are able to discuss and have their concerns addressed (11). The integral position of the generalist clinician (for example, a GP in the UK) enables them to tailor their advice to the needs of the individual in front of them. A clinician might engage in active curiosity about a patient's wellbeing, spotting opportunities to invite a patient to participate in local activities; relate their clinical conversations periodically to these experiences; or even engage directly in social prescribing activities. However the local opportunities are structured, managed and accessed, a person-centred consultation is one of the key elements in supporting and integrating the value of social prescribing activities within clinical care.

Social prescribing models can be seen as 'multidirectional'. This is because the process involves looking at the community to understand what, how and when to offer the support available, as well as knowing individual patients to support a personalised, individual approach. This requires a capacity for considering multiple perspectives and inclusive, adaptable, relational generalism. In this context it may be helpful to consider a broader conceptualisation of social prescribing, as serving not just the individual but the community, and in the process connecting the individual with their local community. Social prescribing has the capacity to support one-to-one relationship-centred care, but also strengthen connections between patients, clinicians and the community. This can help clinicians to move beyond traditional tensions balancing advocacy for 'the patient in front of you' and the broader 'public' (see Chapter 8). Rather, this process of connecting individuals with their local communities can in turn further embed the patient and clinician within their community. Movements like Transition (which originally aimed to address community concerns about climate change) reshape local communities to benefit residents in their health and wellbeing (12). For example, by repurposing farms to provide activities for people with health issues and community cafes that use food that would otherwise be wasted by local businesses (12). Efforts made by healthcare systems to nurture and celebrate this community engagement, could have benefits to patients, communities and clinicians alike (13), as demonstrated through the experiences described in the letters in the following section, and the examples presented elsewhere in this book.

Social prescribing as community engagement in action

In the following letter exchange, Jane M (GP) and Jane R (patient), share examples of integrated social prescribing models whereby relationships and community engagement are key.

Dear Jane

We spoke this morning after you had had your appointment with David, the thoughtful, supportive, kind and knowledgeable oncologist you have been seeing in Wellington. I was sorry to hear that you are again thrown into the storm and the turbulence of uncertainty and decision making. I am glad though, that David allows you sanctuary, a real thinking space. Isn't this where care-ful and kind care begins and happens? I think that is the insight which is rising in significance for me, through our conversations, our inquiry together and the work we have both been doing. I have certainly paid lip-service whilst trying to pay real service to this notion but it has been a hazy vision, like a mirage on the horizon. I feel more certain now that the work we have both been doing toward healing ourselves, each other and the land we come from starts with creating places of sanctuary. We need paths of return with a destination to settle into, to rest and mend, to free our minds from the assumptions we make and a place from which health can flow.

We spoke together at the Royal College of General Practice (RCGP) last December, a talk we called, A River Runs Through Us. We both told our personal stories and how like two tributaries they had intersected. We journeyed together in real time and space when we joined the community gardens we were both involved in founding through an adventure we called Story Walks. We realised we were walking the path of the buried Fleet river and you told a story of times gone by when dragons flew over the land. What tears would our dragon shed if she flew over the concretised landscape, grieving for all that had been forgotten? Our walks were a response to the pandemic and recognising isolation in our communities. Noticing fear in those stuck in flats without access to green space and the healing power of the earth. We walked weekly on our days off, inviting others from our community to join us. We made connections between spaces and between people. You and Rod told mythical stories, I shared poems. Sometimes we practised Qi Gong and our group became one moving, breathing organism. Over time others would bring their own stories, music, art and their writing. The Hardy Tree in St Pancras' churchyard became Yggdrasil, the sacred Norse tree connecting all things and our anchor during turbulent times. We learnt more about ourselves, each other and the repair to be found in settling, in noticing, in being quiet and the creativity that comes from this journey. People, place and prayer as Paul Kingsnorth says (14).

We were travelling on another journey together too. You needed a doctor when you found a lump in your breast and so before you moved back to New Zealand, we were in a doctor and patient relationship again. We imagined being in a village together, taking up different roles at different times. With your action research background, we negotiated our way through the complexities of working together in various ways. We agreed to write together. We have asked ourselves questions. What is health? How do you gently shift hierarchies from power-over to power-with? How do we navigate professional boundaries, moving between *doctor and patient, working as co-conspirators, leading and being led? How do we support each other as humans and how do we manage to live positively when you do not know what the outcome will be? And this seems to be a key question in a time of pandemics, climate change and political turmoil. I wondered if I could do this but with your encouragement, I have found a voice I did not know I had. I am not an academic. I am a grounded clinician, who is in the third decade of practice and sitting with her community. Although the industrialised institution of medicine trades increasingly in metrics, data and numbers, my world in general practice is still centred around stories.*

And we both believe in the power of stories. As doctors we are encouraged to keep our own story to ourselves but at the same time we are taught that history is all. That from your first days at medical school, certainly in the clinical setting, that context is all. You need to find out about your patient's experience, what matters to them, where they come from, what they think, what they believe and what their hopes and fears are if you are to make a diagnosis, come to a formulation and have any chance of making a realistic and mutually agreeable plan together. I chose to tell my story in our talk together as I have done in other settings because it has been only by going back to what has shaped me and what matters to me that I have a deeper understanding about health and about what it is to be human. This work has continued with your support and through the action research group you set up of which I continue to be a part. And I am grateful for this in enabling me to take this wisdom into my work. I have come to understand what did not make sense in the medical world I was inhabiting. A drive to narrow our focus on disease, what is wrong rather than what remains strong and all the wider determinants of good health and human flourishing. And I want to participate and contribute to creating the conditions for health for myself, my patients and the wider world.

Working with many others, I helped to create our Listening Space garden in the middle of our busy urban general practice. I call it my little patch of conscientious objection. A green, growing and wild protest against the roaring, fast, crushing machine that the modern world can be. The machine which seems to have run roughshod over the world, taking us all prisoner, switching off our thinking, uprooting us, cutting us off, leaving us feeling powerless, confused and lost. We resort to all sorts of 'medicine', trying to soothe ourselves. Comfort food, alcohol, smoking, drugs – prescribed and not-prescribed, switching off, tuning out whilst tuning into anything that will distract us from the pain of all this. And we're getting sick. And we are often told that if we just try a little harder, make better choices, that things will be OK. But what if it is not individual issues but a wider malaise, a problem with our culture and the story we've been inhabiting that is sick?

We recognised a kinship in each other through our belief that it is possible to live in a different story. This is a story where life is a little quieter, where you can grow, where you can learn the extraordinary lessons provided by gardens, green spaces and being in and with nature. This is where real beauty lies and where grace, kindness and compassion can flourish. And in these spaces, when we quieten, we can learn to be a little less harsh with ourselves and others. You provided sanctuary spaces for young people and their communities within the concrete developments of the inner city. Gardens like the Skip Garden, the Paper Garden and the aptly named Story Garden.

Some of my most joyful times have been spent in the Story Garden. Respite and repair on my days off. A fugitive space, where you could breathe out, be with others, sit around a fire, listen and tell stories, cook and eat together. A place of ease and appreciation.

The other day, I was 'doom scrolling'. I think that is the term. Going through my news feed and feeling hopeless, lost and confused. What on earth have I been doing trying to introduce gardening, craft, sewing, singing and cooking at the practice? What is the point? But as I talked it through, with listening partners such as you, I realised that is the whole point. To provide places of sanctuary, to hold listening and thinking space for each other. A place to ground and settle. To find what is inside that's still strong in the midst of lots that is wrong. I know that's what I need when I feel alone and abandoned, fearful of what the future might hold. A warm space where possibility might come alive again, for me as a clinician as well as for my patients. A place where we might kindle hope together. Perhaps these are the places we might start a journey back to health again?

So now we are on the other sides of the planet but still connected. Yggdrasil's roots weave around the world and continue to hold us like all good stories of old. You are beginning to rewild the wetlands on your family land. We have been thinking together and with others about themes of regeneration. Your cells are regenerating and healing after the storm that the cancer cells brought. My regeneration as a tired and often overwhelmed clinician and the regeneration that might be possible in our communities, our society and the wider world if we quieten, soften and learn to listen.

In solidarity,

Jane

Dear Jane,

I have been doing my own doom scrolling, the awful compulsion to just see how bad things in the world can get. Not swallowing my own medicine, feeling caught in the great addictive swirl of it all. I put away my phone and take a few moments to find silence. Writing of the many layers of our relationship and our work together deserves that … the roots between us sit within the great restorative well of silence. I bring to mind the many times we have walked and talked and explored the ground between us.

In your letter to me you wrote of sanctuary. I felt sanctuary when we first sat together over the breakfast you gave me in the Listening Space garden. It was the beginning of stepping into the enchantments and the challenges of your world and all the work you and others like your social prescriber Jo and your patients have done in and around the garden. There is a Māori phrase for how I felt when I first came into the garden, Te wāhi hei hokinga atu; *the place to return to. For what we did later it was important for both of us to find sanctuary in the wilder parts of Hampstead Heath. It was a time when all was so uncertain in the rising chaos; for you the health pressures of the pandemic and for me the challenges of adapting Global Generation (15) a community organisation to the social justice needs of the pandemic and also the lurking worry that my cancer might return again. There was solidarity in being together and in going slow, one leading and then the other, folding forward and back and round again. Towering trees, great gnarled roots, shoes off in the wet grass and sharp cold stones, fingers of aliveness reaching up through the soles of our feet … a whole world going on there, free of the hurly burly anxieties of our worlds. Time spent like that brought an anchor of trust which we brought into the Story Walks with your patients, other medical professionals along with people connected to Global Generation's Story Garden. We had a kind of plan, but because of the 'nothing to prove' trust we had established, it was able to be a very fluid plan, held between you and I and those who came … some silence, some movement, some conversation, a story and a poem or two and something creative for everyone to do. Each time we met, we saw familiar faces and walked familiar paths. We visited the same trees, a chestnut in Camden Square and of course the ash that is known as the Hardy Tree in St Pancras Gardens, and in the gentle, slower way of being there, we found newness and beauty. We bathed in a feast of, as you wrote, quoting Paul Kingsnorth, people, place and prayer. Prayers came in the many poems you shared and the old stories that gained new meanings as we felt our way with* the earth. The ways we would gently move beneath the trees or stop and enjoy the silence. The fact that our little WhatsApp group has continued over several years is testimony to the power of all that.

We ducked the formulaic evaluation forms that came from the local authority that provided some funding for us. You even more vociferously than me said … 'those forms will make people unwell'. That being said, we often asked ourselves about the benefit of what we were doing, and what it had to do with health and healing. You described how our mornings included things people need to do to live a healthy life. We found our own qualitative ways to support others to write about their experience and we received such encouraging and insightful letters. Val, one of your patients, wrote, 'none of us in this group is hiding or wearing their "title". We come as human beings reaching out – mixed ages, genders, background experiences.' It was great to see a friendship between Val and Pamela as neighbours who had never met develop and the way they worked together to engage with the council to take on the seating and the garden beds in Montpelier Gardens, a local Park. In a similar vein I loved the fact that different members of the Lewis family got involved with Global Generation. Fatma and Tania in the Voices of the Earth (VoE) work (15) and the photography that went with that. Eben encouraged Rod to play the piano again and worked on the VoE Sound Recordings with Theatre Complicité (16). It was the time of the Black Lives Matter protests and as a teenager with a Jamaican heritage, Eben asked me if we could grow sugar cane as a way of telling the story of slavery associated with many plants. It made me think about how the Story Garden could become a contemporary kind of botanic garden, promoting discussion amongst our staff team and the young people we worked with about the darker side of our history. You re-connected TJ and her son Dontae, who live next to the Story Garden, to their family doctor when you invited us to lunch in the Listening Space. Little did we know that Dontae, another young black teenager, would regularly join our Story Walks and that he would gift us the story of Yggdrasil, the world tree with healing roots that reach the whole way around the earth. He grew his own version of that story (16). We associated Yggdrasil and her Noons, the cosmic weaving witches, with the Hardy Tree in St Pancras Church yard; the ash that is dying of chalara dieback disease. Following her roots down deep we began to hear the running of the buried waters of the River Fleet and learnt that it was once known as the Holy River of Wells. A tiny fragment of an epic story that inspired more linking of community work with degraded waterways. For Global Generation the link became the

Heritage Lottery Funded Voices of the Water project. You used what you had to reach out to others, organising a great plant give-away; calling forth a Rising River of Hope. Later I brought the story to New Zealand as part of our work of restoring a Wairarapa Wetland.

We have had several action research style inquiries that we have lightly held between us. The questions came in many forms 'what are the conditions for health and healing?', 'what is the role of sanctuary and how do we find it?', 'how do we stand hopefully without knowing what the outcome will be?' ... 'how do we grow connection and community between different people and between all of us and the natural world?', another way of saying how do we find our way back into a woven universe. In one way or another writing was a way of exploring these questions. This happened at first with the Story Walk participants, then the Fellows (young graduates of Global Generation's programmes) and then between you and I. After seeing the photography exhibition curated by Silvia and the Fellows, it was a brave, generous and for me quite unexpected move you took in suggesting that Cassie, Maedeh and Lucy come and do a mini action research style film documentary about you and your work in the Listening Space. I clearly remember sitting in the Story Garden Yurt with staff from UCL partners who also provided funding. I was happy and proud as Maedeh and Cassie shared their writing and invited the UCL team in to do their own writing. These two young women went on to be Youth Representatives for UCL partners. Then just before I left London a next step you joined our little online action research group that was just forming. It was another opportunity for me to benefit from your 'gentle presence' way of being. Through the immediacy of your writing I learned about other aspects of your world. For me you radically shifted my ideas about the prevailing hierarchy of the medical paradigm i.e. arms length, being above the frailties of humanity, 'I am meant to be the expert'. Bravely worming your way into your own story, potently and vulnerably sharing the cracks and crevices of the back story that has shaped you and your contributions in the world. Over the weeks and months I also heard more about your experiences at work, the unfolding narratives that illuminated parts of your own story, the healing you found through the practice of deep, side-by-side listening. Alongside the accounts of your back story, were the stories of you treating patients mostly not in your consulting room. However, I also know, because I have experienced it, that behind the closed door click of that room, there is trust and intimacy there too. As I write this, I think of you buying tulips in readiness for a home visit and wondering if the rules and regulations of the NHS would endorse this simple act of kindness. The stories were full of navigating porous boundaries, where human meets human. I am thinking of the shuffling story, you covered in pus as you washed and dressed the feet of your down-and-out patient, in her desolate and dirty flat, you arriving home with the smell of tobacco in your hair. You wrote of finding intimacy between the two of you there. Again a levelling of hierarchy.

Then of course there has been my own health story and my relationship with you as my doctor, and whilst you are no longer officially my GP you are still my primary guide in how to navigate my feelings and prepare myself for all the many choices that being a cancer patient brings. The ongoing dialogue with you has given me a macro view, and a curiosity about my experience which has made the inevitable fear manageable. Our conversations have given me time and ways to bring out the best in myself and the doctors here that are enabling us to engage in genuine shared decision making. I think your strength in this is a combination of being there on the same level, deeply and intuitively listening, mostly supporting what I as a patient felt drawn to do and also not holding back on giving opinions when needed. Sometimes this includes additional research on your part and technical interpretation for my benefit. Overall, to use your phrase, you have enabled me to focus on 'what's strong rather than what's wrong'.

When I embarked on chemotherapy, you encouraged me to think about the hedgerow and hillside origins of modern drugs and I felt better about the taxol I was taking, contemplating the capacity of the yew (Taxus baccata); they can regenerate themselves and live for thousands of years. In one of your recent messages to me you quoted Ursula Le Guin, which spoke exactly to how I was feeling at the time: 'Science describes accurately from outside, poetry describes accurately from inside (and) both celebrate what they describe.' We have, I think, with our eyes open, entered into and managed to swim in sometimes tricky and always rich ground. It is a professional relationship that has evolved into a friendship and an endlessly creative collaboration. Riffing off the American physician Victoria Sweet, I think of it as a 'glasses on and glasses off' marriage of pre-modern and modern medicine … the mythic and the scientific. It seems just yesterday the precision and care you took in sharing with me my histology, this last time we found out that the breast cancer had returned. It was the height of the COVID-19 pandemic and I was in the Auckland managed isolation hotel and so we were on Zoom. The early morning call that followed a thoughtful preparatory text, the wall of unstoppable tears that came. The moment when you stopped, took your glasses off and *we just sat together for a few moments, in the overwhelm of it all. Then just before I had the surgery for my mastectomy, you sent me a message; 'the scar will be another tributary of the river that runs through us; an outer marking of an inner journey'. Since then, I have felt fine about the changed shape of my body and I have a beautiful scar.*

In this back and forth swing between being a collaborator and a friend, a doctor and a patient there has been lots of moving between spaces, hierarchies and ways of being between us and managing all the different expectations that go with that. A memorable example of this is that busy London day just before I left London, we met with Saul and Dani Klein (local philanthropists who have subsequently funded both of us to work beyond our usual day jobs). We then met with other GPs Asiya and Clair from the RCGP. At the end of it all you said that you would push your bike home with me and in the darkness we shifted gear and spoke about the cancer that was rising in me again. You gave me all and everything I needed and it was also helpful, thanks to your openness that I knew my story sat within many other even more intense stories you were dealing with in a 'go the extra mile' kind of way. That evening at the end of our walk, you were going to certify as dead one of your patients, a wife and a mother, that you had been supporting.

There are more stories that I can't do justice to in this letter. We carry the lines and characters forward, in Noon-like fashion reweaving words into new contexts; the dragon's tears and the dragon's breath, the great bog of a coat, the bell jar, Rilke and Brother John O'Donnohue, the wild red twin Tatterhood, the rivers that run through our lives, creating as you said on the call the other day, a safety net of meaning making. A net, now woven with strong rope that stretches across both hemispheres.

Now I am on this side of the planet navigating the rewilding of a wetland and the cancer journey again. Each time I come away from an appointment with one of my doctors, I feel gratitude to you for preparing me for those meetings. You have given me the language and the presence of mind for shared decision making. You have helped me find the questions and the strength in myself and you have also shown me how very human doctors are ... something it is all too easy to overlook. I have learnt that in that humanity it is possible to find points of connection and trust in which a space of mystery opens up that is beyond time and instrumentals and all the decisions that need to be made. It is the sacred space in which I think healing happens; I like to think not only for me but in some small way also for the clinician. I know I am one in a long line of people they are seeing that day, and I still wonder, where do the feelings of clinicians go?

So yes it is a tapestry of light and dark, of making meaning of life and death, and of finding new ways to be a patient, a friend and a collaborator that meeting you has brought about and I will always be deeply grateful for that.

In solidarity and love,

Jane xx

Reflections on social prescribing as community engagement

Exploring stories, experiences and meaning-making within social prescribing are crucial, or we risk over-medicalising its scope and expectations, by merely focusing on clinical outcomes. By exchanging letters between them, Jane and Jane have demonstrated how generalist approaches can be used to benefit and enhance the health and wellbeing of local communities. These are examples of how the participants and co-creators of social prescribing activities achieve integration through: relational care; having a (physical) community space to attend to relationships and wellbeing through regular activities; building knowledge of other networks and resources through participation; and shared storytelling, levelling power relations between clinicians and patients and appreciating how and when participation might be fruitful.

Some clinicians may feel reservations about their potential to engage in this work. Some have reported very little formal training in community engagement, health creation and social prescribing, and cite 'lack of evidence' (formal and informal) as being barriers to their engagement (17). As mentioned in Chapter 17, discussing patients' lifestyles and suggesting behavioural changes (for example, physical activity) have been found challenging for many clinicians for reasons such as feeling they lack the skills, knowledge or resources to offer support (18). Another recent study exploring the barriers and enablers to clinicians engaging in social prescribing for individuals with mental health problems, highlighted the need for formal support to enable clinicians to engage with social prescribing effectively (17). Support from colleagues, having access to appropriate resources, and the availability of on-site services and activities have been identified as facilitators for these important healthy lifestyle conversations with patients (18).

Of course these activities require energy, commitment and time, but they are not a replacement or competing demand for clinical care. Where valued and done well, they support a collaboration between patient, clinician and community, and complement disease management, prevention and proactive support of wellbeing. This of course requires resource (for example, investment in time, materials, or staff), but these do not have to be overwhelming or large, and work best when connected to and integrated with the regular rhythm, vulnerabilities and provision of clinical care. This might be a shared space enhancing visibility of those attending, or simply a shared awareness and appreciation of the value and existence of social prescribing activities enabling access and participation. Active involvement and learning about this might therefore take place in a range of ways and spaces, but can inform the routine and ordinary delivery of clinical care simply through curiosity (and even compassion) about the human nature of *self* and *other* in any or every interaction as a clinician and citizen.

Conclusion

This chapter explores how clinicians can support their local community (individuals as well as the community as a whole) in understanding and managing their health and wellbeing. Positioning this chapter from the view of relationships and the interpersonal factors involved in social prescribing highlights the importance of 'lived experience', distributed expertise and connections, and the contextual, situated nature of social prescribing as a practice embedded within a community. The experiences of Jane (GP), and Jane (patient), demonstrate how clinical hierarchies and priorities can be shifted. While there may be reservations for some, clinicians, patients and communities alike have embraced the relational aspects of supporting one another, and actively identified opportunities to reshape and transform local community offerings, be it green spaces in clinical practices, or community cafes, making use of otherwise ignored valuable local assets. This chapter highlights the fluid and intermittent nature of interactions between patients, clinicians and the wider community, and how these relationships can interlink and complement each other well. This 'fluidity' (in terms of time, people, spaces, and so on) is a central pillar (and potential paradox) of generalism.

Challenges for the generalist clinician include being inclusive in their engagement with patients who are underserved by local healthcare systems and who may otherwise struggle to access local services.

This chapter also highlights the challenge of participation and managing boundaries, and how we might address the tension between clinicians being authentic and 'human' versus role playing a clinician without engaging the 'self' (see Chapter 1). This could, fundamentally, be addressed through institutions taking care of staff as well as patients, and how efforts to support patient wellbeing while simultaneously supporting staff wellbeing, complement one another. Supporting spaces for interactions between individuals as people, maximises opportunities to value and exchange each other's expertise; and can empower clinicians, patients and public to collaborate across traditional hierarchies and barriers. We are experiencing health crises nationally and globally that challenge the stability of our futures (for example, COVID-19, the climate crisis), requiring a re-evaluation of our approach to healthcare delivery and design. Now is the time for healthcare systems and providers to work in partnership with healthcare users, particularly historically underserved groups, and share decisions not just with individual patients about their health, but with the wider community about engaging, cost-effective and impactful ways to support their wellbeing. This may be fundamental to promote the next phase in our society's process of recovery from a global pandemic, and looking towards achieving environmental sustainability.

References

1. Polley M, Fleming J, Anfilogoff T, Carpenter A. *Making Sense of Social Prescribing*. University of Westminster; 2017.
2. Drinkwater C, Wildman J, Moffatt S. Social prescribing. *BMJ*. 2019;364:l1285.
3. Buck D, Ewbank L. What is social prescribing? The King's Fund; 2020. Available from: www.kingsfund.org.uk/publications/social-prescribing (accessed 11 December 2023).
4. Fancourt D, Aughterson H, Finn S, Walker E, Steptoe A. How leisure activities affect health: a narrative review and multi-level theoretical framework of mechanisms of action. *Lancet Psychiatry*. 2021;8(4):329–39.
5. Bertotti M, Frostick C, Hutt P, Sohanpal R, Carnes D. A realist evaluation of social prescribing: an exploration into the context and mechanisms underpinning a pathway linking primary care with the voluntary sector. *Prim Health Care Res Dev*. 2018;19(03):232–45.
6. Elston J, Gradinger F, Asthana S, Lilley-Woolnough C, Wroe S, Harman H, et al. Does a social prescribing 'holistic' link-worker for older people with complex, multimorbidity improve wellbeing and frailty and reduce health and social care use and costs? A 12-month before-and-after evaluation. *Prim Health Care Res Dev*. 2019;20:e135.
7. Kellezi B, Wakefield JRH, Stevenson C, McNamara N, Mair E, Bowe M, et al. The social cure of social prescribing: a mixed-methods study on the benefits of social connectedness on quality and effectiveness of care provision. *BMJ Open*. 2019;9(11):e033137.
8. Carnes D, Sohanpal R, Frostick C, Hull S, Mathur R, Netuveli G, et al. The impact of a social prescribing service on patients in primary care: a mixed methods evaluation. *BMC Health Serv Res*. 2017;17(1):835.
9. Aughterson H. Social prescribing for mental health and well-being: mechanisms of action, active ingredients, and barriers and enablers to effective engagement. Doctoral thesis.

UCL; 2022. Available from: https://discovery.ucl.ac.uk/id/eprint/10154892/ (accessed 19 May 2023).

10. Shiell A, Hawe P, Gold L. Complex interventions or complex systems? Implications for health economic evaluation. *BMJ*. 2008;336(7656):1281–3.

11. Husk K, Blockley K, Lovell R, Bethel A, Lang I, Byng R, et al. What approaches to social prescribing work, for whom, and in what circumstances? A realist review. *Health Soc Care Community*. 2020;28(2):309–24.

12. Smith JN, Hopkins R, Pencheon D. Could the Transition movement help solve the NHS's problems? *J Public Health*. 2017;39(4):841–5.

13. Myat J, Hopkins R, Dixon M. Can GP practices become hubs for transition? *J Holist Healthc*. 2020;17(3):4–8.

14. Kingsnorth P. The Migration of the Holy. The Abbey of Misrule. 2022. Available from: https://paulkingsnorth.substack.com/p/the-migration-of-the-holy (accessed 26 June 2023).

15. Global Generation. Global Generation: growing food, people and community for a just world. Available from: www.globalgeneration.org.uk (accessed 11 December 2023).

16. SoundCloud. Global Generation. 2020. Available from: https://soundcloud.com/user-672467656 (accessed 11 December 2023).

17. Aughterson H, Baxter L, Fancourt D. Social prescribing for individuals with mental health problems: a qualitative study of barriers and enablers experienced by general practitioners. *BMC Fam Pract*. 2020 Sep 21;21(1):194.

18. Keyworth C, Epton T, Goldthorpe J, Calam R, Armitage CJ. Delivering opportunistic behavior change interventions: a systematic review of systematic reviews. *Prev Sci*. 2020;21(3):319–31.

12
Making clinical practice and education socially accountable

Sadie Lawes-Wickwar and Jane Hopkins

Introduction

'Social accountability' is the bedrock of clinical practice and the guiding principle which informs clinical care, funding and healthcare organisation. This social contract underpins a relationship with the public. Person-centred care is one central element of socially accountable clinical practice. A central tenet of generalism is a participatory and collaborative approach to clinical practice, learning and research: learning with and from patients and communities. In this chapter we draw on examples from the UK National Health Service (NHS) and particularly policy and practice across England, to showcase examples of social accountability across clinical and educational practice. The NHS England Long Term Plan (1) details a move away from traditional paternalistic models of healthcare delivery towards a more equal and mutually respectful partnership between clinicians and patients. Person-centred care recognises that the majority of healthcare users desire meaningful participation and to be well-informed to make decisions about their health (2). Clinical practitioners are not only expected to deliver diagnostic and therapeutic services but practise, ideally in partnership with patients, in a way that is 'socially accountable'. This means delivering quality healthcare that is equally accessible to all and responsive to the needs of the individual patient and the wider population. In our chapter, we are referring to 'social accountability' in its widest sense as 'citizens' efforts at ongoing meaningful collective engagement with public institutions for accountability in the provision of public goods' (3).

Theoretically, patients should be at the heart of decisions about how healthcare services are designed and delivered '"what matters to someone" is not just "what's the matter with someone"' (NHS Long Term Plan, p.24 (1)). Patients can contribute to clinical practice and generalist education, provided there is genuine buy-in from clinicians and educators. UK organisations, such as National Voices and The Patients Association, have long lobbied for change and a move towards services 'with' and 'by' patients rather than 'to' or 'for' and 'No decision about me, without me' (4). NHS England's 2014 Five-Year Forward View recommended the transfer of greater power to patients and the public in recognition of the added value they bring: 'One of the great strengths of this country is that we have an NHS that – at its best – is 'of the people, by the people and for the people … we need to engage with communities and citizens in new ways, involving them directly in decisions about the future of health and care services' (Next Steps on The NHS Five Year Forward View, p.32 (5)). Despite these recommendations, many agencies must accept that the 'old ways' of doing things are no longer valid, and that patients and the public need to be empowered to contribute to service design and delivery.

Buchman and colleagues argue that social accountability is defined by health and social justice (6). In this chapter, we use the context of family practice as an example of generalist clinical practice, to illustrate the value patients and the public can bring. Family practitioners (GPs) in the UK provide over 300 million medical consultations per year (5) and are often the only 'gateway' to some services such as an initial assessment with dementia services, referral to a Falls Team, or referral to a hospital-based specialist. The work of the family practitioner includes many elements of generalism, contrasting with some other clinical specialists who more narrowly focus on a particular disease pattern or technical skills. Family practitioners have a unique position within the heart of the community. They are viewed as key players in terms of health-related issues, often with an expectation on them to assume a pivotal leadership and informed advocacy role, speaking out on behalf of marginalised communities that historically register poorer access to and uptake of existing services, poorer health outcomes and premature mortality rates.

To achieve a shared understanding of terminology and key issues, we have adopted the term 'patient' throughout this chapter with the caveat that it carries different meanings and reactions to its use. As discussed in Chapter 3, the term 'patient' may be viewed by some as a disempowering word, promoting an image of passive recipients rather than active members within a health partnership. While 'patient' may be a familiar term to healthcare professionals and, on the whole, acceptable to individuals, it will depend on the context. For example, 'client' is more commonly used in social care services and 'patient' was preferred only to the use of 'victim' in the context of cancer survivorship (7). As we move in the UK towards a more integrated health and social care system, use of more inclusive words such as 'citizen' or 'service user' are becoming more accepted. Elsewhere, in countries such as the USA, healthcare users may consider themselves as 'consumers' where healthcare is not free at the point of use.

Social accountability may be partly achieved through the various activities of the patient liaison volunteers, for example a 'Patient Participation Group' (PPG) in the UK. In the context of medical education, social accountability has been defined by the World Health Organization (WHO) as *'the obligation [of medical schools] to direct their education, research and service activities towards addressing the priority health concerns of the community, region and/or nation they have a mandate to serve'* (8). In practice, this might look like inviting patients to share their 'lived experiences' with clinical students, or by co-producing clinical curricula with patients as equal partners in students' learning (9).

The public contributes valuable knowledge, skills and unique experiences to clinical practice and education. In training future practitioners and improving the delivery of services, healthcare should be open to new ideas and innovative approaches, incorporating patient perspectives in the design of services and teaching undergraduate and postgraduate learners. By ensuring that the clinical setting remains a constant 'learning environment', this will not only sustain and improve the clinical skills of practitioners and community of learners, but also contribute to the way the service or provider is viewed by the local community.

Social accountability in generalist healthcare services

To explore ideas about social accountability and generalist healthcare services, we use here the example of UK general practice. In the UK, the family practitioner is often the first point of contact for any clinical concern. They are not merely a gatekeeper to medical and social care services but also play a pivotal role in the life of the community they serve in terms of signposting, advice, support and guidance. This means the statutory, professional and legal duties of family practitioners are wide-ranging and in the UK this includes key areas such as safeguarding vulnerable adults and children, mental health assessments and registering domestic violence. The Public Sector Equality Duty (PSED) under the

Equality Act 2010 holds practices accountable for prioritising services for those patients with protected characteristics. In some regions, such as isolated rural areas or urban areas with high levels of social deprivation, the local GP practice may be only one of a few community assets and as such, a key player in building and maintaining resilient and sustainable communities.

The social accountability of any general practice is judged on the quality of its relationship with the local community. Traditionally, the UK-based GP was more likely to live locally to their general practice, or cottage hospital in rural areas, and were aware of their patients' personal circumstances and the social constraints they encountered on a daily basis. The working practices of today tend to be of a different order. Changes to the NHS and the centralisation of some hospital services have separated the GP from local hospital settings (10). Many GPs now live outside the community where they practise or might not be present in the same practice each weekday due to working patterns (e.g. working longer days or working across sites), family or teaching commitments (11), research interests, or job-related burnout (12). Consequently, they may lack granular knowledge of the community they operate within and there may be fewer opportunities to build trusting and confiding relationships with patients. Learning about the daily social pressures that might negatively impact on their patients' health and wellbeing may become overlooked. It is important, therefore, that explicit attention is given to consider ways to enable social accountability. Patient representatives, who often enjoy established links with trusted community leaders and networks, can help bridge that gap in knowledge and open up vital communication channels between the GP practice and community. This may be necessary if we are to address the inequalities and uptake of health provision amongst underserved communities (13).

Patients can suggest improvements in, and the streamlining of, service delivery through more constructive channels rather than through a complaints procedure. The Patient Participation Group (PPG) in the UK is one formal channel which consists of volunteer patients and their caregivers, an allocated GP and other practice staff, who meet on a quarterly basis (14). The lived experience of coping with chronic illness as a patient or caregiver can provide authentic feedback on what treatments or services are working well, where the gaps are, and how quality of life could be improved. However, the engagement must be meaningful to all participants for the partnership to work effectively. It is vital that protected time is built in for staff to dedicate to the task. Ideally, participants would reflect the diversity of local patient populations with respect to age, ethnicity and socioeconomic status so that the views of patients are varied and include diverse perspectives. Patients can provide a fresh perspective and alternative solutions to intractable problems, gained from their own lived experience and professional backgrounds, such as financial, legal, or information technology (IT). Provided with the right level of support and matched with a task that fits their capabilities and skill set, patient volunteers can undertake a variety of practical roles and deliver the extra layer of informal services that a practice would offer in an ideal world given sufficient time and resources.

In the research field, patient and public contributors are commonly involved in translating scientific materials and summaries into user-friendly and accessible language. At a clinical delivery level, patient volunteers can undertake a similar role reviewing the accessibility of printed documents for distribution and the navigability of the website. Different platforms for circulating information will suit different cohorts and it is important to remember that 'one size does not fit all'. According to the National Literacy Trust, 16.4 per cent of adults in England have poor literacy skills (15), a figure that might impact on the ability of certain patient groups to read and absorb health communications and campaigns delivered by the practice. This may be of particular importance to communities for whom English may not be their first spoken or written language. Involving patients in the design and delivery of key information in culturally appropriate and age-friendly language might ultimately help raise their overall level of health literacy and empower them to make more informed choices (16).

Patient volunteers could support or host events as extra capacity where this would otherwise be a challenge for a busy staff team. For example, patients can partner practice staff to co-produce health promotion events and presentations at the surgery itself or within other local community hubs. Patient leaders may possess well-established links and an in-depth knowledge of formal and informal grassroots resources to promote engagement among historically underserved communities. Close collaboration with respected local community leaders may help build trust and dispel suspicion within patient groups who have traditionally seen doctors, with their considerable legislative powers, as representatives of the 'authorities'. By close collaboration with community leaders, who can effectively target health messages, the uptake of preventive treatments such as immunisation amongst vaccine-hesitant groups could be vastly improved (17,18). Other initiatives that improve patient experience could be achieved through innovative use of the space the clinic inhabits, such as improving a garden area for the community to enjoy (see Example 12.1 and Chapter 11).

Patients can provide invaluable and unvarnished user-feedback as 'critical friends' within patient and staff liaison groups that might, for example, explore the impact of proposed changes in practice procedures or new initiatives coming on stream. A healthy exchange of views can potentially prevent the implementation of ideas or plans that may prove undeliverable, to avoid wastage of scarce and expensive resources, such as unnecessary clinic appointments, missed appointments or failure to adhere to treatment. Patients may also partner physicians, practice nurses or occupational or physiotherapists to host support groups, or to facilitate walking or weight management groups that tackle common chronic health conditions such as hypertension, type 2 diabetes and obesity (See Chapter 17 and Chapter 13).

Example 12.1: Melbourne Grove Practice (a community hub)

Dr Love envisaged Melbourne Grove Practice as part of a community hub which patients could rely on to meet not just their medical issues but to some extent their social needs thereby improving their overall general health and wellbeing. The initiative was launched in January 2016 by 'Potted History', a charitable offshoot of the Wildlife Trust (33). It consisted of the loan of an experienced organiser to set up and run an arts and crafts cum gardening initiative for a group of over-65s patients over eight weekly sessions. Its primary aim was to design and revitalise a somewhat overgrown patch of wasteland bordering the practice and transform it into a beautiful tranquil space for patients to sit and enjoy. However, the underlying purpose of the group was to offer socially isolated older people living with mild clinical depression and anxiety the opportunity to engage in a productive activity along with others in a similar situation.

Dr Love selected suitable recruits during his surgery sessions who he felt might benefit from the activity and referred them to the group's waiting list. Most had either always lived alone, lost a partner or had close family who had since moved far away. They were all now in retirement and many missed the structure and comradeship that work had previously supplied.

As the sessions progressed, mutual trust grew and they all seemed to relish the chance to forge new relationships and friendship networks. When the 'Potted Histories' eight-week involvement drew to a close, the by-now flourishing group carried on meeting with the support of a volunteer 'Patient Ambassador'. The group membership remained relatively stable, consisting of six to eight people all drawn from the diverse local community of East Dulwich. Its profile reflected the practice patient base in terms of faith, gender, class and ethnicity. Their new friendships bridged traditional barriers of class and ethnicity nurtured over their communal lunches comprising dishes brought in by individual members, shared histories and memories, and the exchange of plants and seeds.

Lack of time and staff resources are often cited as an excuse for not actively promoting patient engagement but this group required minimal funding or staff input other than the weekly use of one of the larger consultation rooms and access to the practice's phone, an allocated pigeon hole, free postage and use of their printer.

As the group's confidence grew and the garden delivered to everyone's satisfaction, they branched out into new activities both based within the practice itself but also further afield within their local community, including setting up a local telephone support network, trips to local venues, developing links to other local surgeries including educational and governance activities, and charity and volunteering work.

The clinical outcomes of this self-directed user group of older people were positive with a noticeable improvement in mood for most, increasing levels of both social- and self-confidence, a trusted network of peer support and a greater sense of wellbeing in general.

Social accountability in clinical education

Social accountability is key to the training of the future clinical workforce. This commitment extends far beyond predictive calculations of workforce number requirements. Medical schools, for example, globally are socially accountable to healthcare patients and their caregivers. In the UK, involving patients and carers in medical training is a requirement of the General Medical Council (GMC) (19). The GMC recognises the valuable role patients can play in clinical learning and advises medical schools to ensure learners are exposed to real-life situations where patients are diverse, autonomous and unscripted (19). This is a move away from the early days of patient involvement which reflected the traditional biomedical approach where patients were the subject of clinical observation to illustrate a condition of interest (9). The possibilities, however, reach far beyond passive patient involvement. In the context of generalism, this means asking patients not to simply represent disease-based knowledge, but to share in a broader sense their knowledge of disease and illness, and the impact of these issues and treatments on their lives (see Chapter 3).

There are numerous frameworks describing the ways educators can work in partnership with patients and the public as active participants in clinical education. Helpfully, Towle and colleagues developed a taxonomy (adapted at Table 12.1) encompassing these various frameworks. This describes not only the type of involvement but also the degree involvement may be active and autonomous (9). 'Higher' levels of involvement include patients teaching students, contributing to medical school interviews, assessing students and providing them with feedback, co-designing curricula and assessments for clinical courses, quality assurance, and, at the highest level, involvement in institutional decision-making.

Recent research has identified the types and levels of involvement typically employed in clinical education settings. Patients shared their experiences with learners (that is, Level 3 in Towle's taxonomy) more often than being 'teachers' (in a traditional sense with presentation slides, and so on) or assessors (Level 4) (9,20). In very few instances the institution is committed to patient involvement at the highest level. For example, the systematic review mentioned above found only two studies reporting patients as education partners involved in curriculum development – that is, Level 5 (20). This suggests that the highest levels of strategic involvement are not frequently implemented by medical schools, or at least not reported in the empirical literature, although there are good examples from across the UK. For example, a 'Primary Care Experts by Experience Group' at UCL oversees the institutional strategy for enhancing the role of patient and public involvement (PPI) in medical education (see Educational example: 'Experts by Experience Group at UCL'). Also, the Doubleday Centre for Patient Experience at the Manchester Medical School coordinates a collaboration of academics and patient leads at medical schools across the UK known as the Doubleday Medical Schools Patient Partnership Collaborative.

Table 12.1 Taxonomy of patient and public involvement in clinical education. Adapted from Towle et al. 2010

Degree of active patient involvement in the learning encounter	Duration of contact with learner	Opportunities for patient agency during the encounter	Education for the patient	Patient involvement in planning the encounter and curriculum	Institutional commitment to patient involvement in education
1. Patient case/ scenario	None	N/A	N/A	None	Low
2. Patient in a clinical setting	Encounter-based	None	None	None	Low
3. Patient shares his or her experience	Encounter-based	None- Low	Brief, simple	None	Low
4. Patients are involved in teaching/ evaluating students	Variable	Moderate	Structured, intensive	Low-moderate	Low-moderate
5. Patients as equal partners in learner education, evaluation & curriculum development	Moderate-extensive	High	Extensive	Moderate-extensive	Moderate
6. Patients involved at the institutional level in addition to patient-teacher(s) in education, evaluation and curriculum development	Extensive	High	Extensive	High	High

Educational example: Experts by Experience Group at UCL

The Primary Care Medical Education team in the Research Department for Primary Care and Population Health (PCPH) at UCL hosts an Experts by Experience (EbE) group focused on primary care and community teaching. This group inputs into the primary care teaching strategy, reviews teaching content and processes, and supports some teaching sessions for example through sharing their experiences or assessing students. The group discusses how future learning can be shaped by patient and public priorities and identifies a range of opportunities for educational research to support this.

COVID-19 posed challenges for medical schools globally. In April 2020 there was an urgent need to redesign modules for teaching to take place remotely. For UCL's MBBS degree this meant moving community and primary care placements in Year 1 and 2 online (via video conferencing software, such as Zoom), while maintaining patient and carer input and involvement. The Primary Care EbE Group reviewed our plans for virtual teaching sessions where patients and carers were planned to be involved. In practice, this included the group contributing content for, and reviewing invitations sent to patients for involvement in remote teaching sessions and how patients might want to connect to sessions. We updated our guidance for placement providers and students based on advice from EbE contributors. There was also a suggestion to offer training in the relevant technology (such as Zoom) to address some of the accessibility needs of people from diverse backgrounds (for example, those less familiar with technology). This consultative process ensured the continued involvement of patients and carers in sharing their experiences with medical students in this era of remote learning.

The positive impact of patient involvement on learners has been well documented. Listening to patients sharing their 'lived experiences' can increase empathy, improve communication and learners' appreciation of person-centred care (20). Patients and caregivers themselves report increased personal satisfaction and a sense of reward in contributing to the education of future clinicians (9,21–23). There is limited evidence available, however, of the benefits of PPI at higher levels, and the impact of learning from patients on later practice or patient outcomes: an important direction for future research.

Enabling a shared understanding of terminology and practice in relation to PPI in clinical education is crucial to enable meaningful involvement and engagement among local communities. For example, 'simulated' or 'virtual' are arguably ambiguous terms that can have different meanings depending on the context. They may be used to describe educational activities where actors or others follow scripts to depict patient clinical issues; clinical computer systems; or, in the era of remote learning, situations where patients join the teaching sessions online (for example, over video conferencing) (24,25). However, the use of the term 'patient' attached to these phrases could be potentially misleading, particularly where nobody with lived experience of the condition(s) portrayed is involved in developing the teaching session. These terms are often poorly described in the literature, meaning studies can lack quality and in-depth findings. The lack of consensus over terms to describe PPI in clinical education can also serve as a barrier to driving forward the field of clinical education research (25).

When involving the public in clinical education, it is important to consider the participants' preferences and information needs. Fortunately, there is a growing body of research reporting patient perspectives in respect to their involvement in clinical learning. These highlight the importance of ensuring consent is informed and repeatedly checked throughout the encounter and to establish confidentiality and privacy agreements (22,26,27). For online teaching activities involving patients and carers the approaches are less clear, students can join remote clinical consultations, or experts by experience participate in a virtual institutional meeting. It is only by identifying a patient's needs beforehand, that we can establish whether technology serves as a barrier to their involvement during this era of digital learning and area worthy of further exploration to ensure clinical education remains socially accountable to the people it aims to serve.

Resources required for socially accountable practice

Some level of pump-priming resourcing, albeit minimal, may be necessary on the road towards demonstrating social accountability within clinical practice and education. Within an institution such as a medical school setting, the need for protected staff time should be recognised and set aside to coordinate Patient and Public Involvement (PPI) activities. In a clinical setting, the chair or coordinator of a patient liaison group should be granted reasonable access to administrative facilities such as a dedicated email address, use of a telephone and, if available, of space(s) to hold public meetings or group activities. A dedicated PPI space in a clinic newsletter or on its website could advertise forthcoming meetings of interest, complete feedback surveys, post PPG meeting minutes and opportunities to participate in research studies or even a teaching or specialist help role. For example, it is recommended in the UK that GP practices hosting medical students highlight how and at what stage patients may be approached for involvement in clinical learning (27).

Funding for PPI contributors undertaking an active role within a clinical setting or teaching clinical learners is important to consider. In the UK, the cost of patient liaison groups was historically built into a GP's contract but is now incorporated into their contractual obligations (28) although not necessarily ring fenced for that very purpose. Public contributors undertake a variety of roles within clinical research, teaching and across the NHS in general with each task requiring a different skill set, depth of expertise and level of experience. The complexity of the task tends to be 'rewarded' on a sliding scale in line with guidance published by various bodies. In the case of research, PPI is now a condition of research funding by the National Institute of Health Research (NIHR): *'Payment guidance for researchers and professionals'* (v.3, 31.8.22) identifies five different levels of financial recognition, cover for caregivers, travel and subsistence expenses. *'Working with our Patient and Public Voice (PPV) Partners – Reimbursing expenses and paying involvement payments'* (v.2) suggests NHS recommended rates for PPI activity within secondary care settings, but the representatives' time and effort is at the time of writing not universally recognised within the primary care sector.

Rewarding patient input with money or shop vouchers may also encourage a greater degree of involvement on the part of those on low incomes or benefits, but pecuniary motives are not always the primary driver. Cash payments may be declined because they interfere with benefit entitlement or tax thresholds. Many may volunteer for purely altruistic and philanthropic reasons, for example to 'give something back' to the NHS. Others, particularly the over-65s, have discovered the tangible physical and mental health benefits of volunteering and the sense of self-worth and validation engendered (29). It is worth bearing in mind that while there are national standard rates for involvement in research in the UK, guidance for other types of involvement (for example, teaching) and at a primary care level is largely absent.

To achieve the desired level of social responsibilities, healthcare leaders and service users alike need to commit themselves to a shared set of values and principles (see Table 12.2).

Table 12.2 Facilitators of PPI in clinical service and education co-design

No	Facilitators of PPI and Co-design in Generalism
1	The entire organisation (e.g. GP practice, university) is committed to a partnership of equals with mutual respect, trust and appreciation of the value each stakeholder, including patients and caregivers, brings to the delivery of healthcare services and education.
2	Willingness to undertake meaningful co-design and co-production between clinicians, educators, learners and patients.
3	The organisation views patients not as passive recipients of healthcare provision but active agents in the management of their own health and wellbeing given appropriate help and information.
4	The generalist clinical organisation (e.g. GP practice) is an agent for change and one of the key actors in building resilience within the local community it serves.
5	The whole healthcare community, including staff, patients, caregivers and clinical learners, work towards becoming a constantly evolving learning environment that draws on each other's skills, knowledge and expertise.
6	Willingness of the clinical community and educational institutions to actively listen and be open to new ideas and change.
7	Acknowledgement that ownership of the clinical and educational institutions is shared not just between the clinicians, federations and workforce but also by patients and the public who invest in the service as taxpayers and consumers of its end product.
8	A shared vision of health and its delivery, agreed by all stakeholders of clinical practice.
9	Recognition that patients bring a valuable hinterland of expertise, knowledge, useful skill sets, lived experience of ill health or disability and are welcomed as 'assets' and listened to in the spirit of 'critical friends'.
10	All stakeholders are united in their determination to tackle healthcare inequalities within their locality.

Challenges to active patient and public engagement

Listed below are a few common barriers that prove a hindrance to the full participation of underserved groups and interfere with achieving social accountability (Table 12.3).

Table 12.3 Barriers to PPI in co-designing clinical practice and education

No.	Barriers to PPI and Co-design in Generalism
1	Available funding streams to reward and reimburse PPI contributors for their time and incurred expenses.
2	The availability of key staff to coordinate PPI activities or provide resources to support PPI leads to host activities within the practice or institution.
3	Access to and confident skills in using appropriate technology to take part in remote meetings and to be able to communicate, interact and access information online.
4	Lack of guidance to support the delivery of PPI activities.
5	Use of terminology that effectively excludes PPI contributors and the wider public such as shorthand technical terms, language and acronyms.

Where's the guidance for involving patients in clinical services and education?

Rules can constrain meaningful involvement. Guidance, however, can highlight the rights and imperatives to support PPI participation, inviting conversations for change and reifying its importance, while enabling local adaptability to meet local needs. Guidance about PPI activity in the research field is widely available. There are fewer texts describing the range of ways in which patients and caregivers might be integrated into generalist practice and education. Much of this guidance derives from statutory bodies such as Healthwatch and the Care Quality Commission (CQC) working on behalf of the public to scrutinise and monitor community and secondary health provision. However, this does not necessarily relate to public and patient activity in health and education, and monitoring and scrutiny do not in themselves support meaningful change. Inclusive, adaptive and creative approaches are therefore required to support future expansion of PPI in clinical education spaces.

Diverse representation

In the UK, family practice sits firmly within the context of the local community it serves, be that predominantly an affluent suburb, a remote rural area or an area with high levels of social deprivation. Family practice priorities and working practices are shaped to respond to the particular health needs of that community. The recruitment of a patient liaison group whose membership closely mirrors the profile of the local population in the task of guiding the organisation, must be a key priority. In the UK, patient volunteers tend to be invariably white, from higher social classes and older (28), this over-representation possibly the result of free time, resources and the social confidence to devote to the task. If patient volunteers are to truly represent the 'voice' of the wider patient base, then closer attention needs to be paid when recruiting individuals. A range of characteristics needs to be included, namely age, race, gender, faith, disability, lower educational attainment, worklessness, deprivation, or lack of fluency in spoken or written English, in order to capture differing points of views and avoid any creeping bias or misrepresentation. Exposure to the wider social determinants of health and social care within a diverse community is essential for learners on placement to help develop their communication and personal skills as future clinical practitioners. But how can representatives of historically underserved groups be supported to take advantage of opportunities to participate in the co-design of services and education of future generalist clinicians? It is crucial in order to be socially accountable, that clinical practitioners need to actively listen to and take into account the views and feedback of 'under-represented' communities from trusted patient advocates. Only then can accessible and welcoming services be best targeted and delivered in user-friendly and culturally appropriate language. One solution to secure higher levels of engagement might be hosting mobile workshops at community hubs (30), alternating the times and days of the week of patient participation group (PPG) meetings to better suit the employed or those with childcare or caregiver responsibilities, or else holding virtual meetings online.

Resources

Limited staff, funding and resources are invariably cited as reasons for failing to actively promote or embed patient engagement, although this need not be the case. The sole exception might be a PPG quarterly meeting attended by the representative clinical practitioner, manager and patients. It acts as the 'official' forum where views can be exchanged and collaborative thinking and planning can take place. The physical space afforded by the clinic in respect to its flexible use, floor size and facilities will also dictate the degree to which it can support the growth of its programme of patient engagement. As mentioned earlier, if available, the innovative repurposing of a clinic's underused spaces, such as its boundary curtilage, can provide opportunities for local community groups.

The investment of just a small amount of initial time and resources could arguably pay dividends over the long term in meeting social accountability commitments.

Digital inclusion

We are living in an era of rapidly increasing digital and technology-based healthcare delivery. Remote technology has the potential to enhance PPI in clinical practice and teaching, but we know from research assessing remote primary care in the UK that online meetings and consultations may prove a barrier for certain groups. In the UK, remote consultations with a GP are predominantly accessed by younger working adults (31) while older patients prefer telephone or face-to-face consultations. However, it is important to keep in mind that 'one size does not fit all' (32). Social media may be suitable to reach younger patients and some may prefer meeting remotely if given the choice, while others may always choose a face-to-face encounter. Consequently, the particular preference of an individual wishing to be involved needs to first be established and alternative choices offered. This also applies to preferences about the effective dissemination of important information in a 'hard copy' format for those not online or unable to access websites, online newsletters or use a smartphone.

Conclusion

The values and qualities that patients' and caregivers' lived experiences and expertise can bring to healthcare service design and education is invaluable. Social accountability is about social justice (6), empowering patients, caregivers and the public to engage in the accessibility of services and the education of the future clinical workforce. In spite of the paucity of central guidance and evaluation, there are excellent examples of local and national initiatives across the UK, like those described in this chapter. To ensure clinical practice and education are socially accountable there may be structural, technological and organisational challenges to overcome. Ensuring patient groups are reflective of the wider patient population must be a priority, offering a voice to seldom-heard, historically poor and often overlooked communities, which might be more difficult in an era of digital healthcare for certain cohorts functionally excluded by lack of access to technical equipment or digital skills. Available resources are also crucial to the long-term success of patient liaison groups, as is the commitment of healthcare and academic staff. Identifying potential barriers and taking practical steps to overcome them could increase the level and depth of involvement and partnership. This will ensure the best experience for all stakeholders concerned with raising the quality of healthcare and education provision and to maximise inclusion of those groups whose health outcomes need to be addressed.

References

1. National Health Service. The NHS Long Term Plan. NHS England; 2019.
2. Chewning B, Bylund CL, Shah B, Arora NK, Gueguen JA, Makoul G. Patient preferences for shared decisions: a systematic review. *Patient Education and Counseling*. 2012;86(1):9–18.
3. Joshi A. Legal empowerment and social accountability: complementary strategies toward rights-based development in health? *World Development*. 2017;99:160–72.
4. Coulter A, Collins A. *Making Shared Decision-Making a Reality*. The King's Fund; 2011.
5. NHS England. Next steps on the NHS Five Year Forward View. National Health Service; 2017.
6. Buchman S, Woollard R, Meili R, Goel R. Practising social accountability: from theory to action. *Canadian Family Physician*. 2016;62(1):15–8.
7. Costa DSJ, Mercieca-Bebber R, Tesson S, Seidler Z, Lopez A-L. Patient, client, consumer, survivor or other alternatives? A scoping review of preferred terms for labelling individuals who access healthcare across settings. *BMJ Open*. 2019;9(3):e025166.
8. Boelen C, Heck JE. Defining and measuring the social accountability of medical schools. World Health Organization; 1995.
9. Towle A, Bainbridge L, Godolphin W, Katz A, Kline C, Lown B, et al. Active patient involvement in the education of health professionals. *Medical Education*. 2010;44(1):64–74.
10. Seamark D, Davidson D, Ellis-Paine A, Glasby J, Tucker H. Factors affecting the changing role of GP clinicians in community hospitals. *Br J Gen Pract*. 2019;69(682):e329–35.
11. Salisbury H. Oh, those lazy, part time GPs! *BMJ*. 2019;367.
12. Iacobucci G. Burnout is harming GPs' health and patient care, doctors warn. *BMJ*. 2021;374:n1823.
13. Gkiouleka A, Wong G, Sowden S, Bambra C, Siersbaek R, Manji S, et al. Reducing health inequalities through general practice. *The Lancet Public Health*. 2023;8(6):e463–e72.
14. Healthwatch Sunderland. Patient Participation Groups: A Best Practice Guide. Healthwatch Sunderland; 2017.
15. National Literacy Trust. Adult literacy. 2017. Available from: https://literacytrust.org.uk/parents-and-families/adult-literacy/ (accessed 19 March 2024).
16. NHS England. Accessible Information: Specification v.1.1. 2017. Available from: www.england.nhs.uk/wp-content/uploads/2017/08/accessilbe-info-specification-v1-1.pdf (accessed 19 March 2024).
17. Lawes-Wickwar S, Ghio D, Tang MY, Keyworth C, Stanescu S, Westbrook J, et al. A rapid systematic review of public responses to health messages encouraging vaccination against infectious diseases in a pandemic or epidemic. *Vaccines*. 2021;9(2):72.
18. Kamal A, Hodson A, Pearce JM. A rapid systematic review of factors influencing COVID-19 vaccination uptake in minority ethnic groups in the UK. *Vaccines*. 2021;9(10):1121.
19. General Medical Council. Patient and public involvement in undergraduate medical education. 2011. Available from: www.gmc-uk.org/-/media/documents/Patient_and_public_involvement_in_undergraduate_medical_education___guidance_0815.pdf_56438926.pdf (accessed 19 March 2024).
20. Gordon M, Gupta S, Thornton D, Reid M, Mallen E, Melling A. Patient/service user involvement in medical education: a best evidence medical education (BEME) systematic review: BEME Guide No. 58. *Medical Teacher*. 2020;42(1):4–16.
21. Dijk SW, Duijzer EJ, Wienold M. Role of active patient involvement in undergraduate medical education: a systematic review. *BMJ Open*. 2020;10(7):e037217.

22. Alao A, Burford B, Alberti H, Barton R, Moloney S, Vance G. Real-time patients' perspectives about participating in teaching consultations in primary care: a questionnaire study. *Medical Teacher*. 2021:1–21.
23. Stacy R, Spencer J. Patients as teachers: a qualitative study of patients' views on their role in a community-based undergraduate project. *Medical Education*. 1999;33(9):688–94.
24. Kononowicz AA, Zary N, Edelbring S, Corral J, Hege I. Virtual patients – what are we talking about? A framework to classify the meanings of the term in healthcare education. *BMC Medical Education*. 2015;15(1):1–7.
25. Lawes-Wickwar S, Lovat E, Alao A, Hamer-Hunt J, Yurtoglu N, Jensen C, et al. Technology-delivered undergraduate medical education involving patients and carers: a rapid systematic review. *medRxiv*. 2021.
26. Howe A, Anderson J. Involving patients in medical education. *BMJ*. 2003;327(7410):326–8.
27. Park SE, Allfrey C, Jones MM, Chana J, Abbott C, Faircloth S, et al. Patient participation in general practice based undergraduate teaching: a focus group study of patient perspectives. *British Journal of General Practice*. 2017;67(657):e260–e6.
28. Gillam S, Newbould J. Patient participation groups in general practice: what are they for, where are they going? *BMJ*. 2016;352.
29. Mundle C, Naylor C, Buck D. Volunteering in Health and Care in England. The King's Fund; 2012.
30. Eccles A, Bryce C, Turk A, Atherton H. Patient and public involvement mobile workshops – convenient involvement for the un-usual suspects. *Research Involvement and Engagement*. 2018;4(1):1–7.
31. Mold F, Hendy J, Lai Y-L, de Lusignan S. Electronic consultation in primary care between providers and patients: systematic review. *JMIR Medical Informatics*. 2019;7(4):e13042.
32. Parker RF, Figures EL, Paddison CA, Matheson JI, Blane DN, Ford JA. Inequalities in general practice remote consultations: a systematic review. *BJGP Open*. 2021;5(3).
33. Wildlife Trust. Potted History at the Centre for Wildlife Gardening. 2016. Available from: www.youtube.com/watch?v=Ykns-T8Ytag (accessed 5 November 2023).

13
Sustainability, health and healthcare

Alice Clack, Frances Mortimer and Kay Leedham-Green

Introduction

> We do not inherit the Earth from our ancestors; we borrow it from
> our children.
>
> Origin unknown (1)

More sustainable approaches to health and healthcare are essential if we
are to continue to provide universal healthcare now and into the future.
What does it mean, however, to create a sustainable healthcare system?
And what does this have to do with generalism? Sustainability requires
envisioning the future and thus requires an honest and careful assessment
of the environmental, workforce, financial, technological and resource
challenges that the future will bring. The principles of generalism articulated in Chapter 1 invite us to explore these challenges from different
perspectives: to identify root causes, to draw on distributed expertise to
innovate and improve, to work collaboratively with colleagues and across
sectors, to involve patients and communities, and to take a strategic view
on what can be changed now with the most impact.

There are strong parallels between the generalist principles that
inform interactions between patients and clinicians and the ways
in which people connect with their local community and environment: working in partnership, offering curiosity and respect, exploring
how different people make meaning or understand particular events,
appreciating diversity and complexity, and negotiating adaptive ways
forward. These are all common and important strategies across clinical and global generalism. Shifting our expectations and habitual
tendencies to objectify people (for example, patients) and nature
(for example, the earth, animals, plants) towards a more subjective

exchange, opens spaces for dialogue about ways in which people and places might be more connected and exist together in mutually beneficial ways. There are wide-ranging social, economic and environmental challenges to the future of healthcare. This chapter focuses on environmental sustainability as a key element of clinical care; however, truly sustainable healthcare, and the principles articulated here, are, by definition, sustainable across all future challenges: workforce, economic and environmental.

In this book so far, we have outlined a generalist philosophy of clinical practice (Chapter 1) and described how generalism can support health (salutogenesis) as well as address illness, for example through Health Justice Partnerships (Chapter 10), social prescribing (Chapter 11), health coaching (Chapter 17), or personalised care (Chapter 18). In this chapter, we discuss how interpersonal and systems-based clinical approaches can enhance planetary health, and indeed how planetary health enhances human health and wellbeing. Through a variety of clinical examples, we show how generalism, at its best, can be one of the most sustainable forms of healthcare and how, through acute sector examples, generalist approaches to complex problems can drive sustainable change more widely.

More broadly, however, we invite you to expand and apply our generalist philosophy to your engagement with the planetary circumstances around you. We are living through one of healthcare's greatest challenges: the degradation of the environment on which all health depends. Developing an understanding of how climate and ecological change impact health, and conversely, how healthcare impacts the environment, is like putting on a new pair of glasses that inextricably alters the way you see the world around you. Each new area of learning is likely to further alter this perspective, and inform the ways in which you integrate planetary health into your personal and professional life. We encourage you to engage with this journey, to access as many routes to change as possible, and to join the growing community of clinicians incorporating sustainability into their work.

Why is sustainable healthcare important?

Climate change is the greatest global health threat facing the world in the 21st Century, but it is also the greatest opportunity to redefine the social and environmental determinants of health.

The Lancet Countdown on Health and Climate Change (2)

The importance of addressing the social determinants of health has been ably articulated by Marmot and colleagues (3). Poverty, low literacy, poor housing and wage insecurity are all known to drive up the healthcare needs of populations and challenge the ongoing sustainability of the services that we provide. The social determinants of health, however, are overshadowed, and indeed compounded, by the projected negative impacts of the climate and ecological crises, which are set to define the future environment in which we provide healthcare and will impact every area of clinical practice (4).

Impacts are already understood to be manifold and include direct effects such as those resulting from air pollution, rising sea levels and extreme weather, and indirect effects such as those resulting from crop failure, population displacement and increased zoonotic infections (4,5). The Lancet Countdown on Health and Climate Change was launched in 2009, and its annual report tracks the impacts of the climate and ecological crisis on health and provides a sobering read (2). The world has already warmed by 1.2 degrees since pre-industrial levels, and the World Meteorological Organization gives a 66 per cent probability of passing 1.5 degrees by 2027 (6). This will destabilise the natural and human ecosystems on which health depends and put additional pressure on health systems worldwide (7).

What is arguably less well articulated is that healthcare itself is one of the key drivers of this crisis, contributing 5 per cent to global greenhouse gas emissions (8). This is equivalent to the footprint of a major country such as Russia or Japan. Thus, to achieve the carbon reduction necessary to limit global heating and avoid triggering irreversible tipping points, healthcare itself must engage in global mitigation efforts to reduce its environmental impact and avoid a vicious cycle. In addition to mitigation, The Intergovernmental Panel on Climate Change (IPCC) 2022 report, 'Impacts, Adaptation and Vulnerability', provides a thorough assessment of the currently observed, and likely future impacts of climate change, and makes it clear that widespread resilience and adaptation will also be required (4) (Figure 13.1).

In addition to its carbon footprint, the health sector has numerous other environmental impacts, which include chemical pollution (9), plastic pollution (10), and air pollution (8). Moreover, unethical supply chain practices, which include the use of child labour, modern slavery and unhealthy working conditions, contribute to a significant health and environmental burden (11). The damage caused is particularly sobering when we consider the dubious value of a significant proportion of this activity such as the suboptimal, single-use PPE distributed during the COVID-19 pandemic (12).

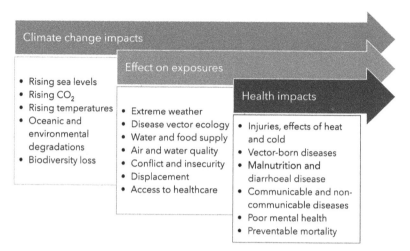

Figure 13.1 Climate change impacts on health. Data source: Centres for Disease Control (76)

Table 13.1 (derived from Tennison and colleagues (13)) gives a breakdown of NHS England's carbon emissions and the distribution of emissions according to service area. Other developed healthcare systems are likely to have similar distributions. This illustrates the resource intensity of acute care compared to other types of activity such as primary care, with the notable exception of primary care prescribing (which arguably averts acute care admissions). The majority of these emissions are indirect emissions as they are not released from within healthcare facilities but are embedded in the production of the materials and medicines consumed. It is therefore the type and quantity of healthcare that we provide that is driving up carbon emissions.

This environmental context creates a clear imperative to adapt our treatment-focused, resource-intensive models of care. The challenge is to develop more resilient and regenerative forms of clinical practice that are environmentally, economically and socially sustainable, while supporting patient and population health outcomes.

Conceptualising a sustainable healthcare system

Sustainable healthcare has been defined and conceptualised in various ways (14). The WHO suggests it is a 'health system that improves, maintains or restores health, while minimising negative impacts on the environment and leveraging opportunities to restore and improve it, to the benefit of the health and wellbeing of current and future generations' (13).

Table 13.1 NHS England greenhouse gas emissions by category, in kt CO_2e, 2019

	Ambulance	Community	Mental health	Acute	Primary care	Non-clinical support activities	Total
Delivery of care							
Building energy	21	150	164	1,900	250	31	2,520
Anaesthetic gases and metered dose inhalers	84	0	0	435	767	0	1,290
Water and waste	16	85	95	883	137	88	1,300
Business travel and fleet	200	100	120	410	60	110	1,000
Supply chain							
Pharmaceuticals and chemicals	5	120	66	2,095	2,750	26	5,060
Medical equipment	16	147	55	1,930	248	128	2,520
Non-medical equipment	38	156	170	1,040	420	137	1,960
Other procurement	100	384	465	2,850	610	1,620	6,030
Commissioned services	3	15	26	90	0	826	960
Personal travel	27	120	350	1,326	536	43	2,400
Total	510	1,280	1,510	12,960	5,780	3,009	25,050

To achieve maximum benefit within the resources available, healthcare needs to achieve what Porter calls 'healthcare value', which he suggests should be considered in relation to patient and population health outcomes, and not simply per unit of healthcare activity, as increased investment in some services can reduce the need for others (15). Mortimer reminds us that financial costs are not the only resources used; environmental and social resources (for example, staff time, community assets, patients and their families) are also relied upon (16). Together, these social, financial and environmental costs constitute the 'triple bottom line' (Figure 13.2 – derived from Mortimer and Elkington (17,18)). Lombardi and colleagues further argue that the social, environmental and financial resources of the triple bottom line have a hierarchy: a sustainable economy is dependent on a sustainable society which is dependent on a sustainable environment (19).

NHS Scotland was the world's first health service to set a strategy for net zero carbon emissions (20) followed by NHS England which has a stated aim of achieving net zero for direct emissions by 2040 and to include indirect procurement emissions by 2045 (21). It is now a requirement for every NHS organisation to develop and act on an individualised Green Plan to achieve these aims. There is an increasingly critical debate, however, that acknowledges a past failure to translate rhetoric on sustainable healthcare into action (22). Policies that have historically focused on financial sustainability alone have failed to acknowledge that social and environmental sustainability also need to be addressed as they drive up healthcare needs and contribute to workforce challenges (23). Financial cuts to health and social care have driven neither efficiency nor sustainability, and may in fact have increased demand (24). It is essential that we take a holistic and strategic approach, and address the integrated drivers of healthcare sustainability which provide co-benefits to people and planet, in addition to affordability.

The UK Centre for Sustainable Healthcare emphasises the need to place patients and health workers at the centre of efforts to create a sustainable health system and to broaden our conceptualisation of environmental sustainability from non-clinical areas such as energy, transport and waste. Mortimer proposes the drivers of sustainable clinical practice, illustrated in Figure 13.3 derived from Mortimer (18)), which offer a holistic approach to improving patient and population outcomes in ways that

$$\text{Healthcare value} = \frac{\textit{Patient and population outcomes}}{\textit{Social, environmental and financial costs}}$$

Figure 13.2   Healthcare value and the triple bottom line. Adapted from Mortimer 2010 (18)

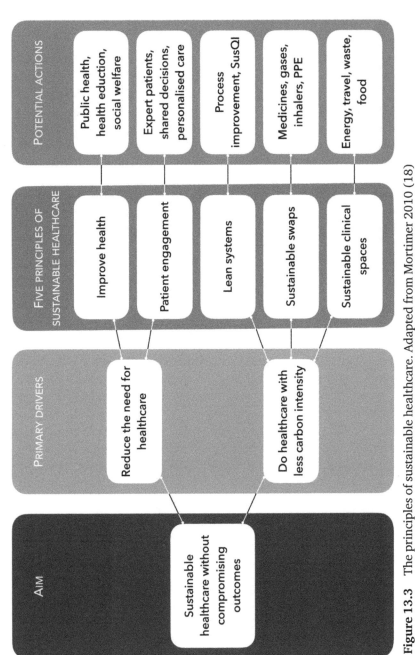

Figure 13.3 The principles of sustainable healthcare. Adapted from Mortimer 2010 (18)

are sustainable. Firstly, and most importantly, by reducing the amount of healthcare that is needed through public health, health promotion and supported self-management, and then secondly, by reducing the resource intensity of the healthcare that is necessary through more efficient clinical pathways, sustainable clinical swaps and estates management (18).

Below, we outline practical examples of how these five principles can support a holistic approach to sustainable clinical practice without compromising the quality of patient care or population health. The intention is not to provide a comprehensive list of what needs to change, but rather, to introduce a range of challenges, while providing a framework to understand and develop solutions. Chapter 14 gives more details on how to embed sustainability into quality improvement 'SusQI' (pronounced Sus-Q-I) as a way of empowering and engaging clinicians in change work.

Principles of sustainable healthcare in practice

> Health inequalities and the social determinants of health are not a footnote to the determinants of health. They are the main issue.
>
> Sir Michael Marmot (25)

Principle 1: Health promotion and disease prevention

'Prevention is better than cure' is a truism embodied in the great public health successes of human history. Despite many examples of progress, however, the challenges of maximising health and preventing disease have often been sidelined by short-term considerations, including corporate interests (26). At a national policy level, climate mitigation has massive potential public health co-benefits and prioritising prevention strategies in clinical pathway design is also key to driving down carbon emissions. Low-carbon healthcare is therefore exemplified by interventions that aim to maximise health and prevent disease, including public health measures such as vaccination; social measures such as housing and education; and health promotion within a clinical consultation such as smoking cessation.

Example 13.1: Prevention of diabetes complications through lifestyle interventions

There is now good evidence that interventions that encourage exercise and low carbohydrate diets in patients with type 2 diabetes are associated with significant reductions in HbA1c blood levels, a reduction in body fat, increased insulin sensitivity and even the remission of diabetes altogether (27,28). Even marginally improved diabetic control through medicines adherence is associated with dramatic long-term reductions in the need for future healthcare services and in the carbon footprint of care (29). This is mediated through the prevention of diabetic complications such as renal failure, cardiovascular disease and diabetic retinopathy. Exercise interventions for diabetes also have other co-benefits including improved cardiovascular fitness and mental health (30).

Despite some criticisms (31), 'lifestyle medicine' is a developing discipline, with an emerging evidence base and academic grounding (see Chapter 17). The British Society of Lifestyle Medicine (32) describes six pillars: healthy eating, mental wellbeing, healthy relationships, physical activity, sleep, and minimising harmful substances and signposts to research and education in the field. It is important, however, to remember that 'lifestyle' is often not a choice, or at least the scope is limited by an individual's circumstances, and to avoid creating value judgements about people whose health is impacted by these factors. Social inequalities, levels of empowerment, public health policy and environmental factors all have profound influences on human behaviour (3). The UK's strategy on food, for example, has the potential to improve health outcomes, social inequalities and the environment, but has yet to be translated into policy (33). The aim, rather, is to engage and inform at both individual and policy levels, so that people become actively involved in decisions and factors that affect their own and others' health.

Principle 2: Patient engagement

Healthcare has historically been framed as something that is done to patients by clinicians; however, the day-to-day work of healthcare, particularly in chronic care, is done by patients and carers who manage their health with only episodic input from professionals. We use the term 'patient engagement' to describe an approach that prioritises the distribution of knowledge and power between patients, practitioners and communities, and which legitimises, enables and encourages patients and carers as active partners. This principle of sustainable healthcare invites engagement not only with healthcare decisions and therapeutic self-management, but also with day-to-day health-related activities. Engagement might be about making meaning differently in a local community setting thus enabling greater involvement with their environment: community gardens, for example, which provide opportunities to grow fruit and vegetables, meet people, and share meals (34). This same dimension of care has been variously described as patient enablement, patient empowerment, patient activation and patient partnership and is associated with reduced needs for acute clinical care, particularly for people living with multimorbidities (35). It is a dimension of generalist care which has the potential to reduce wasted healthcare activity by ensuring services are designed around people's needs, and more importantly, to engage and enable people to maximise their own health through effective self-care. The UK's Personalised Care Institute describes six components: shared decision-making, personalised care and support planning, social prescribing and community-based support, supported self-management, enabling choice, and personal health budgets (36). Personalised care and its core communicative approaches are outlined in Chapter 18.

Example 13.2: Supported self-management and agency in asthma care

Table 13.1 shows how metered dose inhalers contribute 21.8 per cent to total prescribing-relating carbon emissions in UK primary care, or approximately 767 $ktCO_2$ per year. Using the EPA carbon equivalencies calculator (37) this is equivalent to approximately 2 billion car miles per year. This disproportionately large carbon footprint is due to the HFC (hydrofluorocarbon) propellant in some inhalers, not the active medicine. Much emphasis has been placed on encouraging swaps to non-HFC inhalers, or to inhalers with less HFC per puff, through informed choice and the development of guidelines. Inhaler review clinics are also an opportunity to engage patients with their asthma care more generally: do they have the right diagnosis, are they using the right drugs, and are they using their inhaler devices correctly? In the UK, 70 per cent of all inhaler prescriptions are for short-acting reliever inhalers, and around half of UK asthma patients are overusing them (38). This contrasts with Italy where only 46 per cent of inhalers prescribed are short-acting reliever inhalers. Italy's asthma mortality rates in

2019 were less than half of the UK's (39). Sweden has similarly excellent asthma outcomes (39). In 2017, 90 per cent of Sweden's short-acting reliever inhalers were HFC-free, compared to only 6 per cent in the UK (40). Supporting people to switch to dry powder inhalers, which contain no HFCs, can improve asthma control and carbon emissions (41). Even without a switch, optimising inhaler use can significantly improve control and reduce acute admissions (41). Given that poor asthma control in the UK is driving the use of HFC inhalers and acute admissions, it is easy to see how informing people and engaging them in choosing and using their inhalers well has important health and sustainability co-benefits.

Principle 3: Lean systems

Although it is important to ensure that the focus remains on prevention and patient engagement, a sustainable healthcare system also requires attention to how we provide the care that is needed. Much of the scholarship around lean systems comes from industry, where methods have been developed to help businesses identify defects and waste within a process and to implement quality improvement cycles (42). These approaches have increasingly been applied to healthcare in an attempt to improve safety and quality in ways that are more efficient and effective. There are criticisms of top-down quality improvement efforts (22); however, we invite you to imagine the concept of 'lean' differently. Lean process theory was originally rooted in Buddhist philosophy and included respect for people, teamwork, noticing, orderliness and challenge (42). Importantly, 'lean' was not about greater productivity (for example, doing things faster or more intensively); rather, it was about efficiency: encouraging the workforce to notice the way outcomes were achieved and supporting them to continuously improve. A narrow focus on target outcomes tends to generate solutions such as more checking, more protocols and more training. The concept of 'lean', however, focuses on processes and therefore encourages solutions such as making the safe choice the easy choice, stopping low-value patient activities such as unnecessary interventions and tests, and using people's skills to their best effect. Lean philosophy involves defining value from the user's perspective (patients and populations) and changes are collaboratively designed and evaluated by the workers (clinicians). Steps include value chain analysis (studying the system and removing steps that do not add value to patients); finding ways to reduce different types of waste (errors, materials, transport, waiting, space, motion, activities, skills and so on); streamlining processes to reduce variation, improve flow and match demand; and embedding a culture of continuous improvement. Although viewing healthcare through an industrial process lens has been criticised, the application of the principles of lean can draw attention to minimising wasted time, effort and physical resources while simultaneously improving outcomes.

Example 13.3: Reducing wasted activity and enhancing diabetes outcomes

A practice manager noticed that patients at their practice had poor diabetic outcomes compared to national benchmarks, and only 40 per cent of newly diagnosed patients were being referred for self-management education. They invited a trainee to do a SusQI project. The trainee studied the system and found that GPs needed to fill out six pieces of paperwork for each new diagnosis taking up to 30 minutes. They collaboratively designed an improvement which involved a hotkey to automatically complete all six forms. On re-auditing, more patients were getting the right referrals but locum GPs were not aware of the hotkey. This was solved with an automated prompt. Now, 100 per cent of newly diagnosed people get the correct referrals, GPs have less paperwork and patient engagement and outcomes have improved.

Principle 4: Sustainable swaps and low-carbon alternatives

Instinctively, when we consider a low-carbon future, our attention tends to turn towards lower-carbon alternatives to existing practices such as electric cars and wind turbines, rather than the solutions that would drive down carbon requirements, such as active transport and insulation. It is therefore important when considering low-carbon alternatives, that we remember that prevention and supported self-care will usually be more effective and sustainable.

When considering low-carbon alternatives, it is necessary to develop a degree of carbon literacy so that we recognise and focus on key hotspots of carbon emissions (see Table 13.1 above). It is also important to be able to locate and share high-quality evidence on whether a change, for example from disposable to reusable equipment, is an improvement.

Note: it almost invariably is, but the size of the impact varies according to category (43). A simple look-up table for measuring the carbon impacts of various swaps is available in the SusQI Toolkit (44).

Example 13.4: Comparative impacts of two sustainable swaps

If a clinician in the UK supports a dozen people to swap to HFC-free inhalers (saving 422 kg CO_2e per person/year (40)), that would offset an average person's entire annual carbon footprint (5,200 kg CO_2e per person/year (45)). If a clinician swapped from using disposable vaginal specula (88 kg CO_2e per 100 examinations) to reusable (23 kg CO_2e per 100 examinations) (46) they would need to do around 8,000 examinations for a similar effect.

HFC-containing propellant inhalers and anaesthetic gases are key contributors to healthcare's carbon footprint and are therefore considered priority areas for climate mitigation. Reusable equipment has other co-benefits including plastic waste reduction.

Principle 5: Sustainable clinical sites

Although we have focused on the clinical contributions to achieving a sustainable health service, sustainable clinical sites (estate management, general purchasing, energy, travel, food, water, waste management and so on) are also core to achieving carbon reduction targets. Table 13.1 shows how energy use alone represents 10 per cent of the NHS's emissions. In practice, operational resource use often intersects with clinical pathway design and clinical procurement. For example, addressing the environmental hotspots of renal dialysis often involves clinicians working alongside the estates team. Green nephrology has shown that environmentally responsible care is also more cost-effective through reduced waste and power (47).

Example 13.5: Nitrous oxide leaks versus prescribing practices

Anaesthetic gases contribute a staggering 2 per cent to the UK healthcare sector's carbon footprint, the bulk of which is due to nitrous oxide which contributed around 253 kt CO_2e in England in 2019/20 (48). This is equivalent to 650 million car miles per year (37). Alifia Chakera, a clinical pharmacist working in Scotland, decided to audit the use of nitrous oxide and found that clinical usage was not the main problem. Over 90 per cent was lost through poor system design, poor stock management and system leaks (48). Stopping the leaks, for example, by using point-of-care cylinders rather than piped supply, could have significant environmental and economic co-benefits without reducing the availability of nitrous oxide to patients.

This example is a reminder of the importance of taking a holistic approach to emissions reduction and change management, as often the most significant gains are recognised by taking a step away from the problem and considering the change and its solutions within their broader context.

Achieving change

It is easy to feel hopeless with news of climate change. SusQI is invaluable as it gives concrete ways in which we can make a difference rather than just learning about the problem.

SusQI learner (49)

In the introduction, we discussed how an understanding of sustainability can alter the way you see the world around you. In the words of one medical student 'It's made me more aware in my understanding that everything's interlinked ... patient care, my own health, you know, education, treatment, it's all interlinked with sustainability rather than sustainability being this separate thing' (50). Transformative perspective shifts (such as the link between planetary health, human health and healthcare) can sometimes feel uncomfortable and potentially overwhelming without a roadmap for achieving change (51). Conversely, developing a plan is empowering.

We now invite you on another voyage: to explore your spheres of control and influence (Figure 13.4 – derived from Covey (52)), to appraise the routes to change, and to consider joining the growing community of health practitioners working towards a more sustainable healthcare system: one that has a less objectifying relationship with our human and natural resources.

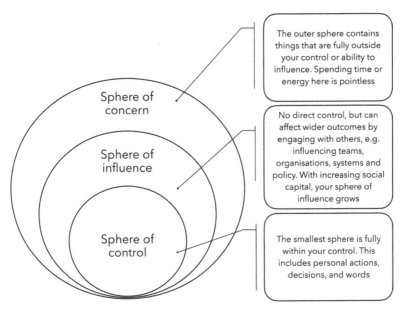

The outer sphere contains things that are fully outside your control or ability to influence. Spending time or energy here is pointless

No direct control, but can affect wider outcomes by engaging with others, e.g. influencing teams, organisations, systems and policy. With increasing social capital, your sphere of influence grows

The smallest sphere is fully within your control. This includes personal actions, decisions, and words

Sphere of concern

Sphere of influence

Sphere of control

Figure 13.4   Covey's spheres of control, influence and concern. Adapted from Covey 1989 (52)

Personal changes

> I think it just really took me aback, like 'wow, the health service plays such a big role in environmental destruction'. I always think that I'm quite a sustainable person generally … I need to do something to balance out.
>
> SusQI learner (50)

The things that are fully within your sphere of control include your personal actions, decisions and words. Hugh Montgomery OBE, professor of intensive care medicine and co-chair of the Lancet Countdown on Health and Climate Change, ends his climate updates by urging the audience to undertake the following seven personal actions, and to encourage seven others to do the same:

1. Use renewable and sustainable sources of electricity and heating.
2. Travel less and, when you do, use active and mass transport.
3. Buy local, seasonal and plant-based foods.
4. Bank with an ethical bank and do not believe the greenwash.
5. Buy less and buy from low environmental impact ethical producers.

6. Vote with climate as your priority and write to your MP to tell them that is what you are doing.
7. Contribute to the development of solutions in your work and in your community.

The logic behind individual action is clear. If large numbers of individuals take these steps, then the resulting political and economic impact is magnified and the chances of shaping policy and practice rise. Furthermore, living in a manner that is consistent with your values, reduces the cognitive dissonance between beliefs and actions, and increases one's authenticity as a climate advocate. Successful movements require mass mobilisation, and in practical terms, Prof Montgomery is using his influence to create a movement for change and to engage us in recruiting to it.

Although it is clear that mass engagement and the action of individuals can effect change, there are accepted limitations to this approach. The first is a recognition that although individuals have an important role in successful movements, it is their role as part of a group that is powerful. Acting alone risks a sense of futility, isolation and disillusionment, and can be negatively viewed as virtue signalling. Furthermore, simple lists of actions can overlook the multiple barriers that can frustrate and restrict engagement. For example, it may be costly to convert to renewable energy if you are reliant on a gas boiler and difficult to buy locally if this produce is not available where you shop.

Importantly, the failure to be a model environmentalist must not prevent individuals from participating in environmental work, or become a bat to beat them with when they do. Likewise, the responsibility of each of us to act individually should not distract from a government's responsibility to create a low-carbon and sustainable society in which environmentally aligned decisions are structurally encouraged.

Changes to individual clinical practice

> Everyone can do something, even if it is a little change. Every patient encounter is a chance to change something.
>
> SusQI learner (49)

It can be difficult to integrate the principles of sustainability into a health service that has been designed without considering environmental impacts. It can also feel uncomfortable raising climate concerns in a workplace that is already struggling to cope with multiple other pressures.

How does someone who wants to practise sustainably continue without frustration or moral injury?

Part of this process is simply to apply the principles of sustainable healthcare to your own practice and to share what you are doing with colleagues. The principles are all considered good clinical practice: having health-promoting conversations, engaging people in effective self-management, sharing knowledge and decisions, critically considering the tests and treatments we recommend, noticing and stopping wasted or low-value activities that do not contribute to patient or population outcomes, choosing less environmentally damaging options wherever possible, and advocating for sustainable clinical spaces.

The potential for spreading change and, importantly, the support one receives to sustain change work can be enhanced by joining a community of practice, such as the growing network of clinical environmental groups on the Centre for Sustainable Healthcare's clinical networks hub (53). Personal change is always possible and your own actions might just tip the balance to shift norms through role modelling away from commercial and compartmentalised interests, to more holistic and integrated efforts and approaches.

Changes to local services and systems

You've got that 'QI head' on your shoulders, asking 'What can I do? What can I improve? Why is this the way it is?'

SusQI learner (54)

SusQI integrates the triple bottom line into quality improvement efforts through stakeholder engagement, value chain analysis, and environmental and human resource stewardship. Changes are evaluated to see if they provide health benefits as well as triple bottom-line benefits (social, economic, environmental). It has been validated in multiple UK health settings and is now embedded and spreading internationally (49). The freely available SusQI Toolkit (55) offers resources for supervising and undertaking projects and ready-made workshop materials for educators. Examples of successful SusQI projects are growing rapidly, and sustainability has been shown to be a motivating factor when engaging teams with change (49).

Generalism invites different lenses on complex problems: thinking about what you are trying to achieve as well as how to do it. This 'double loop' reflection (56) can change the focus of a service and drive service innovation. The WHO defines health service innovation as 'a novel set of behaviours, routines, and ways of working that are discontinuous with previous practice, are directed at improving health outcomes, administrative efficiency, cost-effectiveness, or users' experience and that are implemented by planned and coordinated actions' (57). Numerous innovations, including GP telephone triaging systems and 'See and Treat' Clinics, reflect a drive towards efficiency with a reduction in the environmental impact as a co-benefit, for example through reduced travel. It is, however, essential that improvement and innovation are not completed in silos, and that organisations work to maximise the success factors that are critical to the spread of the most impactful work (58).

The following example is from secondary care and illustrates how a generalist lens on a complex problem can have dramatic impacts.

Example 13.6: Early mobilisation in cardiac intensive care

The University Hospital Southampton NHS Foundation Trust, as part of a hospital-based SusQI initiative, employed a therapy technician to facilitate a twice-daily exercise programme for post-operative patients, including motorised passive movement therapy for those who were intubated (59). 238 patients were recruited into the programme over 24 months, with significant reductions in length of ventilation (−3.54 days/patient), length of CICU stay (−5.5 days/patient) and total length of hospital stay (−7.79 days/patient). Carbon savings, based on the reduced intensity of care, were calculated at 48.5 tCO_2e. Cost savings were estimated at £1.26m ($1.69m). Additional social and health benefits arose through the reduction in length of stay and the prevention of muscle wastage.

Changes to clinical and institutional governance

We came up with a 12-point [sustainability] plan that we would like the university to integrate into the curriculum, expecting them to say 'Yes, we will look at integrating three or five over maybe a five-year period, but ...' After that meeting, they agreed to integrate all 12 points, which is fantastic.

SusQI educator

In addition to individual improvement and innovation projects, institutional and clinical governance needs to support a culture of sustainability and expectation for action. This means engaging with regulatory bodies and institutional leadership so that they formally recognise climate-related threats, and articulate their roles and responsibilities in environmental mitigation, adaptation and advocacy.

Progress has been made, much of it initiated by small groups of individuals. Examples include the Planetary Health Report Card (60) and the climate change and health scorecard (61) which put pressure on organisations by publicly evaluating them. Institutions are also using their collective influence by publicly and jointly declaring a health emergency – for example, through the São Paulo Declaration on Planetary Health (62) or the Academic Health Institutions' Declaration on Planetary Health (63). There are also many groups that work at a national and international level to lobby, educate and produce guidance on carbon mitigation.

Bringing these scorecards and declarations to the attention of institutional leaders is a potential strategy for individuals and groups to advocate for policy change, and has, in the case of the Planetary Health Report Card, been associated with improved year-on-year sustainability content in the UK as measured by the scorecard (64).

Changing society

> And so it's almost like trying to help my future self – if I can make a difference to these problems now, then I'm going to not have to deal with that as much in the future.
>
> SusQI learner (49)

Healthcare has a strong history of campaigning and health advocacy (see Chapter 10). This has helped to create institutions such as the World Health Organization, and frameworks such as the UN's Sustainable Development Goals that seek to maintain and improve the health of the societies we live in. However, institutions and frameworks are often products of conflicting conceptions of good health and healthcare, financial constraints, competing interests and political pressure.

Health advocacy, including campaigning for policy change, has historically achieved major public health improvements, from mandatory advertising on the harms of smoking, through laws banning female genital mutilation, to the implementation of drink driving laws, seat belts and safe alcohol limits. Each area of gain has, however, required a shift in public perception to create what are now culturally accepted norms. Creating a sustainable healthcare system requires a similar cultural shift, such that health workers, their patients and leaders, develop a perspective in which environmental sustainability is understood to be fundamental to human survival. The good news, as discussed above, is that many environmental solutions mirror public health goals, for example, healthier plant-based food, home insulation and a reduction in air pollution.

> Health professionals and their organisations must support and learn from the schoolchildren's [non-violent direct] action, finding more effective ways to help people and politicians understand that climate change is by far the biggest threat human health has ever faced.
>
> Robin Stott, UK Climate & Health Council;
> Richard Smith, former editor BMJ;
> Rowan Williams, former Archbishop of Canterbury;
> Fiona Godlee, editor-in-chief *BMJ*
> 2019 (65).

Although there has been some progress in highlighting the impacts of the climate and ecological emergency, the reality remains that global greenhouse gas emissions continue to rise at an alarming rate (Figure 13.5) and, thus far, competing economic and political interests have sidelined environmental concerns (66). There have been many national and international promises on climate mitigation: the Rio Declaration in 1992, the Kyoto Protocol in 1997, the Paris Accord in 2015, and no fewer than 27 UN Framework Conventions on Climate Change (COP-27 in 2022). Commitments have historically fallen short of what is necessary to limit global warming to 1.5 degrees, and action has lagged behind the promises made (67). Communities globally are already suffering, yet despite this reality, the actions taken by governments and the attention of the media are insignificant compared to shorter-term threats such as the COVID-19 pandemic.

Driven by this inaction in the face of the escalating pace of climate breakdown, protest movements are understandably demanding a more urgent response. Many health workers have joined climate-related protest movements, and as consultant psychiatrist Dr Juliette Brown stated, following a direct action during a record heatwave: 'This week may see the hottest day on record in the UK, putting my patients, people with dementia and serious mental illness, at very high risk from heat stress. It's absolutely my professional duty to sound the alarm' (70). Non-violent civil resistance has a long history with many notable successes (71);

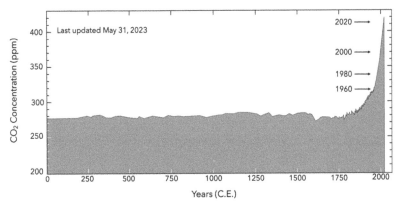

Figure 13.5 The Keeling Curve global atmospheric carbon dioxide concentrations. Scripps Institution of Oceanography at UC San Diego. Available at https://bit.ly/3R79TwJ, CC BY 4.0 (68,69)

however, it should be acknowledged that the safe space for climate activism is narrowing or even non-existent in many countries, and activists frequently face arrest, imprisonment and violence (72).

Amitav Ghosh (73) links our current environmental crisis with colonial perspectives which perceive land and people as resources and commodities to be utilised, owned (and even abused), rather than respected and collaborated with. These latter perspectives view human beings not as dominating over and controlling their environment, but as being part of their environment. This interrelation between place and people is more prevalent in ancient cultures. For example, in Aboriginal culture, meaning is attributed to nature, enhancing connections and a sense of responsibility to work with and care for local and broader ecosystems. Previously positioned by colonial narratives as 'primitive', we are increasingly learning about the power and importance of stories (see Chapter 11), relational continuity with nature and respect for diverse ways of knowing.

Educational approaches

> Education is the most powerful weapon we can use to change the world.
>
> Nelson Mandela (74)

Increasingly, national and international health-education associations and governing bodies have recognised the need for climate-literate health workers who can engage in creating a sustainable health system that is fit for the future. For example, the Association for Medical Education in Europe (AMEE) has issued a consensus statement (14) which sets out a 'vision for educating an interprofessional healthcare workforce that can deliver sustainable healthcare and promote planetary health'.

Clinical education has historically focused on apprenticeship-style learning: senior clinicians mentoring their trainees towards pre-set accreditation standards. Education for sustainable healthcare, however, is different: junior learners, who arguably have the greatest stake in a sustainable future, are driving educational change; seniors are learning alongside juniors; and learners are engaging not because they have to pass examinations, but because they want to see change (49). Learning is not the end point of education, but rather, an ongoing and continual process for the betterment of health and healthcare. Education for sustainable healthcare is inherently practical, requiring a focus on identifying and measuring environmental impacts and developing and implementing strategies to improve them. Assessments that support this type of learning involve practical project work rather than tests of abstract knowledge.

Example 13.7: Near-peer SusQI education at Bristol Medical School

Philippa Clery, a foundation-year trainee, learned about the principles of sustainable healthcare and quality improvement as an undergraduate. On entering clinical practice in Bristol, she wanted to introduce SusQI to medical students there. She teamed up with the Centre for Sustainable Healthcare who provided resources (55), and help with the evaluation. SusQI was the highest-rated session within the clinical practice learning hub. Learners appreciated the opportunity to discuss their values and to learn from near-peer project examples. Challenges included needing time for project work, and strategies to mitigate clinical hierarchies when initiating change. There are now opportunities for student-led projects within the curriculum, and sustainability champions to support in-practice projects. Philippa won the JASME Foundation Innovation Prize for medical education in 2021 (75).

Conclusion

We have shown that the principles of generalism are ideally suited to working with complex problems that are situated in a specific context, and therefore can be used to inform approaches to change. Generalism invites us to bring multiple lenses to a problem; to work holistically; to explore root causes as well as immediate threats; to work collaboratively with patients, experts and colleagues to create potential solutions; and to continuously notice, evaluate and improve in ways that are agile and responsive to contextual constraints and resources.

Finally, as you reflect on the rest of this book, we invite you to consider how generalism, at its best, is potentially one of the most sustainable forms of clinical practice: preventive, proactive, participatory, agile, collaborative and holistic. These are important ways in which we can apply generalism not only in the clinical workplace but also beyond: with our patients, our communities, and across our environments and spaces for living and working.

References

1. 'We do not inherit the Earth from our ancestors; we borrow it from our children' – Quote Investigator®. 2013. Available from: https://quoteinvestigator.com/2013/01/22/borrow-earth/ (accessed 9 June 2023).
2. Romanello M, Di Napoli C, Drummond P, Green C, Kennard H, Lampard P et al. The 2022 report of the Lancet Countdown on health and climate change: health at the mercy of fossil fuels. *The Lancet*. 2022;400(10363):1619–54.
3. Institute of Health Equity. Fair Society, Healthy Lives – The Marmot Review. 2010. Available from: https://policycommons.net/artifacts/2297843/fair-society-healthy-lives/ (accessed 18 March 2024).
4. Pörtner H-O, Roberts DC, Adams H, Adler C, Aldunce P, Ali E et al. Climate Change 2022: Impacts, Adaptation, and Vulnerability. Contribution of Working Group II to the Sixth Assessment Report of the Intergovernmental Panel on Climate Change. Potsdam-Institut fur Klimafolgenforschung; 2022 Sep. Available from: https://policycommons.net/artifacts/2679314/climate-change-2022/ (accessed 20 March 2024).
5. Costello A, Abbas M, Allen A, Ball S, Bell S, Bellamy R, et al. Managing the health effects of climate change: Lancet and University College London Institute for Global Health Commission. *The Lancet*. 2009;373(9676):1693–733.
6. World Meteorological Organization (WMO). WMO Global Annual to Decadal Climate Update (Target years: 2023–2027). WMO; 2023.
7. IPCC. Summary for policymakers. In: Global Warming of 1.5°C: IPCC Special Report on Impacts of Global Warming of 1.5°C above Pre-industrial Levels in Context of Strengthening Response to Climate Change, Sustainable Development, and Efforts to Eradicate Poverty. Cambridge University Press; 2022. pp. 1–24. Available from: www.cambridge.org/core/books/global-warming-of-15c/summary-for-policymakers/31C38E590392F74C7341928B681FF668 (accessed 20 March 2024).
8. Lenzen M, Malik A, Li M, Fry J, Weisz H, Pichler PP, et al. The environmental footprint of health care: a global assessment. *Lancet Planet Health*. 2020;4(7):e271–9.
9. Ortúzar M, Esterhuizen M, Olicón-Hernández DR, González-López J, Aranda E. Pharmaceutical pollution in aquatic environments: a concise review of environmental impacts

and bioremediation systems. *Front Microbiol.* 2022;13. Available from: www.frontiersin.org/articles/10.3389/fmicb.2022.869332 (accessed 20 March 2024).

10. Silva ALP, Prata JC, Walker TR, Duarte AC, Ouyang W, Barceló D et al. Increased plastic pollution due to COVID-19 pandemic: challenges and recommendations. *Chem Eng J.* 2021;405:126683.

11. Trueba ML, Bhutta MF, Shahvisi A. Instruments of health and harm: how the procurement of healthcare goods contributes to global health inequality. *J Med Ethics.* 2021;47(6):423–9.

12. Conn D. Department of Health writes off £9bn spent in England's Covid PPE drive. *The Guardian.* 2022. Available from: www.theguardian.com/politics/2022/feb/01/department-of-health-writes-off-9bn-spent-in-uk-covid-ppe-drive (accessed 28 March 2023).

13. Tennison I, Roschnik S, Ashby B, Boyd R, Hamilton I, Oreszczyn T, et al. Health care's response to climate change: a carbon footprint assessment of the NHS in England. *Lancet Planet Health.* 2021;5(2):e84–92.

14. Shaw E, Walpole S, McLean M, Alvarez-Nieto C, Barna S, Bazin K, et al. AMEE Consensus Statement: Planetary health and education for sustainable healthcare. *Med Teach.* 2021;43(3):272–86.

15. Porter ME. What is value in health care? *N Engl J Med.* 2010;363(26):2477–81.

16. Mortimer F, Isherwood J, Wilkinson A, Vaux E. Sustainability in quality improvement: redefining value. *Future Hosp J.* 2018;5(2):88–93.

17. Elkington J. Accounting for the triple bottom line. *Meas Bus Excell.* 1998;2(3):18–22.

18. Mortimer F. The sustainable physician. *Clin Med Lond Engl.* 2010;10(2):110–1.

19. Lombardi DR, Porter L, Barber A, Rogers CDF. Conceptualising sustainability in UK urban regeneration: a discursive formation. *Urban Stud.* 2011;48(2):273–96.

20. Scottish Government. NHS Scotland climate emergency and sustainability strategy 2022 to 2026 – draft: consultation. 2021. Available from: https://webarchive.nrscotland.gov.uk/20211202194701mp_/http://www.gov.scot/publications/nhs-scotland-draft-climate-emergency-sustainability-strategy/ (accessed 22 May 2023).

21. NHS England and NHS Improvement. Delivering a 'Net Zero' National Health Service. 2020. Available from: www.england.nhs.uk/greenernhs/wp-content/uploads/sites/51/2020/10/delivering-a-net-zero-national-health-service.pdf (accessed 15 October 2020).

22. Boyle S, Lister J, Steer R. Sustainability and Transformation Plans. How serious are the proposals? A critical review. London South Bank University; 2017.

23. Cameron G, Alderwick H, Bowers A, Dixon J. *Shaping Health Futures.* The Health Foundation; 2019.

24. Appleby J, Galea A, Murray R. *The NHS Productivity Challenge: Experience from the front line.* The King's Fund; 2014.

25. Michael Marmot, Interview. Available from: http://epimonitor.net/Michael_Marmot_Interview.htm (accessed 22 May 2023).

26. Brandt AM. Inventing conflicts of interest: a history of tobacco industry tactics. *Am J Public Health.* 2012;102(1):63–71.

27. Thomas D, Elliott E, Naughton G. Exercise for type 2 diabetes mellitus. *Cochrane Database Syst Rev.* 2006;(3). Available from: https://doi.org/10.1002/14651858.CD002968.pub2

28. Goldenberg JZ, Day A, Brinkworth GD, Sato J, Yamada S, Jönsson T et al. Efficacy and safety of low and very low carbohydrate diets for type 2 diabetes remission: systematic review and meta-analysis of published and unpublished randomized trial data. *BMJ.* 2021;372: m4743.

29. Fordham R, Dhatariya K, Stancliffe R, Lloyd A, Chatterjee M, Mathew M et al. Effective diabetes complication management is a step toward a carbon-efficient planet: an economic modeling study. *BMJ Open Diabetes Res Care.* 2020;8(1):e001017.

30. Madden KM. Evidence for the benefit of exercise therapy in patients with type 2 diabetes. *Diabetes Metab Syndr Obes.* 2013;6:233–9.

31. Nunan D, Blane DN, McCartney M. Exemplary medical care or Trojan horse? An analysis of the 'lifestyle medicine' movement. *Br J Gen Pract.* 2021;71(706):229.

32. British Society of Lifestyle Medicine (BSLM). Transforming healthcare through lifestyle medicine. Available from: https://bslm.org.uk/ (accessed 22 May 2023).

33. Dimbleby H. National Food Strategy: The Plan (Part Two: Final Report). 2022.

34. Hume C, Grieger JA, Kalamkarian A, D'Onise K, Smithers LG. Community gardens and their effects on diet, health, psychosocial and community outcomes: a systematic review. *BMC Public Health.* 2022;22(1):1247.

35. Deeny S, Thorlby R, Steventon A. Briefing: Reducing emergency admissions: unlocking the potential of people to better manage their long-term conditions. The Health Foundation; 2018.
36. Personalised Care Institute. The Personalised Care Curriculum. 2020. Available from: www.personalisedcareinstitute.org.uk/wp-content/uploads/2021/06/The-personalised-care-curriculum.pdf (accessed 20 March 2024).
37. United States Environmental Protection Agency. Greenhouse Gas Equivalencies Calculator. 2024. Available from: www.epa.gov/energy/greenhouse-gas-equivalencies-calculator (accessed 21 March 2024).
38. Wilkinson AJK, Menzies-Gow A, Sawyer M, Bell JP, Xu Y, Budgen N et al. An assessment of short-acting β2-agonist (SABA) use and subsequent greenhouse gas (GHG) emissions in five European countries and the consequence of their potential overuse for asthma in the UK. *Thorax*. 2021;76(Suppl 1):A19.
39. Institute for Health Metrics and Evaluation. GBD Results. 2019. Global Burden of Disease (GBD) Study. 2019. Available from: https://vizhub.healthdata.org/gbd-results (accessed 23 May 2023).
40. Janson C, Henderson R, Löfdahl M, Hedberg M, Sharma R, Wilkinson AJK. Carbon footprint impact of the choice of inhalers for asthma and COPD. *Thorax*. 2020;75(1):82.
41. Woodcock A, Janson C, Rees J, Frith L, Löfdahl M, Moore A et al. Effects of switching from a metered dose inhaler to a dry powder inhaler on climate emissions and asthma control: post-hoc analysis. *Thorax*. 2022;77(12):1187.
42. Chiarini A, Baccarani C, Mascherpa V. Lean production, Toyota production system and Kaizen philosophy. *TQM J*. 2018;30(4):425–38.
43. Keil M, Viere T, Helms K, Rogowski W. The impact of switching from single-use to reusable healthcare products: a transparency checklist and systematic review of life-cycle assessments. *Eur J Public Health*. 2023;33(1):56–63.
44. Centre for Sustainable Healthcare. Measuring Impact. Available from: www.susqi.org/measuring-impact (accessed 30 May 2023).
45. Statista. UK: per capita CO_2 emissions 1970–2022. 2024. Available from: www.statista.com/statistics/1299198/co2-emissions-per-capita-united-kingdom/ (accessed 21 March 2024).
46. Donahue LM, Hilton S, Bell SG, Williams BC, Keoleian GA. A comparative carbon footprint analysis of disposable and reusable vaginal specula. *Am J Obstet Gynecol*. 2020;223(2):225. e1–225.e7.
47. Rajan T, Amin SO, Davis K, Finkle N, Glick N, Kahlon B, et al. Redesigning kidney care for the Anthropocene: a new framework for planetary health in nephrology. *Can J Kidney Health Dis*. 2022;9:20543581221116215.
48. Chakera A. Driving down embedded emissions from medical nitrous oxide. *BMJ*. 2021; 375:n2922.
49. Spooner R, Stanford V, Parslow-Williams S, Mortimer F, Leedham-Green K. 'Concrete ways we can make a difference': A multi-centre, multi-professional evaluation of sustainability in quality improvement education. *Med Teach*. 2022;44(10):1116–24.
50. Marsden O, Clery P, D'Arch Smith S, Leedham-Green K. Sustainability in Quality Improvement (SusQI): challenges and strategies for translating undergraduate learning into clinical practice. *BMC Med Educ*. 2021;21(1):555.
51. Meyer JHF, Land R. Threshold concepts and troublesome knowledge (2): epistemological considerations and a conceptual framework for teaching and learning. *High Educ*. 2005;49(3):373–88.
52. Covey SR. *The Seven Habits of Highly Effective People*. Simon and Schuster; 1989.
53. Sustainable Healthcare Networks Hub. Available from: https://networks.sustainablehealthcare.org.uk/ (accessed 30 May 2023).
54. Clery P, d'Arch Smith S, Marsden O, Leedham-Green K. Sustainability in Quality Improvement (SusQI): a case-study in undergraduate medical education. *BMC Med Educ*. 2021;21(1):425.
55. Centre for Sustainable Healthcare. SusQI Toolkit | Sustainable Quality Improvement. Available from: www.susqi.org (accessed 1 June 2023).
56. Argyris C. Double loop learning in organizations. *Harv Bus Rev*. 1977;55(5):115–25.
57. Nolte E. How do we ensure that innovation in health service delivery and organization is implemented, sustained and spread? World Health Organization; 2018. Available from: https://eurohealthobservatory.who.int/publications/i/how-do-we-ensure-that-innovation-in-health-service-delivery-and-organization-is-implemented-sustained-and-spread (accessed 20 March 2024).

58. Leedham-Green K, Knight A, Reedy GB. Success and limiting factors in health service innovation: a theory-generating mixed methods evaluation of UK projects. *BMJ Open.* 2021;11(5):e047943.
59. Sustainable Healthcare Networks Hub. SusQI Project Report – Early Mobilisation in Cardiac Intensive Care. Available from: https://networks.sustainablehealthcare.org.uk/resources/susqi-project-report-early-mobilisation-cardiac-intensive-care (accessed 30 May 2023).
60. Hampshire K, Islam N, Kissel B, Chase H, Gundling K. The Planetary Health Report Card: a student-led initiative to inspire planetary health in medical schools. *Lancet Planet Health.* 2022;6(5):e449–54.
61. Cooke E, Cussans A, Clack A, Cornford C. Climate change and health scorecard: What are UK professional and regulatory health organizations doing to tackle the climate and ecological emergency? *J Clim Change Health.* 2022;8:100164.
62. Myers SS, Pivor JI, Saraiva AM. The São Paulo Declaration on planetary health. *The Lancet.* 2021;398(10308):1299.
63. Association of Faculties of Medicine of Canada (AFMC). Academic Health Institutions' Declaration on Planetary Health. Available from: www.afmc.ca/initiatives/planetaryhealth declaration/ (accessed 9 June 2023).
64. Planetary Health Report Card. Medicine. Annual Summary Reports. 2023. Available from: https://phreportcard.org/medicine/ (accessed 14 June 2023).
65. Stott R, Smith R, Williams R, Godlee F. Schoolchildren's activism is a lesson for health professionals. *BMJ.* 2019;365:l1938.
66. Brulle RJ. Advocating inaction: a historical analysis of the Global Climate Coalition. *Environ Polit.* 2023;32(2):185–206.
67. Clémençon R. 30 years of international climate negotiations: are they still our best hope? *J Environ Dev.* 2023;32(2):114–46.
68. Keeling RF, Keeling CD. Atmospheric monthly in situ CO2 data: Mauna Loa observatory, Hawaii. Scripps CO2 Program Data. 2017;
69. Rubino M, Etheridge D, Thornton D, Allison C, Francey R, Langenfelds R, et al. Law Dome ice core 2000-year CO2, CH4, N2O and δ13C-CO2. v1. 2019;
70. Doctors for XR [@DoctorsXr]. Consultant Psychiatrist Juliette Brown says: 'This week may see the hottest day on record in the UK, putting my patients – people with dementia and with serious mental illness – at very high risk from heat stress. It's absolutely my professional duty to sound the alarm' https://t.co/VEw93ziZpN. Twitter. 2022. Available from: https://twitter.com/DoctorsXr/status/1548618419272138753 (accessed 9 June 2023).
71. Chenoweth E. *Civil Resistance: What Everyone Needs to Know®.* Oxford University Press; 2021. Available from: https://books.google.co.uk/books?id=zEEgEAAAQBAJ (accessed 21 March 2024).
72. Council of Europe. Commissioner for Human Rights. Crackdowns on peaceful environmental protests should stop and give way to more social dialogue. Available from: www.coe.int/en/web/commissioner/-/crackdowns-on-peaceful-environmental-protests-should-stop-and-give-way-to-more-social-dialogue (accessed 24 June 2023).
73. Ghosh A. *The Nutmeg's Curse.* University of Chicago Press; 2021.
74. Mandela N. 'Education is the most powerful weapon we can use to change the world.' From address by Nelson Mandela at launch of Mindset Network, Johannesburg. 2003.
75. Association for the Study of Medical Education (ASME). JASME and ASME are delighted to announce the winner of the Foundation Innovation Prize 2021. 2021. Available from: www.asme.org.uk/winner-2021-fip/ (accessed 9 June 2023).
76. Centres for Disease Control. Climate Effects on Health. 2022. Available from: www.cdc.gov/climateandhealth/effects/default.htm (accessed 2 March 2023).

14
Generalist approaches to quality improvement

Rebecca Mackenzie and Nitisha Nahata

Introduction

This chapter highlights the limitations of traditional reductionist approaches in improving healthcare quality and advocates for the adoption of socially and complexity-informed approaches. It emphasises the complex and socially determined nature of healthcare systems and the need for qualitative, sociological and mixed-methods approaches to gain a deeper understanding of improvement processes. In doing so, it emphasises the importance of collaborative change processes, local tailoring of interventions, and flexible research methods. It also calls for future research to focus on refining these approaches, building a stronger knowledge base, and disseminating social and complexity-informed approaches to improve both outcomes and sustainability in healthcare improvement.

A healthcare system is an organisation of people and resources (for example, training, buildings, equipment and technology), which work alongside other systems to deliver care which meets the health needs of a specific population (1). Quality healthcare systems are those which identify and strive to increase the chance of achieving patients' and populations' desired health goals, as well as minimise the chance of adverse outcomes. They also optimise care to maximise patient and population outcomes in relation to available resources (2).

Healthcare quality is important because avoidable patient harm unfolds without it (3,4). Examples include the palliative care patient who is overtreated and denied quality of life in their last days because services failed to understand their wishes; or the cancer patient whose disease turns from curable to untreatable because of poor access and delays in diagnosis and treatment. Some commercial priorities can position quality healthcare as technologically complex, or high-cost. However, most accept quality healthcare to be safe, sustainable, person-centred, effective, accessible, continuous, timely, efficient and equitable (2).

In the UK, pressure to increase healthcare quality has grown because the gap between actual and ideal standards of care has widened. On one side, scientific advancement continues to broaden diagnostic and treatment horizons while, on the other side, there are real and perceived reductions in standards of care, such as recurrent high-profile scandals, longer waiting times, rising health inequalities, poor access, lack of continuity and worse patient outcomes (3,5,6). Adding to this pressure is the need for services to modernise and become more sustainable given the scarcity of economic, environmental and social resources (3).

The healthcare quality crisis in the UK and elsewhere is multifactorial, although largely driven by demand outstripping capacity. A growing, ageing, multimorbid population has increased the size and complexity of demand, while capacity has been unable to keep up due to inadequate investment in key infrastructure including workforce, buildings, equipment and technology (4,5,7,8).

Yet, in addition to the amount of people and resources contained by the system, how they are facilitated, organised and utilised also impacts the quality of care. Determining how best to do this and improving processes, through the development of evidence-based policies and practices, has been the objective across various research fields, including healthcare services research, implementation science, quality improvement (QI) and improvement science (Figure 14.1) (4,7,9).

Health services research is a multidisciplinary field that examines quality of care by assessing access to, and the use, costs, organisation, financing and outcomes of healthcare services to produce new knowledge about the structure, processes, and effects of health services for individuals and populations (9). Health services research draws contributions from multiple fields with the same aim of improving the quality of healthcare, including implementation science, improvement science and QI; each using different techniques and methods. Implementation science seeks to find a systematic approach to getting evidence-based practice embedded into routine practice through identifying and overcoming barriers and facilitators, in addition to using QI techniques (10). Accordingly, QI techniques are a set of iterative and structured methods to identify and tackle specific quality problems within healthcare systems, and originate from methods used to improve quality in industry,

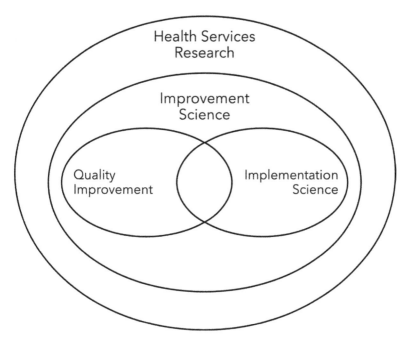

Figure 14.1 Relationships between research fields for improving healthcare. © Rebecca Mackenzie

the military and aviation (10,11). Improvement science is an emerging field focusing on systematically and rigorously exploring how best to improve the quality of care through evidence and, in many ways, encompasses the latter two fields (11).

Historically, such practices have promised straightforward solutions through reductionist approaches, which are based on mechanistic models. For example, by distilling systems down to their component parts to find linear causal relationships; or assuming component parts of the system are rational, predictable and interchangeable (3,12,13). By analogy, these approaches are the equivalent of a mechanic who dismantles a car to find and replace a faulty part.

Such practices also conclude that improvement approaches are generalisable and can be applied to other systems. In the analogy, a spanner used to fix one car can easily be used to fix another. In doing so, the context in which care is provided is not recognised, alongside the complex reality of healthcare system behaviour and the potential effects on quality outcomes. As such, many improvement efforts are ineffective, inefficient and, sometimes, counterproductive; especially in more complex circumstances (3,12,14).

In reality, healthcare systems are highly unique, similar to 'biological' entities or 'ecosystems'. They are composed of self-organising, interdependent components which act in accordance with their own set of deeply ingrained internalised rules. This means components can be unpredictable and difficult to influence, as well as resilient and adaptable (3,12,14). Unlike a car part, an experienced healthcare professional with years of experience cannot be interchanged for another without having a significant impact on the functioning of the system. Moreover, care outcomes are the sum of the dynamic relationships between components across the system as a whole. Therefore, reducing systems to individual components fails to capture the nature and extent of actionable variables (3,12,14).

While reductionist methods might work in more controlled, simple environments, an individualised, socially minded and complexity-informed approach is needed for more complex healthcare settings. In response, researchers have been turning to social and complexity science which – originating jointly from systems theory and cybernetics in the twentieth century – studies the properties and behaviour of complex adaptive systems (CAS) (12,15).

CAS are systems composed of individual 'biological' agents with the freedom to act in ways that are not always predictable, and whose actions are interconnected. They evolve over time, adapt through self-organisation in response to feedback loops and various stimuli, and are characterised by uncertainty, unpredictability and emergence. Examples of CAS include the economy, the immune system and even a colony of termites (14,16). Healthcare systems share these characteristics and can also be described as CAS, which offers a more realistic model for the study of healthcare quality improvement (Figure 14.2) (12,17,18).

While the development of complexity-informed practices is in its infancy, there are several existing approaches which naturally align with the CAS model, as well as many suggestions for how complexity and social science might inform future improvement practices. In this chapter, we will examine these in relation to the stages of an improvement project, with the assumption that readers have some pre-existing QI knowledge and experience. For readers who are at the beginning of their QI journey, we have listed some introductory material in the resources section. We will begin with the process of identifying an improvement goal and assessing quality, followed by priming healthcare systems for improvement and, finally, designing interventions, implementation and evaluation.

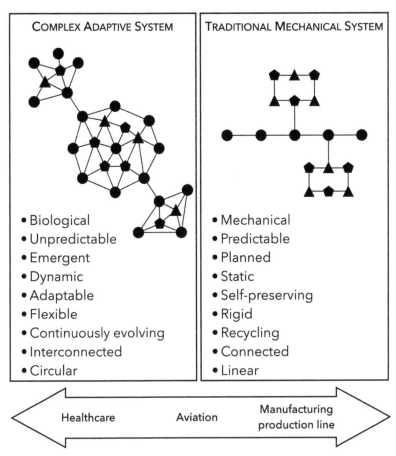

COMPLEX ADAPTIVE SYSTEM	TRADITIONAL MECHANICAL SYSTEM
• Biological	• Mechanical
• Unpredictable	• Predictable
• Emergent	• Planned
• Dynamic	• Static
• Adaptable	• Self-preserving
• Flexible	• Rigid
• Continuously evolving	• Recycling
• Interconnected	• Connected
• Circular	• Linear

Healthcare   Aviation   Manufacturing production line

Figure 14.2 Complex adaptive systems (CAS) versus traditional mechanistic systems. © Rebecca Mackenzie

Identifying improvement goals and assessing quality

The first step in any QI project is to identify an area for improvement and review current performance. Traditionally, healthcare professionals and policymakers have focused on defining 'good quality' by what is easily measurable and more certain, such as biomedical markers of disease (17). However, it is now recognised that the values which inform quality can differ within a population. Since the ultimate goal is to provide insights that can inform decision-making and improve patient outcomes, evaluation methods and questions that help decision-makers find a truly meaningful improvement goal need to be prioritised, as well as ethical and political issues that heavily influence the quality of healthcare (19).

Finding the quality outcomes which matter most to people is important because improvement goals can then be prioritised, thereby increasing care value and reducing improvement waste. This is paramount given the scarcity of social, economic and environmental resources, and in the pursuit of healthcare sustainability (20). Improving QI practices also increases the sustainability of healthcare by maximising the efficiency and effectiveness of care, reducing the need for care, and by optimising the implementation of interventions which reduce resource consumption (20,21). To help improvement teams consider sustainability throughout the improvement process, the 'SusQI' framework was developed (Table 14.1) (20). More information on healthcare sustainability and the SusQI framework can be found in Chapter 13.

Qualitative data

In order to find a meaningful improvement goal, people's 'stories' which illustrate how they experience healthcare need to be taken into account, alongside their perspective of trust and attitudes within the healthcare system. The intention is to uncover 'hidden' and tacit intelligence on patients' and populations' desired health goals, and understand what quality means to them (Example 14.1). Only then can potential barriers to achieving this be identified and overcome (19). Narratives of care experience can also help to identify multiple contingent factors, which in combination, have led to an adverse outcome.

Table 14.1   The SusQI framework – how to incorporate sustainability into the QI process

QI project stage	Sustainability consideration
Setting goals	Maximise value whilst minimising resource consumption and environmental impact during goal setting
Studying the system	Study entire systems and scan for social, environmental and economic resource use
Designing the improvement effort	Design interventions which, firstly, minimise the need for healthcare activity and, secondly, the environmental impact of residual activity
Measuring impact/ return on investment	Capture social, environmental and economic impacts, value added and overall outcomes through measurement

Example 14.1: Exploring patient perspectives on healthcare quality

Kelly et al. describe a community art project in East London involving academics, health professionals, and women from the local Bangladeshi community. Through textile workshops, the researchers created a safe environment for sharing of participants' narratives and experiences of key health issues. By creating time and space for storytelling, important and detailed information on care quality was shared, something which cannot be captured through quantitative means (22).

Equally, recording narratives from the professional perspective is pivotal, as staff values and professional norms influence staff attitudes and approach to co-design of services. This information can be gathered through traditional qualitative interviews (Example 14.2), or more creatively through means of 'narrative clinical supervision'. The latter involves 'retelling' of the patient's story through the professional lens, whereby the clinician challenges the patient's underlying beliefs and interpretations by asking targeted clarifying questions (19).

Example 14.2: Exploring how clinicians understand and assess healthcare quality

Farr and Cressey used grounded theory qualitative, in-depth interviews with 21 members of staff (including clinical and non-clinical members) from a Primary Care Trust (PCT) to explore how they understood and assessed quality in everyday practice. Instead of quantitative and biometric markers, they found that staff assess quality through a myriad of qualitative, social, emotional and relational aspects of care such as professional experience, tacit clinical knowledge, personal standards and values, and conversations with patients and families (23).

The importance of gathering more nuanced, qualitative data also comes to light when examining the day-to-day practices of maintaining and improving quality in healthcare settings. For example, the concept of 'trust' was found to be built on more than just the doctor–patient relationship and included assurances of consistency and predictability in all aspects of patient care. Similarly, the act of 'coding' of medical notes in primary care surgeries was discovered to not only consist of recording specific data, but was shaped by staff interpretation and judgement. These findings were only identified by analysing the ethnographic data in a context-specific manner, to provide richer and more relevant insights.

Employing socially informed approaches to collecting data could lead to more 'illuminative', multi-perspective outcomes and measures that may be unintended. This clears the stage for a process where collected care quality information is not merely used to derive a conclusion, but instead instigates discussion. We explore the uses and types of sociological evaluation methods in more detail in the final subsection of the chapter (19).

Real-time data

For collected data to have maximum impact, it should be provided in a timely fashion and to the appropriate people, such as those who can impact change based on the results. Moreover, the information needs to be measured, acknowledged and actioned in 'real time', in contrast to the traditional linear, time sequential approach. Complexity science is valuable in this area as it can be used to investigate the reverberating interactions amongst the components in a health-based CAS. As a result, information is constantly evolving and measurement methods need to mirror this. One possible approach is emulating feedback loops, where change in one part of the system is transmitted to the rest (12).

Imperfect data

The challenge in using real-world data sets is that they are often imprecise, unpredictable and broad due to their inherent nature. Employing standard data analysis methods to analyse them could produce flawed and suboptimal results, potentially risking the data being either over-interpreted, or dismissed entirely. Instead, it would be more valuable to adopt an emergent approach that recognises the imperfection of the data and strives to incorporate it productively into QI efforts (7).

For example, Wolpert and Rutter examine how the legal system approaches imperfect data. The UK courts require different standards of evidence depending on the severity of the consequence of a decision made using the evidence, ranging from 'beyond reasonable doubt' (used for criminal cases) to 'on the balance of probabilities' (for civil cases)

(24). Further research applying these techniques in healthcare settings is necessary, as well as exploring effective methods of leveraging pluralistic data sets to drive meaningful and impactful QI initiatives (7).

Viewing variation differently

Traditional QI practices, based on mechanical models, view variation in how healthcare systems perform and operate 'negatively'. This approach hopes to minimise poor performance and encourage the uptake of practices associated with quality of care. However, while this applies to practices which are widely agreed and contain a level of certainty, such as the use of hand hygiene in clinical settings, such a negative approach may be less applicable to more uncertain practices. Given the idiosyncratic nature of healthcare systems, eliminating variation for less certain practices can be difficult to implement and suffocate emerging, locally devised practices which have the potential to exceed quality expectations. For instance, nationally mandated service frameworks or detailed guidelines.

Instead, complexity-informed approaches will have a more nuanced view of variation, and equal attention will be paid to areas of high *and* low performance. This will enable the spread of learning from successful practices, for example, by studying the practices of surgical teams with low post-operative infection rates as well as those with high rates (25).

Priming healthcare systems for change

An important common attribute of successful health improvement initiatives is the readiness and capacity of the healthcare system to absorb and integrate changes. Priming an organisation for innovation and transformation requires assessment, followed by a multi-level approach at both the individual and leadership level. We can think about this as the various ingredients needed to build a 'learning health system', defined as one in which 'science, informatics, incentives, and culture are aligned for continuous improvement and innovation, with best practices seamlessly embedded in the delivery process and new knowledge captured as an integral by-product of the delivery experience' (14).

Assessing readiness for change

Healthcare systems, similar to homeostatic systems, are primed to maintain the status quo. This can manifest as organisational resilience to external stimuli, but may also be characterised as inertia and resistance to change. On the other hand, when a homeostatic system is far from equilibrium, a cascade of actions are triggered which return the system to its steady state. In this regard, events which displace healthcare systems from their equilibrium point can act as tipping points for change, where small influences can have a great impact (16,26). For example, the COVID-19 pandemic resulted in the largest uptake of telemedicine that has ever been seen before, overcoming years of resistance to its widespread uptake (27). Assessing a system's point of equilibrium, and timing improvement efforts accordingly can, therefore, be useful in harnessing the homeostatic and adaptive capability of healthcare systems (26).

Another important aspect in recognising a system's readiness for change is identifying local restraints which can hinder progress. For instance, through studying 22 evidence translation projects, Reed et al. found that significant energy was often required to overcome dependent issues relating to people, processes or structures, or to resolve existing problems with 'usual care', before the original project focus could be realised (3). Furthermore, by analysing surveys from 56 innovation projects, Leedham-Green et al. demonstrated that a highly significant factor in projects achieving their intended value was having the right number of staff with the relevant expertise, time and energy (28). As such, investing time in analysing systemic issues before improvement efforts can increase the chance of success.

Participatory culture, adaptive capability and use of information and technology

Participatory culture involves organisational efforts to motivate its members to proactively engage in change efforts. It also requires a culture where members are encouraged to intuitively tailor the suggested change to their local organisational context (14).

In order to skilfully undertake this task of customising the change design, the workforce needs to be educated in adaptive capability (as opposed to just competence), where they are trained to react flexibly to change, develop new theories and continually build their performance. These skills are best learned through non-linear, process-driven techniques, in which the syllabus is dynamic, based on learning needs, includes allocated time for reflective study, and may also involve group-based exercises such as facilitated case discussions or role play (7). Moreover, this requires the creative use of technologies, both for learning capability *and* for applying those skills to change initiatives. These should, therefore, be made widely available and easily accessible (7,14).

Distributed leadership

Distributed leadership is about enabling leaders to cultivate a way of thinking within healthcare systems which acknowledges the evolving connections and interactions between various components of the system, as well as their collective strength to be greater than the individual components. The most effective way for these different parts to work in synchrony towards a common goal is through sharing the responsibility of management and leadership (14). This can be done by transparent sharing of outcomes, as well as pre-agreed 'minimum specifications' which provide direction, boundaries, resources and permissions for a particular performance aim instead of top-down, complicated and rigid plans. As such, minimum specifications permit innovation and creative thinking where various stakeholders can make their own judgements. They also allow stakeholders to modify changes to their local context while maintaining the targets of the whole system, and to optimise the use of local resources (14,25).

Designing interventions, implementation and evaluation

Once an improvement goal has been identified and evaluated, and the system primed for change, the next phase can begin. An improvement project then involves designing an intervention, implementation and, finally, evaluation.

Designing interventions

An intervention is an action taken which aims to improve a particular outcome. This can take the form of a new policy, practice, service, pathway, procedure or treatment. Interventions can be simple or complex depending on the number of components, people affected and behavioural changes required. Moreover, interventions can be identified and selected from existing policy or practice, or be developed based on knowledge of the problem in relation to the context and available evidence. Regardless, the degree to which interventions are successful strongly relies upon their characteristics (17).

Firstly, interventions must have a plausible mechanism of action. Interventions used or developed elsewhere might be supported by evidence of their effectiveness; however, advances in QI research have shown that context matters, and transferability of effectiveness across different contexts cannot be assumed. As a result, the National Institute for Health Research (NIHR) and Medical Research Council's (MRC) framework for developing and evaluating complex interventions refers to interventions containing an underpinning programme theory. This describes how an intervention is expected to work, and under what conditions. Not only is a programme theory important for describing an intervention's active ingredients, but it helps to demonstrate how the intervention can be refined and adapted to the local context without hindering its fidelity (17). Interventions which are more adaptable, while maintaining their fidelity, will have an increased chance of being widely adopted (12,17).

The programme theory can be illustrated through the use of diagrams, such as a driver diagram, which is a visual representation of an intervention's cause and effect. For instance, in North West London, a large regional project aiming to investigate the impact and application of QI methods demonstrated how programme theory can be shown through use of driver diagrams, or 'action effect diagrams' as they prefer to call them, using an example from a project implementing a chronic obstructive pulmonary disease (COPD) care bundle (Figure 14.3 (29)). The diagram was useful in guiding implementation and evaluation efforts. The authors, however, highlight the importance of revising the diagram throughout the development of an intervention, as new information becomes available about strengths and weaknesses of theorised causal relationships. Co-production was also vital, involving all relevant stakeholders (e.g. staff, patients, senior management and academics) to reduce conflict, align motivations and aid communication and understanding between stakeholder groups (29).

In addition to effectiveness, interventions must also be feasible. This is determined by ease of intervention implementation and evaluation, and cost. Feasibility trials and evaluation assessments are increasingly done to establish if an intervention can or should be done, how it can be done, and how an intervention's cost and impact can be measured (12,17,30). Since feasibility is context dependent, it is important these assessments are performed within the intended healthcare system. Once feasibility of an intervention has been determined, its true value can be estimated. This can help stakeholders calculate the acceptability and sustainability of an intervention (Example 14.3) (17,28,29).

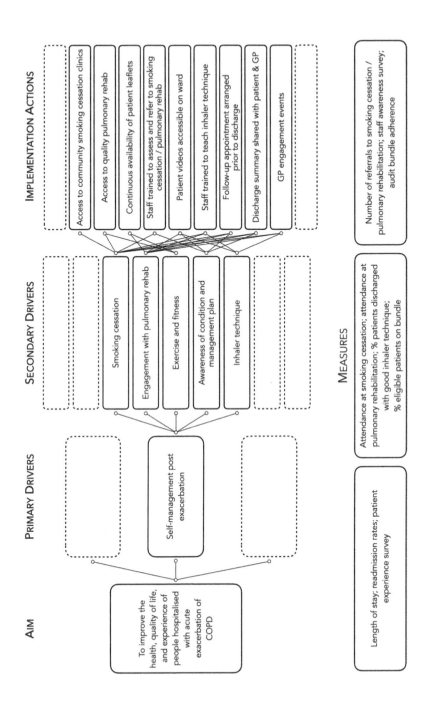

Figure 14.3 Example driver diagram for a COPD improvement initiative implementing a new care bundle. CNS, Clinical Nurse Specialist; GP, general practitioner; PR, pulmonary rehabilitation. Reproduced from Reed et al. 2014 (29) with permission from BMJ Publishing Group Ltd.

Example 14.3: A feasibility study

Researchers in Canada utilised feasibility assessment to test a new evidence-based pulmonary embolism (PE) diagnostic protocol to increase rates of diagnosis and reduce use of unnecessary imaging in three emergency departments (EDs). They uncovered a major measurement barrier which they were able to overcome, which was finding an electronic database able to provide timely data. However, they were unable to overcome this barrier at one of the three ED sites, making implementation unfeasible (31). The exercise, therefore, was critical in identifying local restraints and in preventing a huge waste of time and resources.

Designing an intervention which is both effective and feasible within healthcare systems can be challenging, and increases with the complexity of the intervention, quality problem and healthcare system. This is because they involve more components which are intricately interwoven and behave unpredictably (17,29). For example, the NASSS framework (Non-adoption, or Abandonment of technology by individuals and difficulties achieving Scale-Up, Spread and Sustainability), which provides a systematic means of analysing the adaptability and scalability of medical technologies, predicts that successful implementation is dependent upon the complexity of the condition, the technology and the adopter system, in addition to other factors such as the technology's value and wider organisational and contextual setting (18).

Complexity science and sociological approaches advocate techniques which embrace these complexities, instead of attempting to eradicate or control them (7). For instance, by using collaborative, participatory and bottom-up models for the selection, design or adaptation of interventions. These include participatory adaptation, facilitated evolution, 3S scale-up infrastructure, breakthrough collaboratives and evidence-based co-design (Table 14.2 (14)). Such models enable emergence of successful interventions, self-organisation and adaptation at the local level, and are broad approaches which help manage complexity and conflict in a productive, creative and reflexive manner. In other words, they overcome unsurmountable or hidden barriers to effectiveness and feasibility by encouraging those who form the system (and know it best) to take a leading role in designing interventions (12,13,14).

Table 14.2 Complex and socially informed models for designing interventions

Name of model (author, year)	Key components	Comment
Participatory adaptation (Øvretveit, 2010)	In the context of international health, use of decentralised planning, pragmatic modification and improvement facilitators to adapt the operational details of an intervention to local circumstances.	Proposed as a flexible way of achieving standardisation, replication and accountability while also respecting emergence and adaptation at the local level.
Facilitated adaptation (Øvretveit, 2010)	Local sites are supported to develop the capacity to find, adapt and develop practice and models of care that tackle the challenges they face, with no external expectation placed on how problems are framed or which solutions are to be adopted. Draws on the concept of resilience (defined as a system's capability to recover from internal tensions and external shocks).	More radical approach than participatory adaptation. In one example, the goal of preventing HIV/AIDS in a low-income African community was achieved through a community development initiative, which provided women with an independent income.
3S scale-up infrastructure (Øvretveit, 2011)	A combination of strategic leadership, innovation culture, high-quality data capture systems, and adaptive facilitation.	These should not be viewed as mechanical tools to be applied deterministically to 'solve' complexity (though formulaic versions of the breakthrough collaborative model exist). Rather, they are broad approaches that might be used creatively and reflexively to manage complexity.
Breakthrough collaboratives (Øvretveit, 2011)	Provision of resources, infrastructure and impetus for inter-organisational exchange of resources, stories and ideas oriented to achieving an improvement goal – typically through periodic collaborative workshops.	
Experience-based co-design (Bate and Rober, 2006)	In collaborative workshops and in preparatory and follow-up work together with staff to identify emotional 'touch points' in the patient journey and redesign the service in a way that centres on improving the patient experience.	Not explicitly focused on complexity, but follows many of the principles of effective change in complex systems – notably self-organisation, collective sense-making, and harnessing conflict productively.

Implementation

After an intervention has been designed and its feasibility tested, it needs to be implemented and embedded into routine practice. Previously, it was assumed that interventions would travel from 'bench to bedside' in a linear, stepwise manner, and those backed by evidence of their effectiveness would be automatically adopted by front-line staff. In this regard, a mechanical 'pipeline' model to implementation was taken for granted. However, it is now starkly apparent that implementation is far more complex, with many evidence-based practices experiencing tortuous, unpredictable and paradoxical journeys (12).

As a result, implementation science has begun using the social and complexity science lenses, including the CAS model, to build more effective implementation methods. These models accept the complex and socially determined nature of embedding interventions into practice, and view implementation as an ecological process (14,17). For instance, implementation tends to occur over a long period of time in an iterative and recursive manner, not dissimilar to evolution (Example 14.4) (7,12).

Example 14.4: Agile, adaptive implementation

Braithwaite et al. describe the implementation of a graded warning system to prompt rapid review of deteriorating inpatients. This case study demonstrates the iterative, recursive and long-term nature of quality improvement efforts. Previous attempts to introduce rapid response systems had failed but a tipping point was reached after the tragic preventable death of a teenager. The ultimately successful implementation was the result of years of momentum-building, and agile adaptation in response to feedback. This resulted in a system that worked and was successfully spread across 225 hospitals in New South Wales, Australia. Each step, however, required extensive preparatory work and continual revision in response to feedback as the implementation unfolded (12).

In this regard, it is important to factor in the necessary time and resources required for implementation and relax expectations accordingly. Long et al. promote the importance of embracing emergent outcomes and being flexible in adherence to predetermined implementation plans.

They go on to recommend adaptive use of implementation methods and reflexive mixed methods to match ever-changing research contexts (13,17).

For example, during a research project implementing a simulation model to aid decision-making for a senior leadership group overseeing a large public mental health service in Australia, researchers altered the focus of their simulation modelling in response to the state government changing its strategic priorities towards planning for population growth. Subsequently, greater modelling outputs in this direction resulted in a successful lobbying bid for increased mental health funding released by the state government (13). This case illustrates the unpredictable course of implementation processes shaped by both wider contextual factors and the unique characteristics of the adopter system. Each implementation effort, therefore, requires an individualistic approach instead of aiming towards universal formulae (7).

Implementation approaches also need to be socially informed, given all interventions require behavioural change of some sort in order to become incorporated into routine practice. Such approaches seek to understand and influence the social factors which affect stakeholder adoption. For example, how and why people perceive an intervention in particular ways, or how internalised rules, mental models, motivations and agency alter behaviour (13,14).

Considering the degree to which social factors influence outcomes in human CAS, some researchers posit that a delineation should exist between the theory underlying CAS containing humans, and those containing other types of biological entity (for example, animals or cells); with the former being the realm of social complexity theory, and the latter of classical complexity theory. For example, while agents contained within classical CAS are solely motivated by survival, humans within CAS are motivated by their particular end-goal, which is often emotionally and cognitively influenced. This adds an additional layer of complexity to CAS involving humans, warranting the incorporation of socially informed approaches over ecological ones alone (13).

Social factors are predicted to differ depending on the level of abstraction on which they occur, with varying rules for individuals (micro), organisations (meso) and society as a whole (macro) (13,14). While the individual is governed by local rules and regulations, as well as informal practices and traditions, organisations are governed by wider societal forces such as public expectation, politics, laws, policies and commercial and other interests (13). Taking this into account, in order for an intervention to be adopted into routine practice and 'normalised', it either needs to align with existing individual, organisational and societal rules, or disrupt these and make the case for new ones (25).

Aligning an intervention with existing social rules or behavioural 'attractor patterns' contained by healthcare systems can be helpful in avoiding resistance to change (25). For example, Greenhalgh and Papoutsi discuss the social factors behind successful implementation of a technical checklist for the insertion of central venous catheters. The implementation effort was led by respected university leaders and aligned with what a 'good' intensive care unit was deemed to be. As a result, the checklist was adopted in over 100 intensive care units in America, resulting in huge reductions in the rates of catheter associated infection (14). However, determining a system's social rules can be challenging and requires robust interviewing strategies alongside stakeholder candour (13).

On the other hand, disrupting existing social rules during the implementation phase requires individuals to adapt (14). One way of easing this process is to allow individuals the space to self-determine how interventions can be incorporated and encourage collaborative working. This can be done by setting 'minimum specifications', as discussed in the previous section of the chapter (25).

Additionally, certain frameworks have been developed which aim to analyse the necessary social processes for adoption of interventions. For instance, normalisation process theory outlines four steps which individuals and teams do in order to integrate new behaviours and normalise them, including coherence (or sense-making), cognitive participation (or engagement), collective action (work done to enable the intervention to happen) and reflexive monitoring (formal and informal appraisal of the intervention's value) (14,32). The framework has been used to explore reasons for non-adoption and alter implementation processes accordingly, or to abandon them altogether (32).

Evaluation

While evaluation of an intervention is the final phase of an improvement project, its consideration and planning occur throughout (see Chapter 4 re: planning research; also Chapter 17: evaluating complex interventions), and any measures are ideally embedded at the planning stage. In the first section of this chapter, we explored assessment of the primary outcome, or improvement goal, and much of what was discussed there also applies here. However, evaluation of interventions in complex healthcare systems needs to consider more than the primary outcome and effectiveness of the intervention alone. Analysis also needs to focus on *how* the intervention leads to improvement, as well as under what circumstances, its impact on the rest of the system, and its resource consumption. Only then will information be gained about an intervention's active ingredients, necessary conditions, value and sustainability (13,14,17).

Process measures capture the quality of the implementation process and whether or not the intervention is being implemented as expected. They are, therefore, useful in explaining observable outcomes, in addition to other dependent and contextual variables (17). To select process measures, it is important to have a strong understanding of an intervention's mechanism of action and, as mentioned previously, a driver diagram can be helpful for this purpose (17,28). For example, in the driver diagram used in a project implementing a COPD care bundle (Figure 14.3), they were able to demonstrate the percentage of initial and completed patients. In addition, they were able to evaluate upstream effects through measuring the number of smoking cessation referrals, inhaler technique observations and number of pulmonary rehabilitation attendances (29).

Balance measures have typically been used to measure the impact of an intervention elsewhere in the system. Traditionally, these have been restricted to measuring predictable, linear (usually negative) outcomes in isolated parts of the system. However, given the social and complex nature of healthcare systems, balance measures also need to capture how the intervention alters the functions, relationships, behaviours, social rules and emergent outcomes of the system as a whole (14,17). To capture this type of often nuanced information, better use needs to be made of sociological, qualitative and mixed evaluation methods, such as ethnography, case studies, times-series analysis, social network analysis and social surveys (Table 14.3) (Example 14.5) (13,14,17).

Finally, changes to complex systems are likely to generate unintended as well as intended outcomes. Some of these may be beneficial, such as feelings of belonging through improved teamwork. Others may be less beneficial, such as additional burdens on patients or staff. Illuminative approaches to evaluation invite the evaluator to assess both processes and outcomes through a fresh lens, identifying work 'as done', rather than 'as imagined', and outcomes 'as experienced' rather than 'as intended' (38,39).

Table 14.3 Socially informed evaluation methods and their descriptions

Method	Description
Ethnography	Ethnography is a qualitative research method in which a researcher – an ethnographer – studies a particular social/cultural group with the aim to better understand it. An ethnographer actively participates in the group in order to gain an insider's perspective of the group and to have experiences similar to the group member. In writing an ethnography, an ethnographer creates an account of the group based on this participation, interviews with group members, and an analysis of group documents and artefacts.[33]
Case study	A case study is an intensive, systematic investigation of a single individual, group, community or some other unit in which the researcher examines in-depth data relating to several variables.[34]
Actor-network theory	Actor-network theory (ANT) focuses on the connections that are being made and remade between human and non-human entities that are part of the issues at stake. It goes beyond boundaries that are usually set: ANT does not stop the investigation when it enters contexts or so-called underlying structures. Tracing back connections can be done by (participatory) observation, document analysis, or in-depth interviews.[35]
Social network analysis	Social network analysis (SNA) is a collection of methods and tools that can be used to study relationships, interactions and communications through visualisation and mathematical analysis. SNA visualisation renders relationships between actors in social networks by graphs known as sociograms. SNA mathematical analysis quantifies network parameters on individual actor levels, as well as group levels, using graph theory concepts such as actor distance and the number of interactions.[36]
Social survey	Social surveys collect mainly quantitative but also qualitative data from (usually representative) samples of people, by means of their verbal responses to uniform sets of systematic structured questions presented either by interviewers or in self-completion questionnaires.[37]

Example 14.5: Participatory processes and expansive exploration

Auto-ethnography was used to analyse evidence translation in complex systems via 22 QI projects, which were carried out in North West London over a five-year period. By using auto-ethnography, the researchers were able to gain proximity to the system and build long-term relationships with participants. In turn, this facilitated detailed observation of the system over an extended period of time. This enabled more candid accounts of how the system operated, what unfolded, and the reasons why. As such, they developed a deeper understanding of the complex and socially dependent factors for change, and were able to generate an explanatory and predictive framework for approaching evidence translation and improvement in healthcare (3). Similar methods include the 'researcher-in-residence' model, which sees health service researchers embedded within service-based teams attempting to improve the quality of care (40).

Conclusion

The improvement of healthcare quality can be a slow and challenging process because of the complex and social nature of healthcare systems. In this chapter, we have explored how traditional, reductionist approaches, built on mechanistic models, have fallen short in providing realistic insights into how healthcare systems behave. To date, this has limited our ability to build more effective improvement methods, and harness some of the resilient and adaptable properties of healthcare systems.

However, a paradigm shift is happening and researchers are starting to embrace social and complexity-informed approaches, which have been built on learning gained from the fields of social and complexity science. These approaches include greater use of qualitative, sociological, reflexive and mixed-methods approaches to identifying improvement goals, assessing quality, designing and implementing interventions, and evaluating their impact (see also Chapter 4).

Social and complexity-informed approaches also recognise that improvement occurs as a result of the unique dance between the adopter system, intervention, wider context and improvement process, and that an individualistic approach to improvement is required. Furthermore, they recognise that change happens in a recursive, iterative and long-term manner. Therefore, it is important to prime healthcare systems for continual improvement; adopt collaborative and co-productive change processes to gain expert insights and stakeholder buy-in; embrace local tailoring of interventions and use of feasibility assessment; allow necessary time and resources for improvement; and embrace flexible research methods and emergent outcomes.

Future research needs to focus on refining these techniques and building a stronger knowledge base on which improvement methodologies are appropriate in particular circumstances, such as population characteristics, context (primary versus secondary care), resource availability, potential impact and intervention type. Additionally, given systems are composed of people, future research must examine how best to connect, utilise and facilitate the people within systems, build capability, and embrace the concept of learning health systems. There also needs to be greater dissemination of social and complexity-informed approaches and training within mainstream QI curricula and practices. This should help healthcare teams increase the sustainability of changes and reduce improvement waste, which is particularly important given the current healthcare climate. Finally, we must continue to develop better data collection techniques, technologies and system-based models, given their associated workload benefits, and ability to both catalyse improvement and help teams understand systems.

Further resources

Introductory QI material:

- Institute for Healthcare Improvement's (IHI) Open School Improvement Capability course (41).
- NHS England's Quality, Service Improvement and Redesign (QSIR) College program and resources (42,43).
- NHS England Improvement Fundamentals Course (44).
- A Trainee's Guide to a Quality Improvement Project (45).
- The Health Foundation Quality Improvement Made Simple (46).
- Sustainability through Quality Improvement (SusQI) Toolkit (47).

References

1. White F. Primary health care and public health: foundations of universal health systems. *Medical Principles and Practice.* 2015;24(2):103–16.
2. Busse R, Panteli D, Quentin W. An introduction to healthcare quality: defining and explaining its role in health systems. In: Busse R, Klazinga N, Panteli D et al. *Improving Healthcare Quality in Europe: Characteristics, effectiveness and implementation of different strategies.* European Observatory on Health Systems and Policies; 2019. Available from: www.ncbi.nlm.nih.gov/books/NBK549277/ (accessed 21 March 2024).
3. Reed JE, Howe C, Doyle C, Bell D. Simple rules for evidence translation in complex systems: a qualitative study. *BMC Medicine.* 2018;16(92).
4. Dixon-Woods M. How to improve healthcare improvement – an essay by Mary Dixon-Woods. *BMJ.* 2019;367:l5514.
5. Fraser SW, Greenhalgh T. Complexity science: coping with complexity: educating for capability. *BMJ.* 2001;323(7316):799–803.
6. Murray R. The health and care system is in crisis: what should (and shouldn't) be done? The King's Fund. 2022. Available from: www.kingsfund.org.uk/blog/2022/08/health-and-care-system-crisis-what-should-and-shouldnt-be-done (accessed 21 March 2024).
7. Greenhalgh T, Papoutsi C. Studying complexity in health services research: desperately seeking an overdue paradigm shift. *BMC Medicine.* 2018;16(95).
8. Ward D, Chijoko L. Spending on and availability of health care resources. The King's Fund. 2018. Available from: www.kingsfund.org.uk/publications/spending-and-availability-health-care-resources (accessed 21 March 2024).
9. Thaul S, Lohr KN, Tranquada RE. A Working Definition of Health Services Research. National Academies Press; 1994. Available from: www.ncbi.nlm.nih.gov/books/NBK231502/ (accessed 21 March 2024).
10. Bauer MS, Damschroder L, Hagedorn H, Smith J, Kilbourne AM. An introduction to implementation science for the non-specialist. *BMC Psychology.* 2015;3(1).
11. The Health Foundation. Improvement science. The Health Foundation; 2011. Available from: www.health.org.uk/publications/improvement-science (accessed 21 March 2024).
12. Braithwaite J, Churruca K, Long JC, Ellis LA, Herkes J. When complexity science meets implementation science: a theoretical and empirical analysis of systems change. *BMC Medicine.* 2018;16(63). Available from: www.ncbi.nlm.nih.gov/pmc/articles/PMC5925847/ (accessed 21 March 2024).
13. Long KM, McDermott F, Meadows GN. Being pragmatic about healthcare complexity: our experiences applying complexity theory and pragmatism to health services research. *BMC Medicine.* 2018;16(1).
14. Greenhalgh T, Papoutsi C. Spreading and scaling up innovation and improvement. *BMJ.* 2019; l2068.
15. Jayasinghe S. Complexity science to conceptualize health and disease: is it relevant to clinical medicine? *Mayo Clinic Proceedings.* 2012;87(4):314–9.
16. Wilson T, Holt T, Greenhalgh T. Complexity science: complexity and clinical care. *BMJ.* 2001;323(7314):685–8.
17. Skivington K, Matthews L, Simpson SA, Craig P, Baird J, Blazeby JM et al. A new framework for developing and evaluating complex interventions: update of Medical Research Council guidance. *BMJ.* 2021;374:n2061.
18. Greenhalgh T, Wherton J, Papoutsi C, Lynch J, Hughes G, A'Court C, et al. Analysing the role of complexity in explaining the fortunes of technology programmes: empirical application of the NASSS framework. *BMC Medicine.* 2018;16(1).
19. Swinglehurst D, Emmerich N, Maybin J, Park S, Quilligan S. Confronting the quality paradox: towards new characterisations of 'quality' in contemporary healthcare. *BMC Health Services Research.* 2015;15(1):1–6.
20. Isherwood J, Mortimer F, Vaux E, Wilkinson A. Sustainability in quality improvement: redefining value. *Future Healthcare Journal.* 2018;5(2):88–93.
21. Mortimer F. The sustainable physician. *Clin Med (Lond).* 2010;10(2):110–11.
22. Kelly M, Rivas C, Foell J, Llewellyn-Dunn J, England D, Cocciadiferro A, et al. Unmasking quality: exploring meanings of health by doing art. *BMC Family Practice.* 2015;16(1).
23. Farr M, Cressey P. Understanding staff perspectives of quality in practice in healthcare. *BMC Health Services Research.* 2015;15(123). Available from: https://bmchealthservres.biomedcentral.com/articles/10.1186/s12913-015-0788-1 (accessed 21 March 2024).

24. Wolpert M, Rutter H. Using flawed, uncertain, proximate and sparse (FUPS) data in the context of complexity: learning from the case of child mental health. *BMC Medicine*. 2018;16(1).
25. Plsek PE, Wilson T. Complexity, leadership, and management in healthcare organisations. *BMJ*. 2001;323(7315):746–9.
26. Torday J. Homeostasis as the mechanism of evolution. *Biology*. 2015;4(3):573–90.
27. Ahmed S, Sanghvi K, Yeo D. Telemedicine takes centre stage during COVID-19 pandemic. *BMJ Innovations*. 2020;6(4);252–4.
28. Leedham-Green K, Knight A, Reedy GB. Success and limiting factors in health service innovation: a theory-generating mixed methods evaluation of UK projects. *BMJ Open*. 2021;11(5):e047943.
29. Reed JE, McNicholas C, Woodcock T, Issen L, Bell D. Designing quality improvement initiatives: the action effect method, a structured approach to identifying and articulating programme theory. *BMJ Quality & Safety*. 2014;23(12):1040–8.
30. Eldridge SM, Chan CL, Campbell MJ, Bond CM, Hopewell S, Thabane L, et al. CONSORT 2010 statement: extension to randomised pilot and feasibility trials. *BMJ*. 2016;i5239.
31. Germini F, Hu Y, Afzal S, Al-haimus F, Puttagunta SA, Niaz S et al. Feasibility of a quality improvement project to increase adherence to evidence-based pulmonary embolism diagnosis in the emergency department. *Pilot and Feasibility Studies*. 2021;7(1).
32. Murray E, Treweek S, Pope C, MacFarlane A, Ballini L, Dowrick C et al. Normalisation process theory: a framework for developing, evaluating and implementing complex interventions. *BMC Medicine*. 2010;8(1).
33. Kramer MW, Adams TE. Ethnography. In: *The SAGE Encyclopedia of Communication Research Methods*. 2017. Available from: https://methods.sagepub.com/reference/the-sage-encyclopedia-of-communication-research-methods/i4910.xml (accessed 21 March 2024).
34. Heale R, Twycross A. What is a case study? *Evidence Based Nursing*. 2018;21(1):7–8.
35. ScienceDirect. Actor Network Theory. Available from: www.sciencedirect.com/topics/social-sciences/actor-network-theory (accessed 21 March 2024).
36. Saqr M, Alamro A. The role of social network analysis as a learning analytics tool in online problem based learning. *BMC Medical Education*. 2019;19(1).
37. Payne G, Payne J. Social surveys. In: *Key Concepts in Social Research*. SAGE; 2004. Available from:https://methods.sagepub.com/book/key-concepts-in-social-research/n46.xml(accessed21 March 2024).
38. Stufflebeam DL, Shinkfield AJ. Illuminative evaluation: the holistic approach. In: *Systematic Evaluation: A Self-Instructional Guide to Theory and Practice*. Springer Netherlands; 1985. pp. 285–310.
39. Hollnagel E. *Safety-I and Safety-II: The past and future of safety management*. CRC Press; 2018.
40. Marshall M, Pagel C, French C, Utley M, Allwood D, Fulop N et al. Moving improvement research closer to practice: the Researcher-in-Residence model: Table 1. *BMJ Quality & Safety*. 2014;23(10):801–5.
41. Institute for Healthcare Improvement. Get Started with the IHI Open School. Available from: www.ihi.org/education/ihi-open-school/ (accessed 24 March 2023).
42. NHS England. Quality, service improvement and redesign (QSIR). Available from: https://aqua.nhs.uk/QSIR/ (accessed 21 March 2024).
43. NHS England. Quality, service improvement and redesign (QSIR) tools. Available from: https://aqua.nhs.uk/qsir-tools/ (accessed 21 March 2024).
44. NHS Health at Work Network. Improvement Fundamentals. Available from: https://www.nhshealthatwork.co.uk/ohprogrammes.asp#:~:text=Improvement%20Fundamentals%20is%20a%20programme,support%20individual's%20own%20improvement%20projects (accessed 21 March 2024).
45. Watts D, Limbachia D, Surana N. A Trainee's Guide to a Quality Improvement Project. Royal College of Surgeons. 2021. Available from: www.rcseng.ac.uk/-/media/files/rcs/standards-and-research/standards-and-policy/good-practice-guides/2021/rcs-england-trainees-guide-to-a-quality-improvement-project-2021.pdf (accessed 22 March 2024).
46. The Health Foundation. Quality Improvement Made Simple: What everyone should know about health care quality improvement. 2021. Available from: www.health.org.uk/sites/default/files/QualityImprovementMadeSimple.pdf (accessed 21 March 2024).
47. Centre for Sustainable Healthcare. SusQI Toolkit | Sustainable Quality Improvement. Available from: www.susqi.org (accessed 1 June 2023).

Part IV: Generalist interactions

In the previous three parts of this book, we have discussed the academic, structural and educational approaches that underpin clinical generalism. We conclude with perhaps the most important part: interactional approaches. Building on the generalist clinical consultation described in Chapter 1, we introduce narrative medicine (Chapter 15), prescribing and deprescribing (Chapter 16), salutogenic medicine (Chapter 17) and personalised approaches to multimorbidity (Chapter 18). These bring the concepts of generalism to life alongside practical suggestions for ways in which effective learning might be operationalised.

15
Interactional knowledge

Graham Easton

Introduction

This chapter explores the role of interactional knowledge in generalist
practice and education. Interactional knowledge refers to the knowledge
and skills needed to communicate and interact effectively with patients,
carers, families, colleagues and teams. This chapter focuses on the generalist consultation.

The prominence of evidence-based medicine, protocolised care and
management guidelines are pointers to the historical dominance of scientific over interactional knowledge in modern medicine. This chapter
argues that interactional knowledge is in fact the glue that holds healthcare together; and that generalists in particular must be able to integrate
both these types of knowledge within the consultation to make effective
diagnoses and provide meaningful person-centred care. It also highlights
the importance of authentic collaboration between clinician and patient
in personalising and democratising generalist healthcare. It argues that a
narrative understanding of interactions between patient and clinician is
central to the interpretive model of generalism – the co-creation between
clinician and patient of a personalised account of the patient's experience of illness and a plan for action (1). It explores some of the key narrative capabilities that generalists need in order to navigate uncertain
and complex consultations, including feeling and showing empathy for
the patient, how to identify and listen to stories, and acknowledge their
own personal journeys through clinical practice (2). Using examples
from consultation interactions, it shows how tuning into the subtleties
of language and non-verbal communication in the consultation is central to holistic generalist care, and touches on some key barriers to effective communication including language, culture and hearing or vision

impairment. Finally, the chapter suggests how generalists might adapt these approaches and skills to the new digital remote consulting landscape of phone, video and e-consultations.

Interpretation in generalist consultations

Many problems in generalist healthcare respond well to a simple biomedical approach – for example removing ear wax, a prescription for the oral contraceptive pill, or steroid cream for a stubborn patch of eczema. But one of the prominent features of generalist consultations is that patients often do not present with a single problem, easily definable within a biomedical model of disease. Instead, problems are often undifferentiated and contextual, and they have not been pre-sorted by pathology, organ or system. Generalists are used to grappling with multiple problems, complexity and uncertainty – the so-called 'swampy lowlands' of clinical practice (3) – and when there is no clear diagnosis or treatment (sometimes the case with, for example, 'I feel tired all the time', or 'I just don't seem my normal self'), healthcare professionals still need to support patients in living their lives. How we understand and make sense of our illnesses affects how well we flourish, whether or not healthcare can offer cure or palliation (4), and helping people make sense of their illnesses is a fundamental role of the generalist approach.

The expert generalist, navigating the grey and swampy areas of clinical practice, often needs to integrate the biomedical and the biographical to construct, with the patient, a joint account of illness that meets the needs of both. Reeve has crystallised this facet of generalism in her Interpretive Medicine model (1): for her, generalism is about interpretation of illness, not so much identification of disease. She draws on the ideas of Kvale (5) to characterise generalism in terms of a clinician 'travelling with' the patient to co-create meaning in illness. Attention to this interactional dimension of the consultation, and its integration with the biomedical, goes to the heart of the generalist consultation.

Two voices in harmony in the generalist consultation

In this interpretive role, the generalist clinician needs to 'travel with' the patient, paying close attention to the patient's experiences and interpretations of their illness, while also acknowledging the influence of their own experiences, and not forgetting the essential biomedical aspects of the task. Sometimes this can be a struggle, like rubbing your stomach and patting your head at the same time. Mishler (6) refers to this struggle as a conflict between the 'voice of medicine' (the more technical, biomedical frame of reference), and the 'voice of the lifeworld', reflecting the patient's personal, 'contextually-grounded experiences of events and problems' (p. 104). Too often, suggests Mishler, the voice of medicine dominates the discourse; what the generalist aims for is the two voices in harmony. Both are vital to both patient and professional.

The central role of stories

At the heart of the generalist consultation, then, is this interpretive role, aiming for an account of illness and a plan of action that works for both patient and clinician (7). In order to achieve this complex task, generalists need to be comfortable dealing in stories – the patient's stories, their own professional and personal stories, and the co-created account (or story) that has real meaning for the patient.

As generalists, we are immersed in stories: from the patient's telling of early symptoms, through experiences of treatments and effects on daily life. Every episode of care is interpreted in story form, whether in patient records, letters or chats between professionals, or storytelling in the consultation. The stories in consultations may be brief ('my asthma is worse'), fragmented, or even 'untrue' – but they are still stories, relating events and meanings through the conscious and unconscious choice of words and phrases. Whether seen through the lens of the literary world, psychology or communication, narrative (I will use the term synonymously with story here) is understood as a way for people to organise and interpret their world. Stories are how we try to make sense from the chaos of life. If we accept that the goal of the generalist clinician–patient encounter is to organise and interpret the patient's illness with them, then this narrative perspective is critical to the generalist consultation (8).

More specifically, the generalist needs to have what New York physician and pioneer of narrative medicine Rita Charon has described as 'narrative competence': 'the ability to acknowledge, absorb, interpret, and act on the stories and plights of others' (2, p.1897). This narrative approach represents a fundamental shift from the healthcare professional's more traditional stance of 'needing to solve the problem', to 'needing to understand'. It pays full attention to the wider, socially determined elements of a patient's illness, may be therapeutic in itself (in the telling and in being heard), provides alternatives to over-medicalising and over-prescribing, and can offer the possibility for positive change (9).

In practical terms, for the practitioner this co-creation between the narrator and the listener means listening closely, exploring fears, feelings and emotions with compassionate curiosity; and developing a deeper understanding, not only of the illness experience but also of the patient and of the self. It also means involving the patient in meaningful decision-making, negotiating shared management plans and often re-balancing the power dynamics in the consultation. The example below shows how a narrative approach, underpinned by appropriate communication skills, can achieve a much deeper understanding of the patient and his or her illness, offering a holistic assessment and a plan that has real meaning for the patient. The patient and the doctor work together where possible, to co-create a meaningful account, with the patient fully involved in developing a realistic plan. The patient's worries and concerns have been addressed, they have built rapport through empathy and working together, and the key biomedical aspects have been attended to. This narrative approach may take longer, and is not always warranted or appropriate, for example in an emergency; but on the whole evidence and experience suggests it is time well spent in addressing the patient's problems (1).

Example 15.1: A narrative approach to the consultation

Raj Patel is a 45-year-old headteacher at a primary school who has come to see the clinician about some pain in his chest which he has been getting for the last few weeks.

Clinician (Cn):   Mr Patel? Hello ... how can I help you today?

Patient (Pt):   Well, I don't know if it's anything I should be worried about, it's been a hectic time, but I've been getting these pains in my chest ... [*he is looking intently at the clinician, as if gauging the clinician's reaction*]

Cn: OK ... can you tell me more about them?

Pt: Well they're usually right here [*he points to a specific area on his chest wall, above the left nipple. He keeps pressing it*]. It's very sharp, quite severe actually. And I'll see if I can make it happen now – sometimes if I move my shoulder in a certain way it seems to set it off ... no I can't now, but when it comes it can be pretty terrifying to be honest. D'you think I need some tests or a scan, maybe an ECG?

Cn: Well, let me ask you some more questions so I can get a clear idea of your symptoms, and then we can take it from there perhaps?

The clinician and the patient now need to address the urgent bio-medical aspects of the patient's problem; chest pain is potentially serious and there are important symptoms and signs to explore in order to establish a possible diagnosis and next steps in management. Together, guided by the clinician's open questions and then more specific closed questions about the nature of the pain, what brings it on, what makes it worse or better, any relevant medical history and so on, they quickly rule out pain coming from the heart. To the clinician the story sounds much more like costochondritis – inflammation of the joint between a rib and the breastbone, a much more benign condition. But the clinician feels the patient is on edge; he also noticed the patient's anxious look earlier, and his comment 'I don't know if it's anything to worry about', and that he describes the pain as 'terrifying'. He decides to explore this aspect of the patient's story a bit more.

Cn: Earlier, you said you wondered if this was anything to worry about, and you mentioned the pain can be terrifying when it comes. Chest pain and worry do often go together – do you have any particular worries about this – it really helps me to know?

Pt: Well not really, no. I mean obviously I'm worried it might be a heart attack or something like that? Is it a heart attack?

Cn: No, I don't think it's a heart attack – it doesn't sound at all like the sort of pain that comes from the heart. Hopefully that's reassuring?

Pt: Yes absolutely, that's great to hear. [*For a few seconds the patient gazes thoughtfully into the mid-distance. The clinician deliberately stays silent, giving him space to think.*] My father died, actually, from a heart attack. He was only a bit older than me, in his 50s. He seemed fit and healthy [like me], but he did have a very stressful job running a garage. So obviously I want to make sure it's not my heart …

Cn: Yes of course, I'm sorry to hear about your father. You mention
     he had a very stressful job … can I ask if you have any stress in
     your life at the moment? You said it's been a hectic time?

The clinician has chosen to pick up on the stressful job and the hectic time, sensing that this may be significant. The patient then tells the clinician all about the upcoming visit from the school regulator, and how this is causing a great deal of stress to him and his staff, and how he is concerned that the school's recent performance has not been as good as in previous years and he worries about the school's rating being downgraded. The clinician empathises and explores the wider effects on his family life, his sleep and his mood. They discuss how the recent workload to prepare for the visit means he has also neglected exercise and diet, and he is starting to drink more alcohol. The clinician doesn't try to solve any of these problems, or pass judgement on them, but helps the patient to draw connections between his health and recent stress, and how a benign musculoskeletal problem like costochondritis might cause further anxiety given his experiences with his father and the visit from the regulator.

   The clinician then examines the patient, focusing particularly on the cardiovascular system to provide focused reassurance; and to confirm the diagnosis of costochondritis.

Cn: Well, the examination confirms what I was thinking – this is
     something called costochondritis [*he explains this and answers
     the patient's questions about it*]. And also there is nothing here
     that worries me about your heart. So, shall we think about
     next steps now?

The clinician now invites the patient to work together with him on a plan. They discuss his cardiovascular risk score, and agree that the patient needs to focus on his own health again – especially diet and exercise – and the patient suggests he will cut down on the alcohol. Although they agree that an ECG is not called for today, they also decide that it would be sensible to re-check some basic cardiovascular blood tests like cholesterol and blood glucose given his family history. They agree to meet again after these tests to review how lifestyle changes are going, and how the inspection turned out. They agree a safety net plan; what symptoms to look out for, and when to seek medical help more urgently.

Identifying and analysing stories

If dealing in stories is so central to generalist consultations, it follows that generalists should be able to identify stories and their elements in order to make sense of them. This section will help you to listen more closely for stories and to recognise key story elements and structures.

Any young child can spot a story when they see one. Classical stories often come with familiar signifiers ('Once upon a time ...') and follow recognisable structures; for example, the three-act structure with a set-up (introducing the main character and their challenge or goal), the confrontation (telling how the main character struggles to overcome this challenge), and finally the resolution (which resolves the story somehow). This sort of traditional character-based story structure works very well for Hollywood script writers, or novelists, and seems well-designed to engage an audience emotionally, yet very few of our patients tend to tell stories in this way in consultations.

What is needed is a model of the sort of personal, informal, storytelling that patients tend to use in clinical encounters. One such model is that developed by William Labov, which has been widely used and refined in the fields of sociolinguistics, communication and narrative analysis. It is a useful starting point from which to explore the stories patients tell (although it is important to acknowledge its limitations for this purpose, such as its focus on the telling of stories rather than their co-construction, and how it ignores some crucial aspects of narrative interaction such as non-verbal communication, including the significance of what is left unsaid). William Labov is an American sociolinguist who studied hundreds of natural conversations in New York in the 1960s and 1970s (10) and concluded that fully formed natural personal narratives have six key ingredients (see Figure 15.1 adapted (10)). These include: (1) an abstract, which tells what the story is about through a short summary; (2) orientation, identifying the time, place and people; (3) complicating action, in which the clauses relate the temporal sequence of the event (this happened, then that happened); (4) evaluation, in which the narrator describes the significance of the event or point of the story; (5) resolution, which concludes the story; and (6) a coda, which brings the perspective back to the present moment (11,12).

The strengths of Labov's model lie in providing a clear narrative structure and method for analysis, and its wide acceptance across multiple disciplines. Of course, patients do not always tell fully formed stories, and the elements are not always in this neat order. But it offers learners and educators a common language with which to discuss and analyse the

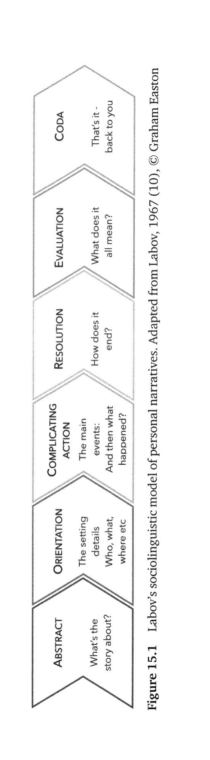

Figure 15.1 Labov's sociolinguistic model of personal narratives. Adapted from Labov, 1967 (10), © Graham Easton

narrative elements of consultations. For example, Labov has described evaluation as 'perhaps the most important element in addition to the basic narrative clause' (11) and Riessman calls it the 'soul of the narrative', telling us what the point of the story is, as well as showing us how the narrator wants to be understood (13). This is a crucial part of the patient's story, it can appear at any point (or even throughout) the story, and is often the element that health professionals have to tease out if it is not forthcoming.

Example 15.2: A consultation analysis using Labov's approach

Clinician [Cn]: Hello. Nice to see you. How can I help today?

Patient [Pt]: Thank you. Well, I've been getting these headaches recently and they just don't seem to be settling down like they normally do. I just can't get rid of them, no matter what I try, so I thought I ought to come and tell you about them. [ABSTRACT]

Cn: OK, well I'm sorry to hear that ... and I'm glad you've come. Roughly how long has it been going on?

Pt: Yes. It's been about a week now – no, it must be more than a week. I think it started around last Monday because that's when I took Jerry to his rehab class. I thought it might have been the long drive that started it off. [ORIENTATION]

Cn: Right. And can you tell me a bit more about these headaches, what they're like and how they're affecting you?

Pt: Well, they're all over here [*points generally to her scalp*]. I can't work out if anything particularly sets them off – sometimes they come during the morning, and sometimes in the afternoon, but they are there, on and off, most of the day. It's not so bad that I can't do anything [COMPLICATING ACTION] – but I do feel exhausted by them; it's just taking it out of me you know? [EVALUATION]

Cn: Yes, I can imagine.

Pt: I do sometimes get headaches – but I've not had them like this before. And not lasting so long – what's that, nearly 10 days now? [COMPLICATING ACTION] It's just that the paracetamol isn't touching it – I can't get rid of them.

> [RESOLUTION] So I thought I'd better come and talk to you about it in case there's something we can do about it you know. [EVALUATION] I'm really hoping you've got a magic potion! [CODA]

However, Labov's model has attracted criticism for its focus on the relationship between narrative clauses rather than the interaction amongst people (12). It also neglects the social and cultural context of storytelling, and prioritises the what over the how of storytelling. Polanyi and others have expanded the Labov model to include the crucial elements of co-creation between teller and listener, acknowledging that they both have a key role in shaping the shared story (14). For example, the task of problem-setting at the start of a consultation hinges on effective co-creation of a shared narrative between health professional and patient. Eggly used this adapted model to identify three further specific narrative types told in clinician–patient consultations, where narratives emerge through the co-constructed chronology of key events, the co-constructed repetition and elaboration of key events, and the co-constructed interpretation of the meaning of key events (8). These co-constructions offer a useful focus for training healthcare professionals in narrative communication skills; for example, checking and clarifying timelines, identifying and elaborating on key events in the story, and exploring and agreeing the meaning patients attach to those key events.

Developing narrative capabilities

Having introduced the basic concepts and value of interactional knowledge for generalists, and the central role of the narrative approach in interactions between patients and clinicians, we will now explore in more detail some of the capabilities generalists need in order to integrate it into their care.

The art of listening

Perhaps the number one capability for generalists is the ability to listen to the patient's story or stories, without judgement, and with compassion and genuine curiosity. GP and family therapist John Launer uses the term 'attentiveness' (15). In clinical communication training we often talk about 'active listening': listening designed to encourage the patient to tell their story, elaborate on it, or develop important aspects. This may also include the use of open questions rather than closed questions, non-verbal encouragement such as head-nodding and eye contact, and the use of 'continuers' such as 'uh huh' and 'go on …'. In one observational study of the effects of doctors' non-verbal behaviour on their patients, researchers found that eye contact and the posture of the doctor were influential in determining what the patient revealed in the consultation (16).

In my own teaching, I often try to persuade medical students and trainee GPs that the key to effective communication lies in being in 'receive' mode more than being in 'transmit' mode. This may sound self-evident, but research suggests that although things may have improved a little in recent decades, doctors still often interrupt patients' initial stories before they have finished telling them (17–19). There are several potential consequences of early interruptions, including denying the patient a chance to offer personal context to their chief complaint, hindering the development of an empathic relationship (20), and increasing the chances of patients only mentioning key problems at the end of the consultation (so-called 'Oh, by the way …' concerns) (18). Clark and Mishler's narrative analysis of two different clinician–patient encounters suggested that interruptions by the clinician throughout the consultation can influence the framing of clinical decisions, and the maintenance of co-operative patient–clinician relationships (21). They also make the point that when clinicians interrupt patients' stories, rather than working together to facilitate storytelling, they are exercising their authority, taking control of what should be a collaborative process. Storytelling in conversation is an interactional accomplishment, requiring finely coordinated activity by both participants (22,23). It is like a dance, where both partners need to be in step with each other, and the generalist should know when to lead and when to follow.

It is true that sometimes constructive interruption may be justified in order to help the patient tell their story when time is running out, or when clarification is needed. And faced with the challenge of dealing with multimorbidity and complexity under time constraints, many generalists may reasonably fear letting – or even encouraging – patients to tell their initial stories in full. There is evidence, however, that with collaborative upfront agenda-setting, consultations do not have to be longer, nor is there an increase in number of problems addressed per visit, and there may be a reduction in the likelihood of 'oh, by the way' concerns surfacing late in the encounter (24). The biomedical knowledge and the interactional knowledge here are interdependent and integrated.

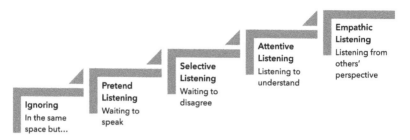

Figure 15.2 The Listening Staircase. Adapted from Prideaux, 2017 (25)

Training for active listening mostly focuses on teachable behaviours such as nodding, making eye contact and using continuers like 'Uh huh' and 'go on'. These are important, but perhaps more important is the listener's mindset, and the quality of the listening when we are with patients. The idea of a listening staircase (25) [see Figure 15.2 adapted from (25)] can be a useful way to think about these aspects; learners seem to identify with it as storytellers. We are often acutely aware of which 'step' on the staircase our listener is standing on. At the lower end, we are not feeling properly listened to, and might decide to close down our storytelling. It is likely we might feel less connected with someone who seems just to be pretending to listen. The higher our listener climbs on the staircase, the more listened to and connected we feel; and the more likely we are to open up.

What we are aiming for in the listening staircase is empathic listening; this demands both attentive listening and empathy as twin approaches.

Empathy as emotional resonance

Clinicians and patients both place a high value on empathic care (26). There is also growing evidence that empathy is associated with improved patient satisfaction, better diagnostic and clinical outcomes, and enhanced patient enablement [defined as the patient's ability to understand and cope with illness and life after a consultation (27)] (26,28). Empathy is a basic component of the therapeutic relationship, and a key facet of the generalist's interactional knowledge.

Empathy is a complex construct, and although it has often been conceptualised solely as a personal attribute, there is increasing focus on its relational, or interactional aspects. Mercer and Reynolds' definition of physician empathy is one of the most frequently used (29). They see it as having three elements: the ability to understand the patient's situation, perspective and feelings; to communicate back that understanding; and to act on that understanding in a helpful and therapeutic way (29). In essence, it involves being able to 'put oneself in another's shoes', and to do this authentically requires what Jodi Halpern, Professor of Bioethics and Medical Humanities at UC Berkeley, calls 'emotional attunement'; a kind of emotional resonance which helps to shape how a clinician imagines another's experience (30).

As the clinician listens to the patient, following the narrative thread of the story, he or she imagines the teller's perspective, and in some way enters into and is moved by the patient's narrative world. Rita Charon suggests that by entering into the patient's world in this way, the clinician has a chance of addressing the common narrative questions that patients often ask, such as: 'What's wrong with me?', 'Why did this happen to me?' and 'What can we do about it?' (2). She goes on to say that although there may not be clear answers to these narrative questions, with narrative competence and courage, the empathic witnessing of patients' stories and co-creating of meaning from them, allows the clinician to attend to other more recognisably clinical tasks such as formulating a differential diagnosis, interpreting tests and physical findings, and ultimately working with the patient to provide effective care (2).

How, though, is empathy a particularly generalist capability? Halpern puts her finger on three crucial reasons, all clearly related to the generalist narrative approach we have discussed (30) (see also patient perspectives on pseudo-person-centred care in Chapter 3). Firstly, emotional attunement helps clinicians to appreciate the personal meanings that patients attach to specific words or phrases; it is an additional tool for noticing which parts of a patient's story are particularly important. This supports meaningful co-creation with the patient, exploring rich story snippets, or encouraging elaboration of others.

This example from John Launer illustrates the point (15):

Among the skills for attentiveness that I find most useful to teach are 'noticing the words we usually ignore' ... I'm always interested in statements such as, 'My headaches are driving me to despair.' Ninety-nine times in 100 we ask about the headaches and never inquire about the 'driving to despair.' Why did that person, consciously or unconsciously, select that exact phrase – and what more will we learn about their life, and possibly even the cause of the headaches, if we're curious about this and ask them to unpack it?

Secondly, non-verbal attunement helps the clinician to focus on aspects of the story that have particular emotional significance for the patient. A change in gaze or body language become powerful signposts of meaning, particularly within a complex or non-fluent story. Interestingly, this works both ways: the clinician's non-verbal behaviour is also considered the most important medium for expressing empathy; in particular, the doctor's direction of gaze and body orientation (31). Thirdly, Halpern suggests that emotional attunement facilitates patient trust and disclosure (30). Clinicians who are emotionally attuned are more likely to match their non-verbal behaviours authentically with patients, and this is vital in encouraging patients to tell their stories in full, to disclose concerns or symptoms, and can even be therapeutic in itself, for example by reducing anxiety.

It is possible of course to 'fake', or act out, mirroring of a patient's body language or words – but patients recognise inauthentic empathy, and authenticity is underpinned by this emotional resonance (32). This has important implications for how educators help learners to feel and show empathy with patients: it is much easier to teach the behavioural aspects of clinical empathy – what to say, appropriate body language or touch for example – than to promote the affective aspects; the emotional resonance that brings authenticity. The risk of focusing too much on behaviours is promoting what is sometimes called 'tick-box empathy', where learners may say and do empathic things, but in an inauthentic way. For example:

Clinician: (delivered in an inexpressive monotone, and little eye contact): 'I am sorry to hear that your wife died recently, that must be very difficult for you. Have you had any bleeding from your back passage?'

Inauthentic, tick-box empathy like this can destroy trust, break rapport and close down patients' stories. Some suggested approaches to developing the more affective aspects of empathy include authentic interactions with patients [dialogue with patients can reinforce the relational aspects of empathy, and as patients reciprocate this can encourage learners to express compassion]; longitudinal interactions with patients over time; role modelling by professionals; and narrative medicine training including creative writing, guided reflection, film and patient stories (33).

There are two further important points to make about empathy in the context of generalism. The first is Roger Neighbour's suggestion that for clinicians, the crucial capability is probably not so much being able to empathise with patients (as opposed to not being able to empathise), but is the ability to switch our empathy on and off as the situation requires (34).

He calls this Crichton's Switch (after the author and former medical student Michael Crichton) (35). In generalist practice, 'there are some clinical situations where hard-nosed clinical skill is all that is required, and others where the very best we can offer is our ability to understand and to empathise' (34).

The second important point is how we measure and assess empathy. Historically, much of the research into clinical empathy has relied on clinician self-report questionnaires, or objective measures by observers. If we accept that empathy is essentially a relational construct, rooted in the interaction between patient and clinician, then it seems self-evident that we should be drawing much more on the patient perspective when measuring it and assessing it. Although potentially reductionist, there is an argument for using validated measures (such as the CARE measure (36), a tool for assessing the patient's perceptions of relational empathy in the consultation) which do take account of the patient's viewpoint when assessing and measuring empathy in learners and clinicians.

Specialised narrative approaches

Close listening and empathy are core dimensions of the narrative approach to consultations, but there is more to it than that. Narrative consulting champion John Launer describes a useful conceptual framework for thinking about a narrative-based approach, called the seven Cs (9), outlined below:

Launer's seven Cs of narrative consulting (9)

Conversations: Conversations do not just describe reality – they can create it. You can think of conversations as interventions in their own right. Launer and his team teach skills for 'conversations inviting change' – exploring connections, differences, new options and new realities.

Curiosity: With curiosity you can invite patients to reframe/reconstruct their stories. Curiosity is neutral – to people, blame, interpretations, facts.

Contexts: This is where your curiosity should be focused – families, history, beliefs, values. What is your context – what do patients expect of you?

Circularity: The idea here is to get away from the linear concept of cause and effect, and unchangeable problems, and instead help the patient to focus on meanings and connections. Circularity conveys the sense that anything in a system is connected with everything else in a non-linear way. Adopting circularity as an approach might involve using circular questions (in other words, based on the words that patients use, and using questions which promote a descriptive rather than explanatory world view).

Co-construction: What you are trying to do with the patient is to create a story that makes better sense for people of what they are going through; a better reality than the present one.

Caution: Do not be unrealistic about your own resources or cover up for the lack of others. Do not upset patients or get scared. Not all consultations are all about stories.

Care: For Launer, this is central to the whole process – without it, nothing else works.

It is worth highlighting two additional approaches at the heart of narrative consulting, which also form part of Launer's seven Cs (37). These are neutrality and hypothesising (38).

Neutrality is about focusing on the task in hand, being mindful and in the moment, and keeping an open mind rather than fixating on specific outcomes or judging particular viewpoints. It represents a counterpoint to active problem-solving (37). Hypothesising is an approach which challenges assumptions: both the patient's and the clinician's, asking questions such as 'How do you explain …?', 'What if …?' and 'Suppose …'. Along with circular questioning, these probes are designed to help patients consider realistic possibilities for positive change, and how they could be achieved (38).

Reflection

Donald Schon (39), Rita Charon (2), John Launer (9) and Michael Balint (40) all highlight the importance of clinicians reflecting on themselves, their patients and the clinician–patient interaction, and effective reflection is so often underpinned by competence in narrative skills. Practitioners who can use a narrative approach to reflect on themselves can better identify and understand their emotional responses to patients, and make sense of their own life journeys and clinical practice: both of which Charon argues allows them to bring what is needed to the caring for sick and dying patients. Self-reflection on personal illness experiences, for example, can promote greater empathy for the experiences of patients. It may also bring greater self-awareness and focus on self-care: increasingly important for today's generalist practitioners.

The power of language

Using words wisely

There are many definitions of generalism, but common to all of them are the principles of legitimising multiple perspectives and priorities, and the concept of distributed power and shared decision-making. These principles are foregrounded in the generalist consultation, where the clinician's interactional knowledge can have huge influence over the power dynamics between patient and practitioner, whether closing down the patient's perspective or actively inviting collaboration. This could be through not listening attentively to the patient, or through non-verbal statements of power (for example avoiding eye contact or through the positioning of chairs); but is often most apparent in our use of language.

Caitríona Cox and Zoë Fritz, researchers from The Healthcare Improvement Studies Institute at the University of Cambridge writing in the BMJ, make a compelling case for paying much closer attention to our choice of words and phrases when talking with, or about our patients (41). Of course generalist clinicians should always tread very carefully when using medical jargon with patients (see Chapter 3). But Cox and Fritz argue that language is about much more than the transfer of information; it has the power to shape therapeutic relationships, influence clinical care, and affect how patients think of their health and illnesses. They conclude that outdated language that belittles, casts doubt, or blames patients is still being used today in written and spoken communication with and about patients, and needs to change (41).

For example, they remind us how the term 'presenting complaint' is so ingrained in clinical training that it is rarely questioned; yet 'complain' has negative connotations and although some have suggested 'problem' or 'concern' as an alternative, many patients do not have either, and simply want to understand more about what is going on. Cox and Fritz suggest using a more neutral term such as 'reason for attendance' which avoids imposing value judgements on the patient (41). Another example they highlight is the use of 'deny' in formal reports of a patient's account – as in 'the patient denies any chest pain', which can hint at untrustworthiness and is often simply inaccurate reporting of the patient's narrative. As one patient states in another research paper: 'I did not deny these things. I said I didn't feel them. Completely different. Language matters' (42). Cox and Fritz go on to describe other examples which can seem to blame patients, such as people being described as 'poorly controlled diabetics', or language which infantilises patients such as 'taking a history' or 'sending the patient home' (41). As modern generalist healthcare emphasises collaboration between health provider and patient, and its rhetoric highlights the importance of partnership, it is surely now time to question many of these outdated words and phrases, and Cox and Fritz suggest some alternatives and a focus for future research on the effectiveness of interventions to change how we use language, and how that might affect health outcomes (41).

Metaphor

Another aspect of language that can play an important part in the interpretive role of the generalist is metaphor. An illuminating study by Skelton et al. attempted to explore how patients and clinicians construct and shape their worlds through metaphoric language: a figure of speech in which a word or phrase is applied to an object or action to which it is not literally applicable – for example, 'the body is a container for the self' or 'he is thick-skinned' (43). They analysed transcripts of 373 UK general practice consultations with 40 GPs to explore how patients and doctors used metaphors. What they discovered was that patients often used very vivid or even dramatic metaphors (for example, 'it feels as if there is something crawling up me like a maggot') perhaps in an attempt to legitimise their presence, or to articulate difficult nebulous thoughts and feelings. Clinicians on the other hand tended to use more literal metaphors (referring to pain in terms of severity rather than as 'burning'), or to describe the body as if it were a machine. Clinicians also tended to use metaphors that see themselves as solvers of problems, and controllers of illness. As well as pointing out the clear implications here for power balance within the consultation, the researchers propose that clinicians may be trying to interpret patients' more vivid and personal metaphors, re-packaging them as emotionally neutral and depersonalised accounts (43). They suggest this might be reassuring for patients, giving them validity and categorising them into manageable states (43). Equally, it could be seen as another subconscious attempt to exert medical power and strip the patient's lifeworld from their illness experience. Whatever the interpretation, it is a salient lesson for generalist clinicians striving for authentic collaboration and patient-centredness – to pay close attention to the metaphors they and their patients choose to use. There may be opportunities, for example, to mirror the patient's metaphors to legitimate the patient's story, improve understanding and perhaps even promote an empathic connection. Equally, it may be helpful to work with a patient to question or develop their metaphor for illness, to explore implications for understanding and lived experience.

Diversity and interactional knowledge

It is impossible to consider interactions from a generalist point of view without also considering the contexts in which they take place, including the cultural and technological ones. Acknowledging and embracing the diversity of the patients we serve is central to effective interactions. The expert generalist needs to be sensitive to cultural influences on communication, for example differences in interpretation of symptoms or health-seeking behaviours, attitudes to patient autonomy, or non-verbal communication. In some cultures for example, eye contact which is too direct or long-lived can be seen as aggressive, and interpersonal space preferences and attitudes to touch can be very different from one culture to the next. To offer person-centred care, generalists also need to be able to adapt to patients whose preferred language is different from their own. This often means being able and willing to work with interpreters to support patient care, either in person or on the telephone. In addition, generalists need to adjust their communication approach to suit patients with specific communication needs, for example a learning disability or hearing or visual impairment, whether through enhanced communication skills or technologies (44).

Interactional knowledge in the new digital landscape

The landscape in which healthcare is delivered has changed dramatically in recent years. Digital remote consulting has long been on the agenda for health services around the world. In England for example, even before the COVID-19 pandemic, the 2019 NHS Long Term Plan stated that by 2023–24 every patient in England will be able to access 'digital first' NHS primary care consultations from either their own GP or a digital GP provider (45), and there was already much political excitement about a new model of digital care delivered by digital health company Babylon Health (46). But driven by the urgent need to reduce face-to-face contact during the COVID-19 pandemic, there was a rapid shift to various forms of remote consultation (defined here as consultations where clinician and patient are not in the same room) – either by telephone, video or by some form of electronic consultation such as text messaging, email or the use of electronic forms, often used for initial triage. Although the dramatic increase in remote consulting during the pandemic has started to level out, remote consulting remains much more prevalent and is likely to remain so (47). Currently most clinical practice around the world involves a blend of remote consulting (by video, phone or text/email) and face-to-face consulting. Much of the existing evidence about clinical interactions has been established in face-to-face settings. So, what does this recent shift towards remote consulting mean for the interactional dimension of generalist care?

It is important to acknowledge the many possible benefits of digital remote consulting, for example in remote or rural settings, where clinicians or patients try to minimise travel (such as time or mobility constraints), have caring responsibilities (48), or for some patients with anxiety or other mental health problems for whom the chance to engage with a clinician without coming into the clinic is a major bonus (49). For many patients [and clinicians], simply being able to consult from home is the greatest benefit. But it is vital that any potential risks and unintended consequences of this 'new normal' consulting landscape are taken fully into account. There is evidence, for example, that professionals and patients have a sense that remote consultations of all sorts have a more transactional nature than face-to-face consultations – a 'call-centre' feel; and this risks losing the interpretive, personalised and collaborative interactions at the heart of generalism (49). So how can we realise the potential benefits of remote consulting while maintaining the benefits of a narrative approach as described above? And how do we avoid undermining spaces for meaningful encounters, by forcing patients to tell biomedical stories of their experience on template proformas, via episodic and asynchronous monologues? Inequity is another major concern, with some patients [often those already disadvantaged by existing health inequalities] lacking the technological confidence, equipment, or connections to access remote consultations (50).

The challenges of remote consulting for interactional knowledge

Although consulting in person and consulting remotely share many similarities (particularly video consulting), remote consulting is not simply a face-to-face consultation with technology bolted on. There are key judgements to make (for example, about consent and confidentiality, and whether remote consulting is appropriate for the specific context (51)), and specific communication approaches to develop.

Here are some practical tips.

Tips on enhancing interactional aspects of remote consultations

General tips for both video and telephone consulting:

- Clear introductions are crucial: introduce yourself, ask the patient how they would like to be addressed.
- Early rapport-building is extra important in remote consultations; think how you might make a personal connection early on.
- Check technology is working. 'Can you hear me? Can you see me OK?'
- Reassure patient about how consultation will work (including what will happen if physical examination is needed), what if technology fails, and probable duration.
- Check if anyone is with the patient and where they are; important for confidentiality but also may affect patient disclosure. Similarly, share if you are with a colleague or learner.
- Ask people with visual or hearing impairment or learning disability or other special communication needs whether this works for them; how would they prefer to consult, what might help?
- Establish early why the patient has organised the consultation at this time, what they may be hoping to get from it, and any concerns they may have – for example, about the technology.
- Summarise: this is a particularly important skill in telephone and video consulting. It allows you to check you have understood the patient's story, and offers a chance for a patient to correct any misunderstandings or mis-hearings.
- Chunking and checking information: if giving information, it is especially important to avoid jargon, and provide small chunks at a time and check that the patient has understood.
- Signposting: video or telephone consultations may be unfamiliar to patients and they are likely to wonder how they will flow. So it is very important to guide the patient clearly throughout

---

by explaining what you are going to do next. For example 'Now I'd like to ask you more about your past medical history', or 'So thanks for describing that for me, that's very helpful. I'd like to now check that I've understood you correctly ...'

- Towards the end, summarise again, inviting patient to add or correct.
- Safety net; anticipate the unexpected and give specific instructions on when to return or seek medical help.
- Clear plan: for example what can the patient expect now, will the clinician see them or phone them? Ideally this should be constructed together with the patient.
- Check if the patient has any questions they want to ask. This is very important in both phone and video consultations in case issues have been missed, or not heard.
- Do you think you have been able to safely assess this patient? What bits of the story are missing? What might make you want to bring the patient in for a face-to-face meeting?

Video consulting tips:

- Make sure the lighting is appropriate and that you have a clear view of each other's faces; facial expressions can provide important communication cues.
- Consider your background; and theirs if appropriate. (You might want to make a [sensitive] comment about a painting or their decor or a pet, to build rapport as you might on a home visit.)
- Eye contact: looking at camera provides eye contact with a patient, whereas looking at a screen allows you to see patient non-verbal cues. You may need to alternate between the two.
- Explain to the patient if you look away on video to write notes for example, or have another screen you need to look at sometimes.
- Show your interest and attentiveness by eye contact (look into webcam) and facial expression.
- If you need to interrupt the patient, try a visual signal such as raising your hand.
- Speak clearly and include regular breaks in speech.
- Taking turns: try hard to avoid talking over each other due to lag/delay. If this happens, address the problem openly and suggest waiting a while after the other person has finished before speaking.

Telephone consulting tips:

- Consider making an early empathic statement – you may need to be more proactive than in a face-to-face meeting due to lack of non-verbal signals.
- Check patient understanding explicitly throughout.
- Be alert for paraverbal cues rather than visual cues (rate and speed of speech, volume and tone, expression, hesitation).
- If appropriate it can help to reflect back to the patient what you have noticed: 'I noticed you sounded very worried when you …'
- Leave space for the patient, for example if you think they might be doing some internal reflection.
- Explain any silences on your part – 'I am just checking your records for a moment …'

Adapted from: Easton, 2020 (59); Neighbour, 2020 (60); NHS England and NHS Improvement, 2020 (61); Neighbour and Stockley, 2020 (62); Greenhalgh et al., 2020 (63).

One of the main challenges of remote consulting lies in the co-construction of a shared narrative: a core task for many generalist consultations. The consultation is a dynamic interaction between two or more people, each giving the other extended turns in the discourse. The shared story is shaped together, through the sorts of prompts, responses and non-verbal communication described earlier. While video consultations allow for some of this nuanced interaction, telephone provides no non-verbal signals, and written consultations offer none at all. To some degree, all forms of remote consulting therefore block many of the vital signals in storytelling – for example, whether someone is really interested in what you are saying, and therefore how much you are willing to reveal, or the subtle visual cues of synchronous face-to-face consultations. One observational study also established some of the significant obstacles to turn-taking during online video consultations (52), which impacted on telling and hearing stories in both directions. The researchers highlighted the importance of joint attention that involves getting camera angles and body position just right and working hard at maintaining appropriate gaze. They observed the need for increased verbalisation in turn-taking to compensate for the reduction of verbal cues on screen. Without the usual verbal [or non-verbal] cues, interruptions are more likely and clinicians have raised concerns about an increase in last minute 'oh, by the way' consultations (48). One study comparing consultation quality in 150 follow-up consultations in UK primary care by telephone, video or face to face, found that both telephone and video consultations were less information-rich than face-to-face consultations, and they also both scored lower than face-to-face consultations across a string of consultation quality indicators such as seeking the patient's own understanding of their illness, shared decision-making and exploring patient concerns (53).

E-consultations using a written template proforma pose a unique threat to the collaborative narrative approach. They are usually asynchronous, and therefore entirely one-sided. Patients have reported that when faced with a free-text box, it can be hard to know how to describe their symptoms without any guidance or help (54). The crucial co-construction of story, including the negotiation of an agenda and shared planning, is missing. Template forms are tempting to help guide patients to tell their story; however, if the templates are designed by clinicians, the risk is that this shoehorns the patient's narrative into a biomedical structure – favouring the voice of medicine over the voice of the patient's lifeworld, as Clark and Mishler might put it (21). More likely to maintain parity in the clinician/patient power balance will be co-design of such templates and processes with clinicians working with patients to design systems that suit both needs.

Remote consulting also challenges the central task of rapport-building and feeling and demonstrating empathy. If generalist care is to be truly personalised and collaborative, it depends on a trusting relationship, developed in large part through an empathic resonance. As we have seen, empathy depends heavily on non-verbal communication in both directions, especially eye contact or gaze. While written e-consultations only permit written expressions of empathy, telephone consultations can allow for picking up on verbal cues and silences, and empathic phrases or noises. Although video consultations do offer the visual element, they pose a challenge here too – the clinician can maintain eye contact by looking directly into the camera, but then risks missing picking up on non-verbal cues from the patient. Experience suggests that flipping from looking at the camera to looking at the patient on screen may be the best approach, but it is not as easy to do both as it is in a face-to-face setting.

A great deal of the research and guidance on remote consulting in UK primary care focuses on practitioner and patient concerns about patient safety. The concern is that without the full range of sensory means of assessment that is available in face-to-face consultations, subtle symptoms or clues might be missed. As an example, when GPs have a 'gut feeling' that a patient might have cancer, they are much more likely to be correct, and those gut feelings seem to depend largely on the non-verbal cues they pick up from the patient (55). To compensate, safety netting is a standard part of remote consultation, including triage (49). Likewise, using interim summaries to check that the patient is happy with any plans, and that the clinician has understood the patient's issues correctly, is vital in remote consultations where there is increased scope for miscommunication. Despite these mitigations, there is evidence that telephone triage and e-consultations can increase rather than decrease practitioner workloads (56), perhaps because clinicians do not feel fully confident that they have interpreted the patient's story effectively, and often because of the inability to perform a reliable physical examination (57).

Finally, the rapid move to remote consulting has the potential to reduce continuity of care, and consequently the sort of personalised care we advocate for generalist medicine (4). One systematic review of mixed studies concluded that there is a 'disturbing lack of empirical research in this area' and emphasised the 'need for real world studies looking at the links between the shift to remote care, continuity and equity' (58). Several studies in the review highlighted the potential for remote approaches to exacerbate inequities of care by reducing relational or episodic continuity for patients, especially for those with complex or chronic conditions (58). Without reliable systems in place to support continuity of care in remote consulting, and individual commitment from clinicians, patients will have to repeat their stories again and again in different forms or on different platforms, and clinicians will have to start afresh each time and work hard to build rapport from scratch.

Ultimately, as with much of generalist medicine, there is no 'one size fits all' answer when it comes to the use of remote consulting. As Greenhalgh says: 'the decision as to whether remote consultation is best for the patient, the practice staff, and the wider community is an ethical, case-based judgement that cannot be over-protocolised' (48). Clinical care will need to ensure practitioners can adapt their narrative competency to the new digital landscape (for example, learning new communication approaches for remote consulting – see the box on p. 349 for practical tips), organisations will need to adjust systems to ensure patients have meaningful choice over how they access clinicians, and patients will need support to get the most from the great potential of remote consulting in all its guises. Patients should have a clear voice in the co-design of processes and proformas designed to support them tell their stories.

Conclusion

In summary, this chapter has explored the central role of interactional knowledge in the consultation between the generalist clinician and the patient. This knowledge is informed by interpretivist and narrative perspectives; especially the co-creation by clinician and patient, of meaningful stories which take account of the patient's experiences of illness as well as the more biomedical aspects. It has outlined some of the narrative approaches and specific communication techniques which generalists can use to make the most of the potential in the consultation for effective, person-centred care. It touches on some of the barriers to effective communication, and ends by exploring the challenges and hopes for remote consulting in terms of its effects on interactional knowledge.

References

1. Reeve J. Interpretive medicine: supporting generalism in a changing primary care world. *Occas Pap R Coll Gen Pract*. 2010(88):1–20, v.
2. Charon R. Narrative medicine: a model for empathy, reflection, profession, and trust. *JAMA*. 2001;286(15):1897–902.
3. Schon DA. Preparing professionals for the demands of practice. *Educating the Reflective Practitioner*. Jossey-Bass; 1987. pp.3–21.
4. Toon P. Towards an Interpretive Patient-Centred Practice. BJGP Life; 2021. Available at: https://bjgplife.com/towards-an-interpretive-patient-centred-practice/ (accessed 21 March 2024).
5. Kvale S. *InterViews: An introduction to qualitive research interviewing*. SAGE; 1996.
6. Mishler EG. *The Discourse of Medicine: Dialectics of medical interviews*. Greenwood Publishing Group; 1984.
7. Levenstein JH, McCracken EC, McWhinney IR, Stewart MA, Brown JB. The patient-centred clinical method. 1. A model for the doctor–patient interaction in family medicine. *Family Practice*. 1986;3(1):24–30.
8. Eggly S. Physician–Patient co-construction of illness narratives in the medical interview. *Health Communication*. 2002;14(3):339–60.
9. Launer J. *Narrative-Based Practice in Health and Social Care: Conversations inviting change*. Routledge, 2018.
10. Labov W, Waletzky, J. Narrative analysis. In: Helm J. (ed.) *Essays on the Verbal and Visual Arts*. University of Washington Press; 1967. pp. 12–44.
11. Labov W. *Language in the Inner City: Studies in the Black English vernacular*. University of Pennsylvania Press; 1972.
12. Langellier KM. Personal narratives: perspectives on theory and research. *Text and Performance Quarterly*. 1989;9(4):243–76.
13. Riessman C. Narrative analysis. In: Huberman AM and Miles MB (eds) *The Qualitative Researcher's Companion*. SAGE; 2002.
14. Polanyi L. Conversational storytelling. *Handbook of Discourse Analysis*. Vol 3. Academic Press; 1985. pp. 183–201.
15. Launer J. The art of paying attention. *BMJ*. 2022;378:o2294.
16. Byrne PS, Heath CC. Practitioners' use of non-verbal behaviour in real consultations. *Journal of the Royal College of General Practitioners*. 1980;30(215):327–31.
17. Danczak A. British GPs keep going for longer: is the 12 second interruption history? *BMJ*. 2015;351.
18. Beckman HB, Frankel RM. The effect of physician behavior on the collection of data. *Annals of Internal Medicine*. 1984;101(5):692–6.

19. Marvel MK, Epstein RM, Flowers K, Beckman HB. Soliciting the patient's agenda: have we improved? *JAMA*. 1999;281(3):283–7.
20. Phillips KA, Ospina NS. Physicians interrupting patients. *JAMA*. 2017;318(1):93–4.
21. Clark JA, Mishler EG. Attending to patients' stories: reframing the clinical task. *Sociology of Health & Illness*. 1992;14(3):344–72.
22. Jefferson G. Sequential aspects of storytelling in conversation. In: *Studies in the Organization of Conversational Interaction*. Elsevier; 1978. pp. 219–48.
23. Polanyi L. *Telling the American Story: A structural and cultural work*. Basic Books. 1989.
24. Brock DM, Mauksch LB, Witteborn S, Hummel J, Nagasawa P, Robins LS. Effectiveness of intensive physician training in upfront agenda setting. *J Gen Intern Med*. 2011;26(11):1317–23.
25. Prideaux B. Leading Change – Why Active Listening Isn't Enough. (The Curious Choice Leader Podcast). Available from: www.bekkaprideaux.com/podcast/why-active-listening-isnt-enough/ (accessed 24 June 2020).
26. Mercer SW, Neumann M, Wirtz M, Fitzpatrick B, Vojt G. General practitioner empathy, patient enablement, and patient-reported outcomes in primary care in an area of high socio-economic deprivation in Scotland – A pilot prospective study using structural equation modeling. *Patient Education and Counseling*. 2008;73(2):240–5.
27. Howie J, Heaney D, Maxwell M. Measuring quality in general practice. Pilot study of a needs, process and outcome measure. Occasional paper. Royal College of General Practitioners; 1997(75):i.
28. Derksen F, Bensing J, Lagro-Janssen A. Effectiveness of empathy in general practice: a systematic review. *British Journal of General Practice*. 2013;63(606):e76–e84.
29. Mercer SW, Reynolds WJ. Empathy and quality of care. *British Journal of General Practice*. 2002;52(Suppl):S9–12.
30. Halpern J. What is clinical empathy? *Journal of General Internal Medicine*. 2003;18(8):670–4.
31. Brugel S, Postma-Nilsenová M, Tates K. The link between perception of clinical empathy and nonverbal behavior: The effect of a doctor's gaze and body orientation. *Patient Education and Counseling*. 2015;98(10):1260–5.
32. Suchman AL, Markakis K, Beckman HB, Frankel R. A model of empathic communication in the medical interview. *JAMA*. 1997;277(8):678–82.
33. Krishnasamy C, Ong SY, Loo ME, Thistlethwaite J. How does medical education affect empathy and compassion in medical students? A meta-ethnography: BEME Guide No. 57. *Medical Teacher*. 2019;41(11):1220–31.
34. Neighbour R. Detachment and empathy. 2016. BJGP Life. Available from: https://bjgp.org/content/detachment-and-empathy (accessed 21 March 2024).
35. Neighbour R. *The Inner Physician*. CRC Press; 2018.
36. Mercer SW, McConnachie A, Maxwell M, Heaney D, Watt GC. Relevance and practical use of the Consultation and Relational Empathy (CARE) Measure in general practice. *Family Practice*. 2005;22(3):328–34.
37. Launer J. Narrative-based supervision. In: *Clinical Uncertainty in Primary Care*. Springer; 2013. pp. 147–61.
38. Zaharias G. Narrative-based medicine and the general practice consultation: Narrative-based medicine 2. *Can Fam Physician*. 2018;64(4):286–90.
39. Schon DA. *The Reflective Practitioner. How professionals think in action*. Basic Books; 1983.
40. Balint M. The doctor, his patient, and the illness. *The Lancet*. 1955;265(6866):683–8.
41. Cox C, Fritz Z. Presenting complaint: use of language that disempowers patients. *BMJ*. 2022;377:e066720.
42. Fernández L, Fossa A, Dong Z, Delbanco T, Elmore J, Fitzgerald P, et al. Words matter: what do patients find judgmental or offensive in outpatient notes? *Journal of General Internal Medicine*. 2021;36(9):2571–8.
43. Skelton JR, Wearn AM, Hobbs FR. A concordance-based study of metaphoric expressions used by general practitioners and patients in consultation. *British Journal of General Practice*. 2002;52(475):114–8.
44. Maru D, Stancel-Lewis J, Easton G, Leverton WE. Communicating with people with hearing loss: COVID-19 and beyond. *BJGP Open*. 2021;5(1).
45. Iacobucci G. NHS Long Term Plan: all patients to have access to online GP consultations by 2023–24. *BMJ*. 2019;364:l87.
46. Iacobucci G. London GP clinic sees big jump in patient registrations after Babylon app launch. *BMJ*. 2017;359:j5908.

47. Murphy M, Scott LJ, Salisbury C, Turner A, Scott A, Denholm R et al. Implementation of remote consulting in UK primary care following the COVID-19 pandemic: a mixed-methods longitudinal study. *British Journal of General Practice*. 2021;71(704):e166–e77.

48. Greenhalgh T, Rosen R. Remote by default general practice: must we, should we, dare we? *British Journal of General Practice*; 2021;71(705):149–50.

49. Mann C, Turner A, Salisbury C. The Impact of Remote Consultations on Personalised Care. The Personalised Care Institute; 2021.

50. Parker RF, Figures EL, Paddison CA, Matheson JI, Blane DN, Ford JA. Inequalities in general practice remote consultations: a systematic review. *BJGP Open*. 2021;5(3).

51. General Medical Council. Remote Consultations. General Medical Council; 2020.

52. Seuren LM, Wherton J, Greenhalgh T, Shaw SE. Whose turn is it anyway? Latency and the organization of turn-taking in video-mediated interaction. *Journal of Pragmatics*. 2021;172:63–78.

53. Hammersley V, Donaghy E, Parker R, McNeilly H, Atherton H, Bikker A et al. Comparing the content and quality of video, telephone, and face-to-face consultations: a non-randomised, quasi-experimental, exploratory study in UK primary care. *British Journal of General Practice*. 2019;69(686):e595–e604.

54. Turner A, Morris R, Rakhra D, Stevenson F, McDonagh L, Hamilton F et al. Unintended consequences of online consultations: a qualitative study in UK primary care. *British Journal of General Practice*. 2022;72(715):e128–e37.

55. Smith CF, Drew S, Ziebland S, Nicholson BD. Understanding the role of GPs' gut feelings in diagnosing cancer in primary care: a systematic review and meta-analysis of existing evidence. *British Journal of General Practice*. 2020;70(698):e612–e21.

56. Campbell JL, Fletcher E, Britten N, Green C, Holt TA, Lattimer V et al. Telephone triage for management of same-day consultation requests in general practice (the ESTEEM trial): a cluster-randomised controlled trial and cost-consequence analysis. *The Lancet*. 2014;384(9957):1859–68.

57. Jones D, Neal RD, Duffy SRG, Scott SE, Whitaker KL, Brain K. Impact of the COVID-19 pandemic on the symptomatic diagnosis of cancer: the view from primary care. *Lancet Oncol*. 2020;21(6):748–50.

58. Ladds E, Khan M, Moore L, Kalin A, Greenhalgh T. The impact of remote care approaches on continuity in primary care: a mixed-studies systematic review. *British Journal of General Practice*. 2023.

59. Easton G. A Guide to Remote Consulting. Teaching materials presented at Barts and The London School of Medicine and Dentistry. 2020.

60. Neighbour, R. Top tips for GP video consultation during COVID-19 pandemic. 2020. Available from: www.youtube.com/watch?v=W5zsEpka2HE (accessed 2 November 2023).

61. NHS England and NHS Improvement. Principles of safe video consulting in general practice during COVID-19. 2020. Available from: https://www.england.nhs.uk/coronavirus/wp-content/uploads/sites/52/2020/03/C0479-principles-of-safe-video-consulting-in-general-practice-updated-29-may.pdf (accessed 21 March 2024).

62. Neighbour R, Stockley S. Ten tips for telephone consultations about COVID-19. BJGP Life; 2020. Available from: https://bjgplife.com/neighbours-ten-tips-for-telephone-consultations-about-COVID-19/ (accessed 2 November 2023).

63. Greenhalgh T, Morrison C, Koh Choon Huat G. Video consultations: a guide for practice. BJGP Life; 2020. Available from: https://bjgplife.com/video-consultations-guide-for-practice/ (accessed 2 November 2023).

16
Prescribing and deprescribing: the generalist's script

Deborah Swinglehurst and Nina Fudge

Introduction

Prescribing is an important part of clinical care. In this chapter we explore how and why prescribing in the generalist context is particularly challenging. It stands to reason that keeping up to date with the technical knowledge required to prescribe safely across the whole spectrum of clinical conditions is difficult. New drugs reach the market all the time. Prescribing guidelines are updated at a dizzying pace. Our computer alerts remind us of the alarming potential for adverse drug reactions (ADRs) and interactions. Prescribing is a risky business!

But the generalist's challenge goes much deeper. Generalists prioritise care of the person over the care of a person's diseases and this brings unique responsibilities. Generalists must attend closely to the particular context of the patient within an institutional context that tends to privilege 'single disease' guidelines and standardised approaches to care. Clinicians may be 'generalists' in the sense that their remit encompasses the full range of clinical concerns, but also 'particularists' in the sense that their unique obligation in each consultation is to the particular patient in front of them. It turns out that general rules often fall short. It also turns out that where medicines are concerned, less is often more.

We begin by setting out the role of the generalist in prescribing in more detail. We then focus on polypharmacy (the use of multiple medicine by one patient) as a way of encouraging you to grapple with some of the complexities of prescribing in generalist practice. Throughout the chapter we invite you to consider what a person-centred approach to prescribing may look like, and seek to equip you with some conceptual tools that will enable you to practise person-centred prescribing. Our examples are situated in general practice; however, the principles are widely applicable across secondary care, particularly geriatrics where the art of 'deprescribing' is acknowledged. We refer specifically to 'doctors' at the start of this chapter, as prescribing is an established part of their professional identity; however, the principles are also important for prescribing clinical practitioners and clinical pharmacists from the wider healthcare team. As more team members become involved in prescribing, the wisdom of knowing when *not* to prescribe, as well as when to, becomes increasingly important.

Prescribing in general practice: an example of generalist work with medicines

Doctors begin their clinical careers as students of medicine. Have you ever considered how interesting it is that the word 'medicine' encapsulates both a foundational discipline and the drugs prescribed? Prescribing is a core medical activity, written into the heart of a doctor's professional identity, right at the start of their professional careers.

The power of medicines lies primarily in a shared belief of efficacy – that is, a shared belief that a medicine may 'work' to achieve a desirable outcome. Without this underpinning assumption of efficacy a medicine would not qualify as a medicine at all (1). But the question of whether and to what extent a medicine 'works' (or might work) for a particular patient is remarkably tricky to answer. Medicines are also capable of causing harm (2). We use the word 'side effect' to describe this potential. This notion reinforces the framing of medicines as fundamentally good. The desirable effect is 'the' effect, but one must accept – on the side – the possibility of different unintended, undesirable effects. Every act of prescribing is therefore an occasion when clinicians must weigh in the balance the serious possibilities of both benefits and harms. To this end, prescribing shares common ground with many of the other practices described in this book, such as ordering investigations, making diagnoses or referrals, and – perhaps most importantly – the communicative contributions through which all of these practices are negotiated. Importantly, a clinician cannot know with certainty that any drug they prescribe will benefit the particular patient for whom they prescribe it. Prescribers practise under conditions of inevitable and inescapable uncertainty.

Prescribing is a complex practice. It brings together the technical (the science, or 'evidence'), the moral (broadly, an intent to ensure that the good outweighs the harm), a quest for meaning on behalf of both patient and practitioner, and a considerable degree of 'know-how' which accrues through a combination of experience and reflection-on-experience. Inevitably it involves dialogue between patient and clinician, without which it is impossible to navigate all these dimensions in a way that enables both parties to agree on a course of action. Achieving the balance then, between 'just enough' and 'too much' prescribing, is no mean feat. Modern medicines, wisely prescribed, can do immense good. But prescribing a drug for a patient that may bring little or no meaningful benefit to them is to expose patients to unnecessary risk of harm. The crux of the matter is how we understand meaningful benefit, and how we go about discerning it. We will unpack this further in the remainder of this chapter.

Prescribing is on the rise. In the UK, most prescribing activity takes place in general practice and approximately 70 per cent is the result of repeat prescribing, when drugs are made available to patients for an authorised period of time without the need for a consultation. A recent UK government report estimated that 10 per cent of drugs prescribed in general practice are 'overprescribed' (3). The evidence supporting this estimate is unclear, but the twin problems of underprescribing (where patients might stand to benefit from drugs which are not prescribed), and overprescribing (where patients may do better with a 'no drug' alternative or are prescribed drugs they do not want or need), are common. The overall direction of travel marches steadily towards ever burgeoning prescribing.

This escalation of prescribing is not a singular problem but goes hand-in-hand with sharp rises in requests for investigations (a staggering 8.5 per cent annually between 2000 and 2015) (4) and the increasing encroachment of market ideology in health care (5). Many systemic factors coalesce including:

- changing demographics (as the population ages, so does the accumulation of chronic conditions);
- policy (for example, financial incentives for prescribing);
- societal trends (for example, decreasing tolerance of risk); (6)
- medicalisation of older age; (7) and
- a thriving pharmaceutical industry with interests in widening indications for products and investing in the potential for profit that lies in 'risk reduction' in the context that risk can never be completely eliminated (however seductive this may be).

This is not an exhaustive list. The key point is that prescribers are only one part of a complex system that includes a wide range of actors.

Prescribing practices and policy can also drive health inequalities, particularly in low- and middle-income countries and for marginalised groups where the availability and affordability of medicine becomes a factor (see Chapter 8).

Generalists face some particularly knotty challenges in their prescribing role. First, the scientific evidence upon which the pervasive logic of 'evidence-based medicine' (EBM) rests is derived from population level studies in idealised trial situations which have poor external validity (the results are difficult to apply in the real world) (7). Many clinical guidelines are based on evidence generated from settings and patient populations that do not resemble most of the patients we see in our clinics. For example, patients in 'gold standard' randomised controlled trials are typically younger and less complex. Patients with multiple long-term conditions, racially minoritised individuals, and patients who are unable to consent to taking part in such trials are often excluded (8,9). This means that guidelines, while incredibly useful, can never offer us any more than a 'general rule'. The application of general rules to particular cases (that is, our patients) demands not only clinical judgement (see Chapter 5) but moral awareness. The moral gravity of the prescribing decision is even more salient when adherence to guidelines brings additional financial incentives, often under the guise of 'quality' (10). Our evidence-based toolkit equips us with useful concepts such as 'Absolute Risk Reduction' (ARR), 'Numbers Needed to Treat' (NNT) and 'Numbers Needed to Harm' (NNH) (although the less useful indicator 'Relative Risk Reduction' continues to predominate in publications) (see also Chapter 5). But even these tools reach the limits of their usefulness when the next patient in a morning clinic has four co-existing clinical conditions, a troubling set of financial and social circumstances, and an already long list of medications. We quickly find ourselves in an evidence desert, with shifting sands beneath our feet and little in the way of signposting.

In the remainder of this chapter we will focus specifically on generalism and polypharmacy. We have selected this focus for three reasons:

• polypharmacy is a common contemporary prescribing challenge, often the result of some of the contextual challenges we have outlined above;
• generalists are regarded as well placed to manage polypharmacy; and
• polypharmacy illustrates very well the complexities that generalists face in their everyday work as prescribers.

Before we turn to polypharmacy, let us introduce you to Dawn.

Example 16.1: Dawn

Dawn, 68, lives alone in a small council flat, her front door opening onto a noisy main road in the inner city. Sometimes she likes to stand there in her dressing gown, watching the world rushing by. But standing for any length of time has become difficult, with her arthritis and COPD competing for her attention. Mostly she sits indoors by her table in semi-darkness, curtains closed, her diary and important papers by her side. Dawn sleeps on her sofa these days as moving between bedroom and living room first thing in the morning when she is stiff is such hard work. She jokes that her flat is full of chairs with nobody sitting on them. Every time the occupational therapist visits she seems to acquire another chair. They are placed strategically around the flat to help her get from room to room in stages.

Dawn has so many medical appointments to keep track of: it seems to be one thing after another. It does get her down sometimes; life can feel like hard work. Hospital, GP, pharmacy, hospital, blood tests, GP. Sometimes she feels she is going round in circles. The singing group is the one thing that really helps. That is where she meets other people like her who are struggling with their breathing and picks up tips on how to manage. *I still can't sing, you know, but I love it and it gets me out.*

Dawn gets out a couple of times a week, but even crossing the main road is enough to make her breathless. It is stressful when the 'little green man' at the pedestrian crossing does not stay 'green' for long enough to see her over to the other side. Sometimes her neighbour pops out to help if he sees her struggling, but Dawn does not like to be a bother to her neighbours. She leans on her shopping trolley which helps her along. There has been talk of a mobility scooter but where would she put one of those with such a tiny flat and no outdoor space to call her own? Dawn's daughter, Sue, visits most days to check she is OK and help with shopping. Sometimes Dawn meets a friend at the local café, but she has very little appetite and feels embarrassed when she has to leave things on her plate. Sue thinks it's something to do with all the medicines her mother takes. Dawn isn't sure, but she is sceptical of her medicines nonetheless, though she does her best to take them. She wonders if her eating problems may be due to the surgery she had a few years ago? Or maybe it is old age? It is so hard to tell what's what with so many conditions and so many pills. If only Jack her little grandson was still around. Life was good. She has definitely not felt herself since he died four years ago.

Dawn's GP invites her to a medication review. The letter asks her to bring her medicines to the appointment. When the day approaches she feels anxious. What if she struggles to get there with her joints playing up the way they are? What if she sleeps in as she sometimes does? She doesn't usually book anything before 10.30 and this appointment is at 10 o'clock. What if she forgets what each medicine is for when the doctor asks? She has lots of questions but doesn't feel she ever gets the answers she is looking for. She thinks one medicine in particular is too strong and doesn't always take it. But she can't imagine the doctor stopping any medicines now. However, she is looking forward to some time with the GP as she worries about the large number of medicines. You can take one thing and it interacts with another. *Sometimes I wonder if they are paid to prescribe all this lot! It doesn't seem right. I don't know.*

She gathers her medicines together. Most of them are on the coffee table within reach of the sofa where she sleeps at night. She has a pharmacy-prepared dosette box, another home-made dosette box, a black sack containing several inhalers and a spacer. Her aspirin is separate; it has to be dissolved in water so she keeps it by the bathroom sink. Her rescue pack of steroids and antibiotics for her chest is in the kitchen cupboard. She sets her alarm for seven o'clock so that she has time to pack them all in her shopping trolley and catch the bus. On her way out she remembers to take a letter which arrived recently from one of her hospital consultants. It was buried under a pile of bills on the kitchen table. She wishes they wouldn't use so much jargon, but maybe the medication review will be a good chance to ask what it's all about without needing to make another trip.

She takes her medicines one by one from her bag and lays them on the GP's desk. First the pharmacy-prepared dosette, then all of the others in turn. It's slow work with her arthritic hands. She walks painfully to her trolley to find her inhalers. She sits and catches her breath. Five minutes in and they have barely begun, but at least the GP's attention is with her and her medicines and not on the computer screen as so often happens with doctors these days! And at least both Dawn and her GP can see what's what as they work through them together.

Polypharmacy: What it is and why it matters

There is no consensus definition of polypharmacy (one review estimates there are 138 definitions!) but everyone agrees that it involves the prescription of multiple medicines to a single patient (11). Polypharmacy is escalating. Older people's use of medication, both prescribed medication and those available for purchase over-the-counter, has increased dramatically over the last 20 years. The number of older people (aged 65+) taking five or more items increased from 12 to 49 per cent. The proportion who do not take any medication has decreased significantly from around 1 in 5 to 1 in 13 (12).

Sometimes polypharmacy can be problematic. The risks of polypharmacy to individuals are well documented and include: medicine errors; adverse drug reactions; cognitive decline; falls; frailty; hospitalisations with increased length of stay; and premature death (13,14). The risks increase as the number of medications increases, with 10 or more items regarded as a pragmatic marker of 'higher risk' polypharmacy (15,16). Wider societal harms of polypharmacy include the environmental and economic impacts of medicine waste through unnecessary prescribing or unused medicines (17–20). Given the risks of polypharmacy to individuals and society, polypharmacy has become a global health safety concern taken up by national and international organisations (3,21,22).

At best polypharmacy may be a necessary response to shifting demographics and a growing, ageing population of patients with multimorbidities; above the age of 65 multimorbidity is the norm. At worst, polypharmacy is an example of clinical overactivity and iatrogenic harm (23,24). Generalists can find themselves caught in a 'polypharmacy paradox' juggling not only many medicines but also conflicting demands on their professional selves (25). They may be encouraged (and financially incentivised) to follow single-disease guidelines in the service of 'quality' while at the same time being encouraged to address the harms of problematic polypharmacy which may emerge directly from their efforts at 'quality' (25).

The complex systemic, cultural and social context in which polypharmacy has emerged as a global safety concern suggests that addressing it will inevitably require system-wide collaboration and innovation. Clinicians are an important part of this system and it may be useful to reflect on what part you can play in addressing this. In the next section we invite you to think about polypharmacy through the lens of patients' experiences. We hope that this will equip you with additional concepts to 'think with' in your prescribing role.

Living with polypharmacy: the treatment burden

When we prescribe medicines we prescribe not only pills, creams, inhalers and so on; we also prescribe work (26). With each additional medication we contribute to the overall workload that we are demanding of patients, sometimes known as the 'burden of treatment' (27–29).

There is not one burden, but multiple burdens and they take several forms. Thinking about prescribing in this way encourages clinicians to shift away from a predominantly 'disease-centred' perspective (and its focus on indications, contra-indications, side effects), towards a perspective that accommodates the person with their many conditions in their social context. It is within this broader social context, and not within the consultation, that patients do most of their decision-making about their medicines (26). Clinicians ignore this at their peril, especially since *these burdens often remain hidden from practitioners* (27). It is only by remembering to think deliberately about these burdens that they are likely to be discovered. As Carl May and colleagues remind us 'we must respect patients for what they do as well as for who they are' (28).

We list some examples of the *kinds of burden* your patient may experience in the box 'Burden of treatment'.

Burden of treatment

Concealment burden. This arises when clinicians fail to provide information in ways that are personalised, meaningful, consistent and enabling of patients and their carers. This is burdensome in that it does not support understanding and may also result in patients and carers seeking information elsewhere (which may or may not be reliable, but always involves effort).

Exclusion burden. This arises when professionals do not fully recognise or acknowledge the expertise and experience that patients and carers bring to managing their own health and medicines. Investing time and effort (the professional work) to ensure meaningful involvement lessens the burden for patients (and is, after all, our job!).

Discursive burden. This refers to the complex interactional work that patients engage in to present themselves as morally good (that is, 'adherent') patients to avoid inviting judgement from their clinicians. The discourse of medicines adherence as a moral 'good' is powerful; patients may feel an imperative to perform as adherent (regardless of the extent to which this is so). This burden can be mitigated if clinicians can engage patients in more candid conversations.

Fragmentation burden. This occurs when patients are seen across a wide range of services. Patients and carers may experience a burden of work (and responsibility) as they try to 'glue' the contributions of different professionals and services together. This burden can be lessened if one professional (such as the GP) has oversight and takes overall responsibility, and if services strive for coordination and collaboration. As primary care delivery involves a widening range of prescribing professionals (for example, nurses, clinical pharmacists) the potential for this kind of burden exists even *within* a single service.

A key consideration for clinicians is whether, how and to what extent a patient (with the support of their social network, such as family and friends) has the capacity to manage the work that is demanded of them. By capacity, we refer not only to cognitive capacity (although this is important) but all the resources patients may draw on to take the actions necessary to manage their medicines into their daily lives. This includes cognitive, practical and social action; it also includes the resources needed to coordinate and appraise these different forms of work (28). Organising polypharmacy is time consuming. It involves devising routines, surveillance of self and supplies, managing priorities and a certain amount of creative experimentation with prescribed regimens. What emerges is often a compromise. Even when patients strive to adhere, their organisational efforts privilege 'living with medicines' over taking medicines 'as prescribed' (26).

As generalists we must therefore be curious about the daily lives of patients, their priorities for their lives, and how their medicines fit into this (or not as the case may be!). It is also important to appreciate that the balance between the work demanded of patients/families and their capacity to address the work does not remain static but changes over time. This means that every occasion of reviewing or reconciling a patient's medication is an(other) opportunity to revisit this balance and seek to mitigate, where possible, the burden of treatment your patient faces. If the balance tips, such that our demands outstrip capacity, then it is likely that patients will be unable to adhere to their medicines. Your prescribing – however well intended or 'evidence-based' – may then contribute to the overall burden of suffering, rather than relieving it, resulting in undesirable outcomes, poorer health and wasted resources.

The medication review

Medication reviews are often promoted as the solution to addressing the problems that being on too many medicines can bring. In the UK, a number of organisations have highlighted medication reviews as the means to address problematic polypharmacy. NICE, the National Institute for Health and Care Excellence, defines the medication review as a 'critical examination of a person's medicines with the objective of reaching an agreement with the person about treatment, optimising the impact of medicines, minimising the number of medication-related problems and reducing waste' (30).

Other professional organisations adopt similar definitions, although they vary in how they position the patient within this encounter and by being more or less prescriptive about what this should entail. In Wales, for example, guidance for delivering high-quality medication reviews suggests five criteria need to be met: involving patients and carers; considering medicines safety; reviewing all prescribed and non-prescribed medicines; reducing waste; and updating patient records and completing documentation (31). In England, a new (2021) contractual arrangement for general practice specifies that patients who are on 10 or more medicines should be identified and invited for a structured medication review (SMR) (32). Patients with fewer than 10 medicines, but whose repeat prescriptions include medicines that are prone to errors or known to contribute to frailty and addiction, are also encouraged to attend for a SMR.

This contractual obligation places considerable expectations on, for example, clinicians in primary care to deliver a review that satisfies policymakers' ambitions for:

- optimising medicines to make best use of medicines and reduce unwanted or inappropriate medications;
- reducing financial waste and environmental harm as a result of unnecessary or unwanted medicines; and
- listening to and addressing patients' concerns, needs and goals in relation to their health and their medicines.

This 'new', structured medication review builds on previous experience of medication reviews delivered within UK general practice settings (both as part of 'best practice' around repeat prescriptions and as part of previous iterations of incentivisation structures for conducting reviews). In the new specification, a longer consultation is recommended (30 minutes instead of the more standard 10 minutes), clinicians are advised to offer a 'personalised and holistic review' of medicines that incorporates patient-defined outcomes, and recognition is given that the person best placed to conduct such a review may include professionals such as clinical pharmacists and prescribing nurses as well as GPs. Their implementation follows the abandonment of incentivised Medicines Use Reviews (MURs) which were delivered in community pharmacy settings but which came under criticism for being delivered inconsistently, lacking personalisation and failing to reach the patients who may most benefit from them (33).

As the name suggests, medication reviews are primarily concerned with medicines. But as generalists, you will know that it is impossible to isolate medicines from a patient's wider needs and concerns. This is particularly the situation when a patient has multiple conditions and is prescribed many medicines. For example, a clinician may invite a patient to consider whether a particular medicine is causing a side effect. But when that medicine is just one of a collection of ten medicines it may be impossible for the patient to discern one side effect from another, or even to discern whether a side effect is a *side effect* at all, or rather a symptom of long-term ill health. Understandably, patients may use the medication review as an opportunity to discuss any or many of their health concerns (a phenomenon that is not limited to medication reviews). Where multimorbidity and polypharmacy are concerned this may be inevitable, and any effort on the part of the clinician to focus specifically on medicines may be quickly thwarted. While this may leave clinicians wondering *What will I (or should I) be dealing with today?* or feeling frustrated at the difficulty of 'getting through' the medication review, we suggest that reconceptualising the medication review in ways that bring the key concern(s) of patients to the fore (that is, considering what matters most to them within this review) may be helpful. Patients gain from this, and in the end, medication reviews are best thought of as an *ongoing process* rather than as a task to complete today; they do not have a clear beginning and end (25).

Organising medication reviews

Given the challenges we have started to outline, how then might clinicians seek to organise the medication review? As with many clinical consultations, the computerised medical record tends to play a significant role. It is usual for clinicians to work their way down a patient's list of medications as they appear on the screen. This can be a limiting way to structure a medication review as the list of medicines on the patient's record is unlikely to align with the patient's priorities or concerns for their medicines (they may simply be alphabetical, for example). One simple way to overcome this constraint is to ask patients to bring their medicines with them to the review (see also Example 9.2: 'Show me your meds, please').

Bringing medicines to the review has three key benefits:

1. *Ensures clinicians and patients are talking about the same medicine*
   Patients and clinicians often have different ways of knowing and talking about medicines (25). Patients often know their medicines by the colour, shape or size of the pill ('the blue one'; 'the big one'), the time of day they take the pill ('the morning one'), and the part of the body or system the medicine relates to ('the one for my knees'; 'the one for cholesterol'). This contrasts to clinicians who know medicines by their generic (chemical) or brand name (the latter vulnerable to frequent change, depending on what the pharmacist dispenses) and who have little contact with the material properties of medicines. Clinicians and patients can spend a lot of time in medication reviews doing nothing other than trying to work out which medicine they are each talking about. Having the medicines on the desk, between you and your patient, reduces the need for translation and minimises the scope for misunderstanding and confusion.

2. *Patients can focus on the medicines they are most concerned about*
   With the medicines immediately visible and to-hand it is much easier for patients to quickly identify those they wish to discuss with you. The medicines (and their boxes) act in several ways to support this. For example, they may remind the patient of specific concerns ('this one is terrible to swallow and always sticks in my throat') or prompt a patient to theorise ('I've been wondering if this medicine may be …?') or to make a request to change their medicines ('do you think I might be able to cut this one out?').

3. *Provides a tangible experience for the clinician of what being on a lot of medicines involves*
   We all know that polypharmacy can be problematic but having the volume of medicines in the room with the patient can really bring home

what being on lots of medicines is like. Seeing the patient interact with their medicines and their packaging, and witnessing their efforts at organising their concerns within the consultation can offer a window into the burden that so many medicines may create. It invites empathy for the very concrete, everyday practice of medicines-taking that is difficult to grasp from a neatly organised list of technical names on a computer screen. In particular, it may open up conversations regarding whether and how the patient has the capacity to manage – within their particular social context – the treatment regimen you have prescribed, and all the work that you are demanding of them.

Deprescribing – the expertise is in the room

Deprescribing is a challenge for clinicians. There is a lot of guidance advising when to start medicines. But decisions around not prescribing or stopping treatments are more complex and the evidence to support these practices is often missing (34). Although some progress is being made in targeted areas in the UK (the 2022 NICE guideline on the withdrawal of medicines associated with dependence is an example) the context of older people affected by polypharmacy is particularly difficult terrain to navigate (35). However, willingness to engage in such decision-making is a necessary contribution to addressing patients' treatment burden. Recent UK multimorbidity guidelines produced by NICE illustrate well the predicament that clinicians face: specific recommendations regarding stopping medicines were only possible for one group of preventive drugs, the bisphosphonates (24,36).

One challenge that deprescribing presents is the question of who is responsible (that is, who has a legitimate warrant) to stop a medicine. The term 'deprescribing' is somewhat unhelpful as it implies an 'undoing' of something important, a withdrawal. Given the close alignment of 'medicine' with medical professional identity (introduced at the beginning of this chapter) it is not difficult to see that this is a delicate manoeuvre if it is not to be interpreted as abandonment or withdrawal of 'care' itself. Generalists are regarded as well placed to tackle polypharmacy (37), but may feel reluctant to stop a medicine they did not start, or may feel the need to discuss the matter with a specialist. This may of course be helpful, but as a generalist working in a community setting, the GP may well be the clinician who knows the patient, their social networks and context best, especially if they have had the privilege of being involved in their healthcare over time. The GP might have recurring opportunities to discuss with a patient their goals and priorities, and to understand how one condition relates to another and how all of their conditions and treatments shape their daily lives. This knowledge is crucial to help the clinician and patient make decisions about starting or stopping a medicine. In this sense, the generalist is the appropriate specialist for supporting patients through this process. Usually this will be a process of small, incremental changes over time.

A dialogue with the patient – rather than a discussion about the patient – is likely to be key to enabling responsible decision-making under conditions of uncertainty. This means appreciating each person as a unique being situated within a context, and requires what has been called an 'ethical affective' – a situated mode of decision-making based on being *for* the other, arising from the quality of the interpersonal relationship (25,38).

Conclusion

In this chapter we have introduced some of the complexities of generalist prescribing, drawn your attention to the social contexts within which professionals' and patients' medicines practices take place, and used the concept of 'burden of treatment' as a way of conceptualising the full reach of prescribing decisions into patients' lives. We hope that introducing you to Dawn has helped to bring to life the daily reality of medicines-taking for older people with multiple conditions. By putting yourself into the shoes of patients like Dawn you may be able to identify some different ways of approaching your medication reviews, which take careful account of whether patients are able, willing and likely to benefit from doing what you are asking them to do when you prescribe a(nother) medicine. Sometimes less is more.

Acknowledgements

This chapter presents independent research funded by the National Institute for Health Research (NIHR) through a Clinician Scientist Award CS-2015-15-004 (DS). Additionally, this research was supported by the NIHR ARC North Thames. The views expressed in this publication are those of the author(s) and not necessarily those of the NIHR or the Department of Health and Social Care.

Further reading

Time to talk *differently* about medicines

A useful public engagement resource designed primarily for patients, including a collection of illustrated fictional stories available to read or listen to, each with discussion points. www.medicinestalk.co.uk

If you wish to extend your learning about polypharmacy in general practice we invite you to try these interactive RCGP e-learning resources (39). You can register for an e-learning account free of charge. The course invites you to think differently about multimorbidity and polypharmacy. There are two introductory screencasts (5-minute presentations with audio) and three 30-minute modules.

- **Screencast 1 – Polypharmacy: it's time to think differently**
- **Screencast 2 – Polypharmacy: thinking differently about the medication review**
- **Module 1 – Polypharmacy, multimorbidity and the treatment burden**
  This module introduces the concept of 'burden of treatment' with a particular focus on how it impacts patients affected by multimorbidity and polypharmacy. You are invited to reflect on how the burden of treatment plays out in the lives of patients and their social networks and to consider how you might apply this concept to improve patient care.
- **Module 2 – Polypharmacy, multimorbidity and the medication review**
  This module asks you to reflect on how you go about doing a medication review. You will reflect on the purpose of medication reviews, what makes a good medication review and how to approach conversations about medicines with patients. You will consider some of the factors which influence how a medication review proceeds.
- **Module 3 – Medicines: whose knowledge counts?**
  This module introduces the concept of epistemic injustice – a form of prejudice that arises from a wrong done to someone in their capacity as a 'knower'. Using polypharmacy as a case example, you will learn how the circulation of epistemic injustice within the health care system disempowers people and can lead to inertia. You will also learn some ways to help challenge epistemic injustice in the context of polypharmacy.

References

1. Whyte S, van der Geest S, Hardon A. An anthropology of material medica. *Social Lives of Medicines*. Cambridge University Press; 2002. pp. 3–19.
2. Smith R. Limits to medicine. Medical nemesis: the expropriation of health. *Journal of Epidemiology & Community Health*. 2003;57(12):928.
3. Department of Health and Social Care. Good for you, good for us, good for everybody. A plan to reduce overprescribing to make patient care better and safer, support the NHS, and reduce carbon emissions. 2021.
4. O'Sullivan JW, Stevens S, Hobbs FR, Salisbury C, Little P, Goldacre B et al. Temporal trends in use of tests in UK primary care, 2000–15: retrospective analysis of 250 million tests. *BMJ*. 2018;363.
5. McGregor S. Neoliberalism and health care. *International Journal of Consumer Studies*. 2001;25(2):82–9.
6. Adam B, Van Loon J, Beck U. *The Risk Society and Beyond: Critical issues for social theory*. SAGE; 2000.
7. Kaufman SR. *Ordinary Medicine: Extraordinary treatments, longer lives, and where to draw the line*. Duke University Press; 2015.
8. Hussain-Gambles M, Atkin K, Leese B. Why ethnic minority groups are under-represented in clinical trials: a review of the literature. *Health & Social Care in the Community*. 2004;12(5):382–8.
9. Taylor JS, DeMers SM, Vig EK, Borson S. The disappearing subject: exclusion of people with cognitive impairment and dementia from geriatrics research. *Journal of the American Geriatrics Society*. 2012;60(3):413–9.

10. Mangin D, Toop L. The Quality and Outcomes Framework: what have you done to yourselves? *Br J Gen Pract*. 2007;57(539):435–7.
11. Masnoon N, Shakib S, Kalisch-Ellett L, Caughey GE. What is polypharmacy? A systematic review of definitions. *BMC Geriatrics*. 2017;17(230).
12. Gao L, Maidment I, Matthews FE, Robinson L, Brayne C. Medication usage change in older people (65+) in England over 20 years: findings from CFAS I and CFAS II. *Age and Ageing*. 2018;47(2):220–5.
13. Avery AA, Barber N, Ghaleb M, Dean Franklin B, Armstrong S, Crowe S et al. Investigating the prevalence and causes of prescribing errors in general practice: the PRACtICe study. General Medical Council; 2012. Available from: https://www.rpharms.com/Portals/0/Documents/Old%20news%20documents/news%20downloads/gmc-report.pdf (accessed 22 March 2024).
14. Sears K, Scobie A, Mackinnon NJ. Patient-related risk factors for self-reported medication errors in hospital and community settings in 8 countries. *Can Pharm J (Ott)*. 2012;145(2):88–93.
15. Guthrie B, Makubate B, Hernandez-Santiago V, Dreischulte T. The rising tide of polypharmacy and drug-drug interactions: population database analysis 1995–2010. *BMC Medicine*. 2015;13(1):74.
16. The King's Fund. Polypharmacy and medicines optimisation – making it safe and sound. 2013. Available from: www.kingsfund.org.uk/insight-and-analysis/reports/polypharmacy-and-medicines-optimisation (accessed 22 March 2024).
17. Boxall AB, Rudd MA, Brooks BW, Caldwell DJ, Choi K, Hickmann S et al. Pharmaceuticals and personal care products in the environment: what are the big questions? *Environmental Health Perspectives*. 2012;120(9):1221–9.
18. NHS Business Services Authority. Pharmaceutical waste reduction in the NHS. 2015. Available from: www.england.nhs.uk/wp-content/uploads/2015/06/pharmaceutical-waste-reduction.pdf (accessed 22 March 2024).
19. Panigone S, Sandri F, Ferri R, Volpato A, Nudo E, Nicolini G. Environmental impact of inhalers for respiratory diseases: decreasing the carbon footprint while preserving patient-tailored treatment. *BMJ Open Respiratory Research*. 2020;7(1):e000571.
20. Bartholomew T, Finikin, S. Tackling overprescribing: a must for climate action. BJGP Life; 2022. Available from: https://bjgplife.com/tackling-overprescribing-a-must-for-climate-action/ (accessed 22 March 2024).
21. World Health Organization. Medication safety in polypharmacy. 2019. Available from: https://apps.who.int/iris/bitstream/handle/10665/325454/WHO-UHC-SDS-2019.11-eng.pdf?ua=1 (accessed 22 March 2024).
22. AGE UK. More harm than good. Why more isn't always better with older people's medicines. 2019. Available from: www.ageuk.org.uk/globalassets/age-uk/documents/reports-and-publications/reports-and-briefings/health--wellbeing/medication/190819_more_harm_than_good.pdf (accessed 22 March 2024).
23. Armstrong N, Swinglehurst D. Understanding medical overuse: the case of problematic polypharmacy and the potential of ethnography. *Family Practice*. 2018;35(5):526–7.
24. Swinglehurst D, Fudge N. The polypharmacy challenge: time for a new script? *British Journal of General Practice*. 2017;67(662):388–9.
25. Swinglehurst D, Hogger L, Fudge N. Negotiating the polypharmacy paradox: a video-reflexive ethnography study of polypharmacy and its practices in primary care. *BMJ Quality & Safety*. 2023;32(3):150–9.
26. Swinglehurst D, Fudge N. Organising polypharmacy: unpacking medicines, unpacking meanings – an ethnographic study. *BMJ Open*. 2021;11(8):e049218.
27. Maidment I, Lawson S, Wong G, Booth A, Watson A, Zaman H et al. Towards an understanding of the burdens of medication management affecting older people: the MEMORABLE realist synthesis. *BMC Geriatrics*. 2020;20(1):183.
28. May CR, Eton DT, Boehmer K, Gallacher K, Hunt K, MacDonald S et al. Rethinking the patient: using Burden of Treatment Theory to understand the changing dynamics of illness. *BMC Health Services Research*. 2014;14:1–11.
29. Shippee ND, Shah ND, May CR, Mair FS, Montori VM. Cumulative complexity: a functional, patient-centered model of patient complexity can improve research and practice. *Journal of Clinical Epidemiology*. 2012;65(10):1041–51.

30. NICE. NICE Guideline [NG5]: Medicines optimisation: the safe and effective use of medicines to enable the best possible outcomes. 2015. Available from: www.nice.org.uk/guidance/ng5 (accessed 22 March 2024).
31. All Wales Medicines Strategy Group. Welsh National Standards for Medication Review. 2020. Available from: https://awttc.nhs.wales/files/guidelines-and-pils/welsh-national-standards-for-medication-review-brief-guide-pdf/ (accessed 22 March 2024).
32. NHS England. Network Contract Directed Enhanced Service. Structured medication reviews and medicines optimization: guidance. 2021. Available from: www.england.nhs.uk/wp-content/uploads/2021/03/B0431-network-contract-des-smr-and-mo-guidance-21-22.pdf (accessed 22 March 2024).
33. Madden M, Mills T, Atkin K, Stewart D, McCambridge J. Early implementation of the structured medication review in England: a qualitative study. *British Journal of General Practice.* 2022;72(722):e641–e8.
34. Mangin D, Heath I, Jamoulle M. Beyond diagnosis: rising to the multimorbidity challenge. *BMJ.* 2012;13(344):e3526.
35. NICE. NICE Guideline [NG215]: Medicines associated with dependence or withdrawal symptoms: safe prescribing and withdrawal management for adults. 2022. Available from: www.nice.org.uk/guidance/ng215 (accessed 22 March 2024).
36. NICE. NICE Guideline [NG56]: Multimorbidity: clinical assessment and management. 2016. Available from: www.nice.org.uk/guidance/ng56 (accessed 22 March 2024).
37. Duncan P, Duerden M, Payne RA. Deprescribing: a primary care perspective. *European Journal of Hospital Pharmacy.* 2017;24(1):37–42.
38. Sellar S. The responsible uncertainty of pedagogy. *Discourse: Studies in the Cultural Politics of Education.* 2009;30(3):347–60.
39. RCGP Learning. Polypharmacy and multimorbidity 2022. Available from: https://elearning.rcgp.org.uk/multimorbidity (accessed 22 March 2024).

17

Embedding health and wellbeing into clinical practice and education

Jessica Ying-Yi Xie, Kay Leedham-Green and
Sara Thompson

Introduction

The promotion of health and wellbeing in clinical education and practice is complex, and yet it is fundamental to generalist forms of healthcare. When done well, it has the potential to address many of the risk factors for common non-communicable diseases driving a more equitable, regenerative and sustainable healthcare system. It is intrinsically participatory as patients must be active partners in addressing their own risk factors for disease and strategies for wellbeing. It requires multiple lenses on complex real-world problems as well as collaborative intersectoral working, and it benefits from longitudinal, relationship-based care.

Much of a healthcare student's early clinical education is likely to centre on learning about how to support people who are unwell. Generalist education, however, also invites learners to engage across a person's life narrative: exploring current and past contextual factors, and imagining and planning for a future centred on what matters to that person.

Chapter 11 articulates how generalists interact with community wellbeing resources such as dementia cafes, park runs, creative arts and community canteens. Chapter 18 discusses the principles of personalised care: working collaboratively with patients and carers to identify and address what matters to them and supporting them in effective self-management. This chapter focuses on how health and wellbeing can be promoted within a clinical encounter, either opportunistically or as part of a personalised care-planning appointment. We also explore some of the educational challenges and strategies for supporting learners in developing the associated capabilities and using them to good effect.

Conceptualising health and wellbeing

There are multiple and sometimes conflicting definitions of health and wellbeing. Although the two concepts overlap, they are not the same. Health has been described variously as (1) an absence of disease or impairment; (2) a state of fitness or an ability to cope with one's activities of daily living; (3) a state of internal and external equilibrium; and (4) a state of complete physical, mental and social wellbeing. Health can be measured both subjectively ('do you consider yourself to be healthy?') and, depending on which definition is used, objectively through metrics such as blood pressure, cholesterol, body mass index or other physiological indicators. Wellbeing, on the other hand, tends to be framed more positively and in more complex ways, encompassing hard-to-measure factors such as happiness, life satisfaction, quality of life and self-esteem. A person in a state of good wellbeing is said to be able to enjoy and contribute to society with a sense of meaning and purpose (5). While health can impact on wellbeing, it is not the only influence. Someone who is objectively unhealthy can also experience a sense of subjective wellbeing which might be influenced by factors such as autonomy, good relationships, a sense of purpose, and social support (6).

In this chapter, wellbeing will be considered through multiple perspectives: those of the patient, the clinician and the learner. Our aim is to demonstrate that wellbeing is relevant to all, yet has a unique meaning to the individual. Worked examples of how wellbeing can be taught and supported in clinical and educational practice are integrated into this chapter to demonstrate the multiple scenarios in which wellbeing can be opportunistically addressed. We will also touch on the role of the healthcare sector in supporting the wellbeing of people with long-term health conditions, as well as the wellbeing of healthcare workers themselves through a culinary medicine educational example.

The consultation: a window of opportunity

The consultation is the ideal setting for healthcare professionals to engage patients in opportunistic or planned discussions about their wellbeing, and ideas, concerns and expectations around this. This is especially the case where relational continuity with people exists, such as in general practice. GPs are therefore in a good position to identify people whose health and wellbeing could be improved with lifestyle changes, optimisation of clinical management and social care, and/or support through any other means, such as community groups or rights and benefits advice (see Chapters 10 and 11). We will explore how the art of generalism can be applied to transform these brief patient encounters into pivotal opportunities to inspire both patients and ourselves as clinicians, and to change our mindset and behaviour to improve wellbeing.

The determinants of health

Health inequalities are unfair, avoidable and systematic differences in health between different groups of people (7). These inequalities can be broadly categorised into intrinsic and extrinsic factors (see Figure 17.1). Intrinsic factors may be considered modifiable determinants of health, as they tend to be behavioural: for example, smoking, diet, alcohol, obesity, taking medicines regularly, exercise and so forth. Rather than being a simple 'personal choice', these 'behaviours' tend to be influenced upstream by extrinsic, wider commercial and socioeconomic determinants. Multiple factors and stakeholders shape possible behavioural 'choices' and opportunities for care. This affects access to (and then quality and experience of) healthcare. Factors include poverty, poor housing, literacy, education, environmental degradation, social isolation and trauma (see also Chapter 11). Treating healthy living merely as a lifestyle choice is therefore likely to meet with limited success. The principles of generalism, however, invite the practitioner to view a patient's health needs through multiple lenses – the biomedical and the behavioural as well as the upstream social, commercial and environmental determinants – and to work collaboratively with people to identify what matters and what might make a difference.

There are, of course, evidence-based guidelines for the management of many of the direct challenges to health such as smoking, alcohol

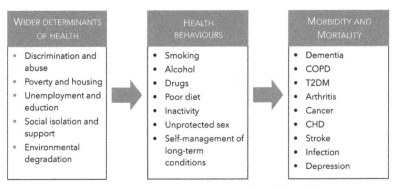

Figure 17.1 The modifiable determinants of health and disease.
© Kay Leedham-Green

dependence, substance misuse, unprotected sex, exercise and dietary inadequacies. There are also wider health-related components to the management guidelines for many long-term conditions such as diabetes and COPD. These guidelines may include specific tests, screening, therapies, referrals and lifestyle advice. Specific health promotion guidelines will change over time and vary between organisations and healthcare systems, and are therefore beyond the scope of this chapter, but they should also inform consultation approaches.

The negative health behaviours in Figure 17.1 can be inverted to become the positive drivers of health and potentially wellbeing: *stopping* smoking, *starting* to exercise, *taking* antihypertensives more regularly, *changing* dietary habits, *stopping* substance misuse, *starting* a hobby, *meeting* up with friends more frequently, *learning* to self-manage and so forth. There is an action verb to each of these positive drivers, suggesting a behavioural lens might be important.

Health and behaviour

So long as the upstream determinants of health are not forgotten, nor a patient's immediate biomedical needs, it can be helpful to explore health and wellbeing through a behaviour change lens. Michie's theoretical domains framework (Figure 17.2), also known as the COM-B model (capability, opportunity, motivation => behaviour change), is a well-established theory that integrates all the potential drivers of a change in behaviour (8). All components of the model can impact on each other, for example, motivation may be increased when a new skill or knowledge is acquired which means the person now has the capability to initiate a behaviour. Importantly, the model includes attending to a person's external social and physical environment (their opportunities), their intrinsic and extrinsic motivations, as well as their physical and psychological ability to undertake the new behaviour. The COM-B model can be used to understand why an intended behaviour, for example stopping smoking, is or is not happening. Perhaps they live with a smoker? Perhaps they are using smoking as a psychological crutch? Perhaps they do not feel the risks are relevant to them? Perhaps they need help managing physical cravings? Perhaps they simply do not want to quit?

The COM-B model can inform a behavioural understanding or diagnosis, which can then be used to personalise an intervention according to its function. Michie's theoretical domains framework also provides a comprehensive taxonomy of intervention functions: education, training,

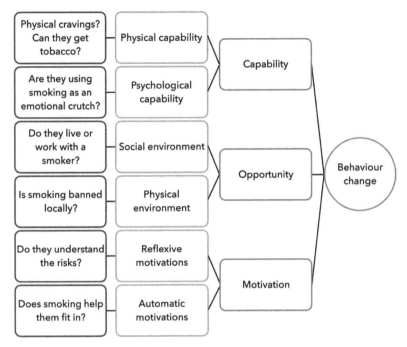

Figure 17.2   Exploring the drivers of a health behaviour (smoking) using the COM-B model. Based on Michie and colleagues' COM-B framework. © Kay Leedham-Green based on Michie et al. 2011 (8)

modelling, environmental restructuring, restriction, enablement, incentivisation, persuasion and coercion. Not all of these are appropriate within a person-centred consultation, but the principle remains: a behavioural diagnosis is needed to inform the intervention function. There is no point in educating someone about the dangers of smoking if they already understand, and are willing to accept the risks; if their main problem is a social trigger rather than physical cravings then nicotine replacement therapy is unlikely to be helpful; if they are using tobacco as an emotional crutch, then that may need to be addressed first.

A complex evidence base

Producing a quantitative evidence base for health and wellbeing interventions within a personalised clinical consultation, as opposed to wider public health and policy, is challenging. Quasi-experimental research might involve randomising patients to one pathway and comparing their outcomes to another. But how feasible is it to randomise consultation approaches? How ethical is it? How can one ensure the control group is effectively controlled? How reproducible is an intervention, particularly if it is based on longitudinal relationship-based care? Instead, the evidence base for health and wellbeing interventions tends to be built on larger cohort studies of clearly defined or system-level interventions, rather than personalised consultation-based approaches. Meta-analyses are also challenging as each study might have a different target population and different outcome measures. Over time, however, it becomes possible to estimate what typical health and wellbeing interventions are achieving, and to make pragmatic adjustments for what might be achievable within a personalised consultation. It is important to remember that the lack of 'hard' quasi-experimental data for health and wellbeing interventions within a clinical consultation reflects the characteristics of personalised care and should not be confused with ineffectiveness: the evidence base is just more complex. Table 17.1 provides example outcomes from health and wellbeing interventions, with contextual notes.

Table 17.1 Example outcomes from health and wellbeing interventions

Intervention	Outcomes	Contextual notes
Smoking cessation	54% of those setting a quit date remain successful 4 weeks later.	National UK statistics[9].
Obesity	46% of those starting a group weight-loss programme lost >5% of their body weight a year later (60% of completers) 23% lost >10% (31% of completers).	Australian, German and UK study exploring free referrals to a commercial weight-loss support group[10].
Alcohol	38% of alcohol abuse-affected individuals and 30% of alcohol dependent individuals who try to quit were successful.	North American data based on a national epidemiological survey[11].
Exercise	A pedometer and 12-week walking diary intervention was associated with significant decreases in both new cardiovascular events and fractures at 4 years. Number needed to treat (NNT) to avoid an event was approximately 60 for a cardiovascular event and 28 for a fracture.	UK-based cohort study[12].

(continued)

Table 17.1 (Cont.)

Intervention	Outcomes	Contextual notes
Wellbeing through social prescribing	Of the 136 participants, 62% were depressed, based on the Hospital Anxiety and Depression Scale before the intervention and 45% after. 93% suffered from anxiety before the intervention, 77% after. Also, significant improvements in validated self-efficacy and wellbeing scales.	Social prescribing in Scotland: meditation and creative arts courses[13].

Structuring a conversation about health and wellbeing

Although the COM-B model is a helpful way of conceptualising the drivers of behaviour change, it is not a consultation model. How does one start a conversation about health and wellbeing? How does one ensure a patient's autonomy and preferences are respected, while still inviting conversations about difficult topics such as obesity, alcohol or loneliness? How does one elicit 'change talk', or tap into people's existing strengths, building on previous successes? How does one maintain forward momentum within a time-limited clinical encounter? How does one generate a plan that is sensitive to a patient's needs, context and wishes? How does one negotiate uncertain engagement or outcomes?

There are a variety of consultation models and communication toolkits to choose from with an array of acronyms such as MI (motivational interviewing), SBIRT (screening, brief intervention and referral), StACC (structured agenda-free coaching conversations), T-GROW (topic, goal, reality check, options, way forward), CIC (conversations inviting change), the 2Es (every patient, every visit), the 5As (ask, assess, advise, assist, arrange) and others (14–19). Some frameworks are more directive than others; for example, a very brief intervention might involve simply advising the person to quit a negative behaviour or adopt a positive one. Others involve more psychologically informed approaches: engaging the patient in reflecting on their own needs and context, asking them to articulate an achievable goal that is important to them, a realistic plan for achieving it, and supporting them through problem-solving, resources and follow-up.

Directive versus coaching approaches

Table 17.2 contrasts a relatively directive 6As approach (20) with a more patient-centred 'coaching' approach (described in more detail in Chapter 18). For this example, we have moved away from a health

Table 17.2 The 6 As, comparing a directive and coaching approach. Adapted from Glasgow et al. 5As (14) and Leedham-Green et al. 6As (20)

The 6 As	A directive approach	A coaching approach
Ask	Are you socially isolated?	Would you like to talk about your loneliness? What are your concerns?
Assess	How often do you interact with others?	Can you take me through a typical day? What do you think the issues are? What do you think might help? [barriers and facilitators to change, COM-B diagnosis]
Advise	Social isolation puts you at risk of depression, anxiety, heart disease and dementia	It sounds as though some of the issues are ... Some potential resources/evidenced strategies include ...
Agree	You should aim to interact with others at least once per day	What is an achievable goal/action that might make a difference to you? What other options are there? Which option sounds best? How and when can you make that happen?
Assist	Here is a diary to track your progress	How confident are you in making that change? What might improve your confidence? Would a [resource/ referral] help?
Arrange	I will see you again in 6 weeks to review	Would you find follow-up helpful? When would you like to come back?

behaviour to a more complex wellbeing problem: addressing the needs of an adult experiencing loneliness.

Example 17.1a: Johan needs more than medicine

Johan is a refugee who has presented with clinical depression which he associates with the loneliness of living in a foreign country and the working restrictions placed on him while awaiting his resettlement papers. After attending to local guidelines on depression, his GP broaches his loneliness through a health coaching approach (see Table 17.2).

Johan says that he is keen to socialise with other refugees as he feels they would understand him. He also misses meaningful work, which he thinks would provide him with opportunities to meet people. Unfortunately, while he waits for his resettlement papers, paid work is unavailable to him. They agree on a referral to their local social prescribing link worker who is familiar with local opportunities.

To be continued ...

The stages of a coaching consultation, from information-sharing to goal-setting, action-planning, problem-solving and follow-up, are reasonably generic across consultation models, as are the core communicative strategies articulated by Miller and Rollnick: open questions, affirmations, reflections and summaries, expressing empathy, rolling with resistance, developing discrepancies and supporting self-efficacy (17). Learning to find the right words at the right time, however, takes time and practice to perfect. Most health coaching courses, for example, take a couple of days to complete, followed by supervised practice; this chapter is intended as an introduction rather than as a replacement for a course.

Promoting change one step at a time

Truly transformative change may need to address deeply ingrained beliefs, motivations, behaviours and contextual barriers. Although practitioners can initiate and stimulate conversations inviting change, the real work of change is done by the patient with the support of their social network outside the consulting room in their own time. One of the features of generalism is the focus on longitudinal approaches to patient needs through relationship-based care, which can be used to advantage in the promotion of health and wellbeing. Follow-up is, after all, a driver *in itself* of sustained behaviour change (21).

The transtheoretical model (Figure 17.3), also known as the stages of change model, articulates the phases that a person might go through, from realising that change is necessary, to planning and initiating change, through to sustaining change and managing relapses (22). This framework allows the practitioner to identify where a person is on their change journey. It can also be used to 'chunk' health-promoting conversations into smaller achievable steps. Focusing on one stage at a time may feel more achievable within a time-constrained consultation. A single consultation might, for example, help to move someone from pre-contemplation to contemplation with the words 'Have you thought of (health or wellbeing topic)? When you last (did x), what worked? How would (change) make you feel?' and inviting them back to discuss it another day. Aiming for a single step at a time allows the patient time to process each step, to do their own research, to discuss with others, and even to attempt change before returning for follow-up. It is key that follow-up is supportive and encouraging rather than directive or admonishing. The latter approach is likely to elicit defensive behaviour and there are always reasons (capability, opportunity, motivation or competing interests) why a behaviour did not occur.

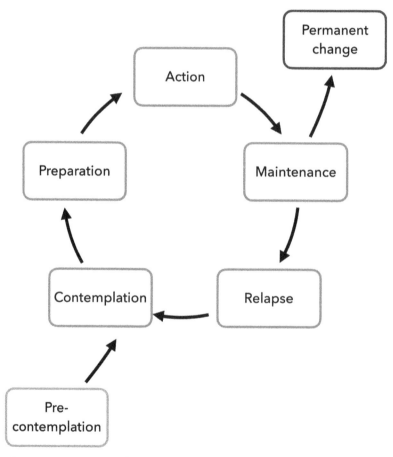

Figure 17.3 Stages of change (transtheoretical) model. © Kay Leedham-Green based on Prochaska et al. 1992 (22)

Broaching complex or sensitive topics

One of our chapter authors ran a training day for 60 general practitioners and practice nurses on person-centred approaches for addressing obesity within a clinical consultation. Their pre-course survey asked participants what they were struggling with, and their post-course survey asked what they found most helpful. The pre-course survey highlighted the level of complexity that these generalists were encountering. Specifically, the association of morbid obesity with factors such as complex childhood trauma, poverty, mobility impairment, binge eating disorder, or ongoing abuse. A large observational study in California found that two-thirds of respondents with morbid obesity were survivors of complex childhood trauma (23). The pre-course survey also highlighted concerns about causing offence or further trauma by raising sensitive issues. The post-training survey identified learning to broach sensitive topics in person-centred ways as the most helpful learning point of the day; the second being how to use coaching rather than directive approaches.

These practitioners expressed differing views on how and when conversations about weight should be brought up within a consultation. Is it ethical to only raise the issue of obesity after pathology such as hypertension, arthritis or diabetes has set in? Is it ethical to raise the issue proactively if it has the potential to offend? Is it ethical to ignore it, given the strong association with eating disorders and abuse? We asked our invited patient advocates and course participants with lived experience of obesity for their views. Can the topic be raised proactively without causing offence? One participant said that they did not like being told they were overweight ('You're not breaking bad news, I do know!'), but that it was a relief to be invited to talk about their concerns as they themselves sometimes found it difficult to start the conversation. Their consensus was that it was appropriate to offer the conversation proactively, but not to impose it: effectively 'asking to ask'. Table 17.3 summarises workshop comments on some of the approaches commonly used to broach obesity.

Working collaboratively

Another feature of generalism is the emphasis on collaborative working. Generalists approach all types of health problems at all stages in life, not because they know everything, but because they work collaboratively and know when (and when not) to draw on evidence-based guidelines

Table 17.3 Critiquing strategies for broaching obesity in a consultation

Strategy	Comments from patient advocates	Impression given by strategy
While you're here, would you mind stepping on to the scales … I'm sorry to tell you that you have an unhealthy BMI (body mass index) …	Sounds like 'breaking bad news'.	Practitioner's agenda.
We need to have a conversation about your weight …	Sounds like a 'telling off'.	Practitioner's agenda.
Can I ask you about your weight? Is this something you would like to talk about today? What are your concerns?	Offering, not imposing, the conversation. Asking to ask. Focusing first on the patient's agenda.	Patient-centred. Mutually engaged.

(see also Chapter 5). This way of working creates a form of dynamic, distributed expertise: patients have a single point of contact, but access to a much wider network of information and healthcare professionals who may be experts in exercise, diet, self-management and other health-related issues.

Example 17.1b: Mukta and Joe work together

Mukta is a busy practice nurse who runs a weekly personalised care-planning clinic for patients with multimorbidities. Each patient gets two appointments, the first is for tests such as mental health screening, blood pressure, blood tests, foot checks, BMI and inhaler checks. After the results have been shared with her patients, they come back for their second appointment, which is where the conversation about what would make a difference happens. Mukta used to avoid asking about wider social issues, even though she knew how important they were, because she didn't know how to help. That was until she met Joe, their local social prescribing link worker.

Joe is an experienced health coach and met Mukta on a course he was running. Mukta is now happy to invite conversations about anything including housing, poverty, heating, nutrition, social care and loneliness. If Mukta can't help her patients resolve something that is affecting their health and wellbeing within her care-planning consultation, if appropriate, she offers a referral to Joe. Joe doesn't solve his patients' problems for them. Instead, he supports them to look together at what it is possible to solve, supported through his knowledge of local and online resources. Joe explains how, if he can't find a resource to suggest, he will offer to link patients with someone who might be able to help. He describes a repair and recycle club for refugees that was set up by Johan (see Example 17.1a) at his local community centre, with the help of a social enterprise grant they applied for together.

To be continued ...

Evaluating health and wellbeing interventions

Although evaluative data can be used in research, the purpose of evaluation is to understand, monitor, or improve a contextualised intervention rather than produce transferable knowledge (24). A very simple outcomes evaluation might ask whether an intervention achieved its stated goals. A more complex 'realist' evaluation might look at who the intervention worked for, to what extent, in which contexts, and why. An economic evaluation might look at the social, financial and environmental inputs in relation to outcomes to determine what value was created for different stakeholders. A participatory action research model might invite patients and carers to work with those delivering the intervention to evaluate its processes and improve it. Evaluation plans should ideally be built into the intervention from the start, involve stakeholders, specifically patients and communities, and follow legal and ethical guidelines for consent, confidentiality, data protection and minimisation of harms. Formal ethical oversight may be required if the results are to be disseminated, for example through publication or conference presentation.

Direct measures of evaluation can be relatively straightforward. For example, frequency of use of a weight-loss or smoking cessation app. However, exploring how, why and when a wellbeing intervention is used (or not) may be more complex. For simple health-related interventions, it may be possible to track physiological markers of morbidity over time such as blood pressure, cholesterol, glycemic control or BMI, or to use self-reported behavioural outcomes such as smoking cessation rates, exercise diaries or medication adherence. Many wellbeing interventions, however, tend to have harder-to-measure outcomes, such as reducing loneliness, increasing someone's sense of purpose, or reducing feelings of overwhelm. An understanding of how an intervention is supposed to achieve the desired wellbeing outcomes (its theory of change) may allow proxy interim measures to be usefully proposed.

Example 17.1c: Johan and Joe evaluate their work

Joe recognises the importance of evaluating the wellbeing interventions he recommends, both at an individual and collective level. He encourages providers of local community groups to do their own evaluation, but he also asks his patients to complete the WHO-5 wellbeing index before and after the intervention (25), with a few qualitative questions before (What are you hoping to achieve? Do you need any special adjustments to help you engage?) and afterwards (What difference did this intervention make to you? What was most helpful about it? How could it be improved for others?). With consent, Joe shares anonymised quarterly data with both the referrer and provider. This, he says, encourages the referrers to refer again, and the providers to continually improve and develop. The quantitative evaluation helps Joe to compare interventions and he combines this with demographic data to monitor inclusion.

Johan designed the evaluation of his repair and recycle club for refugees with his club members, supported by Joe. Many refugees arrived with language barriers. Some were suspicious of authority. Many, like Johan, were looking for friendship, a shared sense of purpose and belonging, as well as new skills. They agreed on a visual record of all the repaired items that have been returned to their community, and an informal attendance register, with a record of why people left the club (relocation, employment, or other).

In this case, the physical outputs of the repair and recycling project are a proxy interim measure for one of their intended wellbeing outcomes: a sense of purpose. Their attendance register is another useful interim measure as social participation in the group is likely to be a precursor of reduced loneliness. Seeing whether people have moved on to employment might also be an indicator of language and skills development, and can be compared with local benchmarks.

Interim proxy measures are useful as they can often be charted over time with minimal burden on participants. There are also a variety of validated questionnaires that can be used to measure complex constructs such as quality of life, happiness and wellbeing; for example, the WHO-5 wellbeing index (26) or the Warwick-Edinburgh Mental Wellbeing Scale (27). Validated questionnaires can often be used as 'before and after' measures to see whether the intervention had an impact, and combined with demographic and qualitative data to understand for whom it worked, and why. Many validated questionnaires also have benchmark data so that practitioners can compare their intervention population with a population mean. This enables providers to check, for example, that the intervention is being used by the people that need it. As a note of caution, validated measures are only as useful and relevant as their underlying constructs. A quality of life index that is based on physical constructs such as chronic pain and mobility is unlikely to pick up changes in social or psychological wellbeing. Evaluation measures should be chosen carefully and collaboratively.

Developing health promotion competencies

The cognitive apprenticeship model (Figure 17.4) is a useful framework for describing the tacit steps from novice to expert in the acquisition of complex skills such as coaching for health and wellbeing (28). Learners typically start by learning *about* the practice including its theoretical and evidential grounding, for example through pre-reading, a presentation or e-learning. Next, they might observe application of theory, modelled by an expert, then try it themselves under direct observation in a safe environment, for example through simulation, expert patients, or role play, and receive personalised feedback. Next, they apply their newly acquired skills with clinical patients, aided by prompts, guidelines and

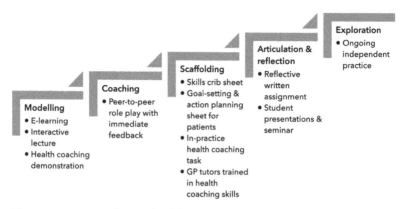

Modelling
- E-learning
- Interactive lecture
- Health coaching demonstration

Coaching
- Peer-to-peer role play with immediate feedback

Scaffolding
- Skills crib sheet
- Goal-setting & action planning sheet for patients
- In-practice health coaching task
- GP tutors trained in health coaching skills

Articulation & reflection
- Reflective written assignment
- Student presentations & seminar

Exploration
- Ongoing independent practice

Figure 17.4   Developing health promotion competencies through a cognitive apprenticeship. Derived from Wylie & Leedham-Green (29)

other scaffolding support, ideally with near-hand debrief support from an expert. Support is gradually withdrawn as the learner gains confidence. Finally, once the learner can articulate what excellence looks like, and critique and reflect on their performance in relation to others, they develop as experts who can independently innovate, improve and educate. Figure 17.4 illustrates how these steps were integrated into an undergraduate health promotion course component at King's College London (29).

There are additional factors that may need to be addressed if a learner is going to integrate discussions around health and wellbeing into their evolving clinical practice. It may not be enough for them to simply develop the right professional competencies, for example, by completing a health coaching course. They also need time and the appropriate environment in which to engage their patients in discussion; to believe that health promotion is an effective use of that time and in their patients' best interests; and that wellbeing and health promotion are part of their professional identity. Mukta's example, above, also illustrates that learners are more likely to act if they are familiar with any available resources, such as link workers, self-help apps and referral options. These requirements for effective clinical practice have been described as role competency, role legitimacy and resource adequacy (20). These are illustrated in Table 17.4, alongside potential educational interventions.

Table 17.4 Challenges and strategies for health promotion in clinical practice

Facilitator	Challenges	Strategies
Role legitimacy • Seeing health promotion as part of their professional identity • Believing health promotion is in their patients' interests	Lack of senior role modelling Judgemental attitudes Fear of offence Despondency	Training seniors in parallel with juniors to enhance role modelling Expert patients who are willing to share their story Learning patient-centred approaches Exploring positive evaluations
Role competency • Knowledge of the evidence base • Ability to use clinical guidelines effectively • Health coaching skills	Knowing what to do Knowing how to do it Knowledge of resources Knowing how to work interprofessionally	E-learning and pre-reading Practical skills workshops Opportunities for practice with feedback Scaffolding tools (see above) Assignments and assessments Interprofessional projects & seminars
Resource adequacy • Opportunities, resources, support • Ease of access to resources	Finding time and headspace Local referral options and protocols Effective therapies	Appointments with protected time for forward planning Chunking: one change-step per consultation Health navigators / link workers Responsive commissioning of local services

Educational example: Integrating culinary medicine education into the core undergraduate medical curriculum at UCL

Culinary medicine at UCL (30), which was introduced into the core undergraduate medical curriculum in September 2019, is a worked example of supporting learners in applying knowledge to clinical practice using elements of the cognitive apprenticeship model (29).

> Let food be thy medicine and medicine be thy food.
>
> Hippocrates

It is well-known that food can be used to navigate the interface between wellbeing and health or illness by preventing, informing, mitigating or supporting management of diseases. This involves healthcare professionals working with patients in partnership to embrace this element of their life as relevant to discuss during a clinical encounter; and to be curious about the patient's story to focus and negotiate areas for potential change. However, healthcare professionals may find it challenging to discuss, or even raise, the subject, given that food can be a sensitive topic. Healthy eating has marketised associations with physical appearance, mental health and self-esteem; it has significance in diverse cultural practices, which may be poorly understood; and there are complex associations with food poverty, insecurity and eating disorders.

Culinary medicine is the art of teaching healthcare professionals about evidence-based scientific principles of nutrition and its application to clinical practice. A bespoke course developed with UCL medical school was designed to focus on general practice-based conversations with patients and is delivered by a multidisciplinary team of healthcare professionals (GPs, dietitians, chefs and patients). The course is delivered to penultimate-year medical students and aims to provide clinically relevant nutrition training on dietary management of chronic disease, such as type two diabetes mellitus (31). Students are encouraged to draw upon experiences of patient encounters during their clinical GP placements to help maximise the relevance and potential connections between theory and practice. The course teaches the role of food and dietary conversations in disease prevention and management, and the interplay of cultural and socioeconomic factors in food availability and diet. Students first complete a session of e-learning before attending a hands-on day of consultation workshops (motivational interviewing, role play and active learning through speaking to expert patients), case-based group discussions and practical culinary skills training in a teaching kitchen. Students are then encouraged to apply their newly acquired knowledge and skills to future patient encounters in general practice, by identifying a patient during their general practice placement, with whom they can talk about food and diet (e.g. a young woman with polycystic ovarian syndrome). The intended learning outcomes are to equip students with the skills to provide holistic, patient-centred care to empower patients to embrace healthier eating. Iterative adaptations to the course were made to address changing clinical need: for example, the SARS-CoV-2 pandemic of 2019 and food insecurities exacerbated by the cost of living. This topic was introduced into the course to highlight the challenges of accessing affordable, healthy and nutritious meals for a greater number of people and the available support services.

This worked example demonstrates the role that generalists play in discussing food with patients, working with patients on a personal level at the interface between the individual and wider society. In the UK, despite the evidence base for improving health and wellbeing through a healthy diet, and the public's support for public health initiatives, the national food strategy has yet to be translated into policy, for example the sugar tax and banning advertising of junk food.

It is also important to note that teaching medical students these skills does not serve to replace the work of dietitians, who are trained professionals. Instead, the aim is to emphasise that recognising ill health as a result of poor nutrition and co-negotiating simple, appropriate dietary strategies is in the scope of practice for all healthcare professionals, and a competency required of UK medical school graduates whatever their chosen career (32). The ability to notice a relevant opportunity for a conversation with a patient about food is a crucial element of the way in which clinicians problem-set. This involves attending not only to issues explicitly brought by a patient, but also related opportunities for health promotion or management of chronic conditions (see also Chapter 1). Equipping healthcare professionals with these skills can only strengthen collaboration between the different members of the multidisciplinary team, with further increased shared understanding and goal setting for improving patient health and wellbeing through dietary changes.

A further reason to support clinically relevant nutrition training for healthcare trainees is the evidence base for health benefits for medical students who learn about healthy eating themselves (30, 33–36). Many students report a positive impact on their own food preparation and use. Thus, through learning how to help patients lead healthier lives, there are mutual benefits for learners.

Conclusion

In summary, embedding wellbeing into education and clinical practice requires fostering a collaborative working relationship between the patient, clinician and learner to establish and achieve mutually agreed goals for improving and/or maintaining a good state of wellbeing. Goal setting should take place in a supportive environment, with access to the wider multidisciplinary team and services as necessary. In this chapter, we have explored examples of how wellbeing can be taught, how collaboration can be supported through various frameworks, and how clinical consultations can be structured using models to inspire change. Ultimately, each individual will bring their own interpretations and values about what good wellbeing looks like. It is the responsibility of the clinician working with that patient to acknowledge and explore this further, and to offer them appropriate and personalised support.

References

1. Engel GL. The need for a new medical model: a challenge for biomedicine. *Science* (American Association for the Advancement of Science). 1977;196(4286):129–36.
2. Huber M, Knottnerus JA, Green L et al. How should we define health? *BMJ*. 2011;343(7817): d4163–237.
3. Sartorius N. The meanings of health and its promotion. *Croatian Medical Journal*. 2006;47(4):662–4.
4. World Health Organization. Constitution of the World Health Organization. 1948. Available from: www.who.int/about/governance/constitution (accessed 10 April 2023).
5. World Health Organization. Health Promotion Glossary of Terms. 2021. Available from: www.who.int/publications/i/item/9789240038349 (accessed 10 April 2023).
6. Ibrahim AF, Tan MP, Teoh GK et al. Health benefits of social participation interventions among community-dwelling older persons: a review article. *Experimental Aging Research*. 2022;48(3):234–60.
7. Williams E, Buck D, Babalola G, Maguire D. What are health inequalities? The King's Fund; 2022. Available from: www.kingsfund.org.uk/publications/what-are-health-inequalities#what (accessed 16 April 2023).
8. Michie S, Ashford S, Sniehotta FK et al. A refined taxonomy of behaviour change techniques to help people change their physical activity and healthy eating behaviours: the CALO-RE taxonomy. *Psychology & Health*. 2011;26(11):1479–98.
9. NHS Digital. Statistics on NHS Stop Smoking Services in England – April 2022 to September 2022. 2022. Available from: https://digital.nhs.uk/data-and-information/publications/statistical/statistics-on-nhs-stop-smoking-services-in-england/april-2022-to-september-2022 (accessed 10 April 2023).
10. Jebb SA, Ahern AL, Olson AD et al. Primary care referral to a commercial provider for weight loss treatment versus standard care: a randomised controlled trial. *The Lancet*. 2011;378(9801):1485–92.
11. Chiappetta V, García-Rodríguez O, Jin CJ et al. Predictors of quit attempts and successful quit attempts among individuals with alcohol use disorders in a nationally representative sample. *Drug and Alcohol Dependence*. 2014;141:138–44.
12. Harris T, Limb ES, Hosking F et al. Effect of pedometer-based walking interventions on long-term health outcomes: prospective 4-year follow-up of two randomised controlled trials using routine primary care data. *PLoS Medicine*. 2019;16(6):e1002836.

13. Morton L, Ferguson M, Baty F. Improving wellbeing and self-efficacy by social prescription. *Public Health (London)*. 2015;129(3):286–9.
14. Glasgow RE, Emont S, Miller DC. Assessing delivery of the five 'A's for patient-centered counseling. *Health Promotion International*. 2006;21(3):245–55.
15. Henry K. Structured Agenda-free Coaching Conversation ('StACC') Model. Know Your Own Health; 2022. Available from: https://kyoh.org/StACC-model (accessed 4 January 2023).
16. Launer J. *Narrative-Based Practice in Health and Social Care: Conversations inviting change*. 2nd edn. Routledge; 2018.
17. Miller WR, Rollnick S. *Motivational Interviewing: Helping people change*. 3rd edn. Guilford Publications; 2012.
18. Rogers J, Maini A. *Coaching for Health: Why it works and how to do it*. McGraw-Hill Education/ Open University Press; 2016.
19. Vendetti J, Gmyrek A, Damon D et al. Screening, brief intervention and referral to treatment (SBIRT): implementation barriers, facilitators and model migration. *Addiction*. 2017;112(Supp.2):23–33.
20. Leedham-Green KE, Pound R, Wylie A. Enabling tomorrow's doctors to address obesity in a GP consultation: an action research project. *Education for Primary Care*. 2016;27(6):455–61.
21. Kwasnicka D, Dombrowski SU, White M, Sniehotta F. Theoretical explanations for maintenance of behaviour change: a systematic review of behaviour theories. *Health Psychology Review*. 2016;10(3):277–96.
22. Prochaska JO, Di Clemente CC, Norcross JC. In search of how people change. Applications to addictive behaviors. *Am Psychol*. 1992;47(9):1102–14.
23. Williamson DF, Thompson TJ, Anda RF et al. Body weight and obesity in adults and self-reported abuse in childhood. *International Journal of Obesity*. 2002;26(8):1075–82.
24. Twycross A, Shorten A. Service evaluation, audit and research: what is the difference? *Evidence-based Nursing*. 2014;17(3):65–6.
25. Topp CW, Østergaard SD, Søndergaard S, Bech P. The WHO-5 Well-Being Index: a systematic review of the literature. *Psychotherapy & Psychosomatics*. 2015;84(3):167–76.
26. World Health Organization. Wellbeing Measures in Primary Health Care/ The Depcare Project. WHO Regional Office for Europe; 1998.
27. Tennant R, Hiller L, Fishwick R et al. The Warwick-Edinburgh Mental Well-being Scale (WEMWBS): development and UK validation. *Health Qual Life Outcomes*. 2007;5:63.
28. Stalmeijer RE, Dolmans DHJM, Snellen-Balendong HAM, van Santen-Hoeufft M et al. Clinical teaching based on principles of cognitive apprenticeship: views of experienced clinical teachers. *Academic Medicine*. 2013;88(6):861–5.
29. Wylie A, Leedham-Green K. Health promotion in medical education: lessons from a major undergraduate curriculum implementation. *Education for Primary Care*. 2017;28(6):325–33.
30. Xie JY-Y, Poduval S, Vickerstaff V, Park S. Cross-sectional questionnaire study to gather the teaching preferences and expectations of UK undergraduate medical students for culinary medicine learning. *BMJ Open*. 2020;10(10):e036410.
31. Unwin D, Khalid AA, Unwin J, Crocombe D et al. Insights from a general practice service evaluation supporting a lower carbohydrate diet in patients with type 2 diabetes mellitus and pre-diabetes: a secondary analysis of routine clinic data including HbA1c, weight and prescribing over 6 years. *BMJ Nutrition, Prevention & Health*. 2020;3(2):285–94.
32. General Medical Council. Outcomes for graduates. 2020. Available from: www.gmc-uk.org/education/standards-guidance-and-curricula/standards-and-outcomes/outcomes-for-graduates/outcomes-for-graduates (accessed 16 April 2023).
33. Conroy MB, Delichatsios HK, Hafler JP, Rigotti NA. Impact of a preventive medicine and nutrition curriculum for medical students. *Am J Prev Med*. 2004;27(1):77–80.
34. Pang B, Memel Z, Diamant C et al. Culinary medicine and community partnership: hands-on culinary skills training to empower medical students to provide patient-centered nutrition education. *Med Educ Online*. 2019;24(1):1630238.
35. Ring M, Cheung E, Mahadevan R, Folkens S et al. Cooking up health: a novel culinary medicine and service learning elective for health professional students. *J Altern Complement Med*. 2019;25(1):61–72.
36. Schlair S, Hanley K, Gillespie C et al. How medical students' behaviors and attitudes affect the impact of a brief curriculum on nutrition counseling. *J Nutr Educ Behav*. 2012;44(6):653–7.

18
Addressing multimorbidity through personalised care

Danielle Nimmons, Emma Hyde and
Kay Leedham-Green

Introduction

Multimorbidity is a term often used as a 'call to arms': to justify more generalist approaches to organisation and practice of clinical care, and similarly
the need to support more generalist approaches to learning and workforce
development. The terms multimorbidity and generalism, however, should
not be conflated and are not synonymous. In this final chapter, we come
full circle, showcasing elements of the generalist principles we describe
in Chapter 1; illustrating some of the challenges and opportunities for
production and use of research and evidence described in Chapters 4 and
5; ways to support learning and assessment described in Chapters 6 and
7; and implementation opportunities and challenges in how we organise
care (see Chapter 8), prescribe (see Chapter 16) and embed patient partnership in clinical approaches (see Chapters 3, 11, 12 and 15). Done well,
clinical care of patients with multimorbidity provides key examples of collaborative (see Chapter 13) healthcare.

    Multimorbidity as a term is often challenged during patient and carer
discussions within clinical encounters or research. Multimorbidity and
related challenges have conversely been a persuasive and influential tool
for change: introducing to a wide audience many of the important concepts
outlined in this book. For example, strengthening person-centred healthcare priorities; 'lean' and sustainable systems to minimalise medicalisation
and treatment burden for patients; and highlighting the tensions created
by linear and compartmentalised approaches to care, which forefront and
prioritise disease-specific notions of 'good practice'. Patients' dislike and the

medical 'success' of this term are connected. We have talked throughout this book about the privilege and preferences attributed to disease-based knowledge: often at the expense of attention to additional knowledge forms (such as experiential knowledge of patient, carer or practitioner). There are myriad definitions for multimorbidity, but all embrace the existence of one or more disease(s). Some, in addition, use the term to mean broader (and often co-existent) issues such as social determinants of health (for example, homelessness, relationship breakdown, debt, loneliness) as discussed particularly in Chapters 8, 10 and 11. But the presence of disease is still the key factor to inclusion (or not) in this umbrella of attention (and potential care) within current clinical practice, research and education.

This chapter, then, examines a subset or instance of generalism. It is not, however, synonymous with, or the totality of, generalist possibilities for practice and learning. The current burgeoning of political attention to multimorbidity is by no means a bad thing. But we urge you as interested readers and participants in generalist approaches to be mindful not to limit your gaze to this disease-focused element of generalism, at the risk of forgetting the myriad additional lenses, knowledge forms and legitimate concerns a generalist encounter might require. Our key tenets of generalism (outlined in Chapter 1) include connecting knowledge; expansive exploration; adaptive implementation; and participatory approaches forefronting partnership and collaborative approaches to working with patients and colleagues. These can apply to patient problems attributable to a disease diagnosis, but also illness or problems with no formal disease label. This chapter showcases, then, ways in which these generalist principles might be examined, learned and implemented for patients labelled with multimorbidity.

A key area of current international interest relates to how generalists care for people with multimorbidity. Multimorbidity, or the presence of more than one long-term health condition, has been called the 'defining challenge' of our era (1) and is important for healthcare systems worldwide. How can rising multimorbidity be managed equitably and sustainably for current and future generations within a resource-constrained environment? How can we support people and carers who live with multimorbidity to live well to the best of their abilities? This chapter focuses principally on how generalism is enacted within a care-planning consultation for patients with multimorbidity to deliver what is known in the UK as 'personalised care'. It also touches on the healthcare systems and community-based resources that support people and carers who live with multimorbidity; however, these are covered in more depth in Chapters 8 and 11.

We invite you to consider how the core principles of generalism afford a different perspective on multimorbidity to the disease-centred approaches around which most healthcare, clinical research and clinical education are configured. Although patients are likely to need episodic input from specialists, this chapter argues that generalism needs to thread and weave through these intermittent encounters with specialists, as well as being complemented by primary care clinicians offering comprehensive, longitudinal, personalised approaches and coordination of care. Throughout the chapter, we will refer to a UK national workforce development programme led by the Personalised Care Institute, describing how it is transforming multimorbidity care through personalised approaches.

Background

Definitions

Multimorbidity has been defined in a number of ways, although the presence of two or more long-term health conditions is commonly used (1). This definition has come under scrutiny for many reasons, not least of which is its relevance to patients. How should comorbidities related to a patient's principal diagnosis be labelled? For example, complications of diabetes? At what point does an acute problem that may or may not resolve, such as pain or depression, become classified as long-term or chronic? The definition uses a simple count of conditions without a focus on one condition over and above the others, despite different conditions impacting people differently. For example, high blood pressure is usually asymptomatic and has little impact on people's lives, while a single diagnosis of dementia or stroke will have a much greater impact leading to greater care use, treatment burden and reduced quality of life. Further terminology and definitions include the use of predefined lists, the term 'complex multimorbidity' (2), 'condition clusters' and 'weighted indexes' where conditions are graded according to severity or impact (3). However, it is unclear if weighted indexes are superior to a simple count of conditions – for instance, when predicting population outcomes (4). While limited data shows certain condition clusters are associated with poorer health and higher healthcare needs, in particular those including mental health (5–7), further research is needed to explore multimorbidity clusters and their effects across different sociodemographic groups (8,9). There are likely to be multiple evolving interpretations of what constitutes a long-term condition. Ultimately, the best way to define what is (or isn't) a long-term condition, and so make decisions about care requirements, is through a conversation between an individual and their healthcare professional.

Prevalence

The prevalence of multimorbidity is complicated by competing definitions, imprecise boundaries between health and illness, fluid disease definitions, and factors that impact on the accuracy of disease surveillance such as access to healthcare, socioeconomic status and study methodology (10). Some studies that include risk factors such as obesity and excess alcohol, estimate prevalence as high as 95 per cent (11), while more commonly used definitions place it at around 23–27 per cent in the UK (12,13). Despite various attempts, a precise unifying definition or monitoring strategy remains elusive (14). A unifying definition is also perhaps unhelpful, given the un-unified nature of people's needs and priorities – including young people with disabilities, tri-morbid survivors of complex trauma, and those with age-related frailty. Whichever definition one takes, the prevalence of multimorbidity appears to be increasing worldwide, driven by ageing populations as well as social, economic and environmental factors (15), although there are criticisms that some of this might be diagnostic creep as ageing, poverty, pain and distress become labelled, pathologised and marketised (14).

Causes and associations

The determinants of multimorbidity include genetics, ageing and the risks associated with clinical treatment. They also include potentially modifiable environmental and social factors such as poverty and poor housing, and 'behavioural' factors such as smoking, obesity, nutrition and alcohol which are all associated with and compounded by low socioeconomic status (4,16). The clustering of certain conditions, such as diabetes with heart failure and kidney disease, suggests that morbidity itself is a risk factor for further morbidity, either related to a common underlying cause, such as poor diet, or one disease causing the next, such as poorly controlled diabetes leading to cardiovascular and ophthalmic complications. Multimorbidity is also a risk factor for reduced mobility and socioeconomic participation, which can lead to frailty, depression and anxiety (17) and increased risk of mortality (18). Those with more than one long-term condition often experience more frequent hospital admissions with longer length of stay compared to those without multimorbidity (19,20). There is evidence to suggest quality of life can be impacted by the severity of conditions (21) and certain combinations of conditions can have larger negative effects on quality of life than expected compared to the sum of each condition considered independently (22).

Mental health conditions also play an important role in multimorbidity. Not only is there evidence that the risk of mental health conditions increases as the number of long-term conditions increases, but also that mental health conditions can increase the risk of further multimorbidity (23). Moreover, symptoms of depression are thought to be predictive of multimorbidity in older people (24). Having physical and mental health conditions can lead to poorer quality of life, worse clinical outcomes and early mortality, compared to those who have physical conditions alone (25).

There is a clear association between increasing age and multimorbidity (12,26), although it is important to note that many young people are also affected (27), and in absolute numbers, there are more people with multimorbidity below the age of 65 years than above (12). The diagnosis is also more common in women (11) and those from low socioeconomic groups, where those in the most deprived areas experience higher levels of multimorbidity compared to wealthy areas, and develop it at a younger age (12). Self-management of many long-term conditions requires time, effort and skills, including literacy (28) and studies suggest low health literacy is associated with the presence of multimorbidity (6).

> [Health literacy] is linked to literacy and entails people's knowledge, motivation and competences to access, understand, appraise, and apply health information in order to make judgments and take decisions in everyday life concerning healthcare, disease prevention and health promotion to maintain or improve quality of life during the life course. (29)

Impacts

Recognised complications of multimorbidity include reduced quality of life, which may be further reduced by increased condition severity (21) or by having certain combinations of conditions (22,30). Fragmentation of care is also potentially increased (31) as is the burden of treatment for patients and potentially their carers, as people may need to self-manage multiple conditions, attending multiple appointments, managing many drugs and engaging with many different healthcare professionals (32,33). Multimorbidity is associated with reduced life expectancy (34,35) and increased use of health services, including primary care and emergency care (19,36,37).

Multimorbidity is associated with polypharmacy and high healthcare utilisation, which leads to higher treatment burden for those affected and potentially increased costs to themselves and/or the healthcare system (37). Few single-condition guidelines explicitly address treatment burden or details on how to prioritise competing recommendations. These are crucial to consider in patients with multimorbidity, in whom treatment burden may become overwhelming (38,39). Multiple long-term conditions tend to result in multiple GP or hospital outpatient appointments, and it can be challenging to navigate healthcare services that are fragmented and designed for people with singular conditions.

Healthcare professionals can experience challenges managing the needs of patients with multimorbidity. This may include having to follow multiple clinical guidelines for one patient, managing conditions outside of their areas of expertise, as well as prescribing complexities (40). The complexity and volume of work and number of patients can also make it difficult, particularly for generalists who tend to provide continuity of care (41).

Researching multimorbidity

The case for a new research lens

Clinical research tends to focus on single diseases and/or clearly defined interventions (42): randomising one set of patients to one clinical pathway and comparing their outcomes to another. Guidelines are then developed based on a synthesis of these quasi-experimental studies. The development of evidence-based management guidelines for multimorbidity, however, is challenging.

Most research evidence focuses on single diseases. While some people with mutlimorbidity might be included in studies, this is rarely explicit. Often, people with multimorbidity are deliberately excluded: they may be too frail, ill or complex. This raises questions about the applicability of research findings to this population (43). Patients may also find themselves excluded from or dropping out of care pathways if services are not designed to address their 'entanglement of physical, mental, and social vulnerabilities' (14). When randomising patients to one arm or another, for example personalised versus non-personalised care, it may not be possible to blind either the patient or the clinician, raising questions of bias. How ethical is it to refuse personalised care in the non-intervention arm? And what is 'usual care' in the control arm? Humans are social creatures, and clinicians are likely to improve their practice based on what they see and hear others doing, so is the control arm ever effectively controlled? Effective multimorbidity interventions are likely to be complex rather than unifactorial, so it may be unclear whether all parts of the intervention are needed. Interventions often require adaptation to meet local or contextual needs, and these adjustments and necessary agility are important to enable and capture in research and evaluation.

How relevant are predefined interventions, or indeed outcome measures, to personalised care? High-level outcome measures, such as 'quality of life' indexes, are necessarily based on proxy indicators. These indicators might well be associated with greater or lesser quality of life, for example chronic pain or reduced mobility, but are these proxy indicators fixed or remediable in patients with multimorbidity, and how accurate are these indices if quality of life improves in other ways or if people have multimorbidity without chronic pain or impaired mobility? Countable outcomes such as death or emergency admission may require very large sample sizes to confidently differentiate between the two arms of a study as the effect size may be small, the frequency of countable events low, inter-person variability high, not to mention problems with the accuracy of reporting or adherence to intervention. Individual confounding factors abound, but so, too, do regional and temporal ones such as the availability or quality of a service in a particular area, pandemics, recessions, geo-political conflicts and environmental changes. Even if confounding factors such as socio-economic deprivation have been adjusted for, how is a clinician supposed to interpret the evidence if their patient or service is situated in an area of socioeconomic deprivation (4)? Although there have been some notable attempts to conduct high-quality trials based on complex interventions for multimorbidity (1), the use of multiple definitions, terminologies and indexes of multimorbidity make it difficult to compare and synthesise evidence across interventions (43).

These research challenges, which are bound within a positivistic deductive philosophy of science, have arguably led to a division within multimorbidity care and a mismatch between the needs of people living with multiple conditions and the resources offered by health systems focused on evidence-based care (44). The lack of evidence for more complex, personalised interventions does not mean that they do not work, just that they are harder to research within the prevailing clinical research paradigm (see also Chapters 4 and 5).

Embracing agility and subjectivity in multimorbidity research

The lack of evidence for multimorbidity interventions has often led to calls for 'more research' without addressing the above epistemological challenges. We argue that multimorbidity requires a different research lens. Instead of researching predefined and marketable interventions, perhaps we should be embracing local differences, allowing for agile evolution of services, and simply researching and optimising impacts locally instead? In addition to clinical trials that use objective measures, such as biomedical markers of disease control or countable events, perhaps we should also focus on more subjective patient-reported outcomes? These could be qualitative descriptions of what worked and why, or well-constructed quantitative patient-reported experience and outcome measures ('PREMs' and 'PROMs') (45).

PREMs, or patient-reported experience measures, have had a bad press (46). Simple ratings such as 'customer satisfaction' or 'would you recommend this service to friends and family' can be skewed by anything from the availability of car-parking to racial discrimination. Goodhart's Law also reminds us that 'When a measure becomes a target, it ceases to be a good measure' as incentivised ratings are easily manipulated by selecting who is asked to provide feedback (47). And fundamentally, there is little point in collecting un-actionable data: how can a global satisfaction rating inform what needs to change?

Although harder to create and use, more carefully constructed measures can pinpoint important areas of excellence or areas to improve. If aggregated over many patients, a validated index such as the 12-point Consultation Quality Index (48) can allow practitioners to monitor how a specific aspect of their practice is evolving over time or in relation to peers, for example shared decision-making, listening skills, or explaining. If combined with qualitative data, carefully constructed and validated PREMs can provide actionable information on how to improve, and whether a change is an improvement. If patient experiences are to be used effectively within research and evaluation, then practitioners may also need support learning to embrace and grow from feedback, which might otherwise feel critical (49).

Whereas PREMs (experience measures) tend to be reported at a single point in time, PROMs, or patient-reported outcome measures, are usually reported before and after an intervention to see if there has been an improvement. Validated outcome measures might be very targeted, for example pain, depression or exercise scales. There are also indices that aim to measure higher-level generic attributes that may be relevant to multimorbidity such as quality of life (50), wellbeing (WHO-5), health literacy (51) and illness perception (52). Patient activation (an individual's knowledge, skills and confidence for managing his/her health and health care) is associated with improved multimorbidity outcomes and is a potential outcome measure for health coaching interventions (53). The PACIC (Patient Assessment of Chronic Care) is a validated measure that integrates PREMS and PROMS to reflect the quality of care experienced by people living with one or more chronic conditions, and has been shown to be highly specific for multimorbidity interventions (54).

The Personalised Care Institute invited patients and carers with experience of multimorbidity from the NHS Peer Leadership Academy for their input on how to evaluate personalised care (55). Participants from diverse socioeconomic backgrounds and with a wide range of conditions and disabilities were interviewed in depth about their best experiences and outcomes of care planning. The resulting themes were honed at a co-creation event involving 40 patients and carers. Their responses are thematically summarised in Table 18.1. Their ideal experiences are very similar to the Consultation Quality Index (48) with the added construct 'feeling supported', which further validates that measure. Their desired outcomes included learning to understand their conditions and treatments, strategies for reducing acute crises, adapting their care to their specific needs, engaging with supportive resources for health and wellbeing, and regaining or retaining some control so that they could engage with living rather than just coping.

Table 18.1   What do people with lived experience of multimorbidity want from their care-planning appointments?

How patients would like to experience personalised care	What patients hoped to gain from personalised care
• Feeling welcomed and respected by healthcare staff • Being invited to talk about what matters to them • Feeling listened to and understood • Being treated as a whole person, not just a case • Feeling cared for, preferably by someone that knows them • Having their concerns taken seriously • Having things explained clearly • Being involved in discussions +/− with their family/carer(s) • Feeling in control of their decisions and plan • Feeling supported	• Understanding of their conditions and/or treatments • Ability to reduce or prevent problems • Ability to problem-solve if challenges arise • Engagement with health and wellbeing • Access to helpful resources and support • Ability to adapt to their personal circumstances and needs • Ability to act on their own ideas and preferences • To feel more in control and less overwhelmed • Ability to focus on what matters to them rather than just coping

Generalist approaches to multimorbidity

Replacing someone's knee is a complex process. Titrating someone's pain medication is a complex process. Even arranging a meeting can be a complex process. These processes, however, all have clearly defined outcomes. Everyone involved can see whether you have got it right or wrong. Addressing multimorbidity, however, can be considered a 'super-complex' problem. Not only are the processes complex, but the outcome is also not clearly defined. What is a priority from one perspective, may be different from another. Even for the same problem, the healthcare practitioner, the patient and their family/carer may have different perspectives on what is a good outcome.

We articulated the core concepts of generalism in Chapter 1. These include:

- Participatory values and practices: respecting and inviting the views and strengths of patients and carers.
- Embracing and integrating multiple ways of thinking and paradigms of knowledge.
- Leveraging distributed expertise by working collaboratively.
- Agile and responsive systems and processes.
- Working pragmatically and sustainably to address what matters to people and what is necessary for population health.

These principles have led generalists to design integrated services that are centred around people rather than diseases; to respect patients and carers as experts in their own needs and priorities, with their own strengths and problem-solving abilities; to work collaboratively with patients and carers to identify and address what matters to them; to work collaboratively across sectors, consulting specialists and guidelines as needed; and to focus sustainably on the determinants of health as well as disease. In Chapter 5, we looked at the different ways in which evidence informing decision-making about management and prevention of osteoporosis is framed and produced, focusing for example differently on cost-effectiveness, or patient outcomes. Here we use a similar decision about osteoporosis prevention to explore participation and engagement within decision-making (see Example 5.1).

Example 18.1: Funmi

Funmi (she/her) is a 79-year-old retired administrator. She is frail, mobilises with a frame, falls regularly, and was recently admitted to hospital with a wrist fracture. She has urinary incontinence and occasional faecal incontinence following adjuvant chemotherapy for breast cancer five years ago and gets angry and distressed if she is unable to get to the bathroom on time. She has a history of self-harm, drinks alcohol to excess, has moderate hearing loss and mild memory loss. She has always lived alone and wants this to continue. She has weekly visits from her brother who has anxiety, a specialist continence nurse, and a daily carer who makes her lunch and does her laundry. Her carer says Funmi often refuses her medicines and lunch.

Funmi's brother phones the practice social worker who coordinates her care. He says Funmi has received an appointment for a bone density scan from the local hospital following her recent fall. He is concerned that the letter says she should come alone using hospital transport, but he doesn't think she will attend unless he goes with her. After a brief discussion, he agrees to bring Funmi to the practice so that they can go through the options together.

Her brother says that Funmi would be confused and distressed without him and explains the risk of incontinence if she is left waiting without easy access to facilities. Funmi is a bit annoyed about the scan as no one discussed it with her. The social worker calls the GP in for advice on the risks and benefits of the bone scan. The GP calculates Funmi's fracture risk and explains that she meets the NICE intervention guidelines for bone protection without the scan. They agree to cancel the scan.

The GP then asks Funmi whether she wants to discuss bone protection. Funmi says she wouldn't want any medicines as she has 'given up'. The GP explains that bone protection might halve her risk of another fragility fracture. Funmi agrees this is something she does want to avoid. They agree on an annual intravenous infusion at the local hospital, which, although slightly less effective than regular oral medication, she is more likely to tolerate. The GP then asks Funmi whether she would like to discuss her mood or drinking. Funmi roundly refuses.

After the GP leaves, the practice social worker opens the discussion up and asks Funmi 'What matters to you, and what would make a difference?' After a pause, Funmi says a new hearing aid would make a difference. Her previous one is no longer helping and doesn't fit very well. This is causing social isolation and worsening her mood. Her brother says he is more worried about her falls which are increasing in frequency. He explains that Funmi often spends the night on the floor as she doesn't want to disturb him by pressing her personal alarm (which defaults to his phone) and she can't get up alone. They agree on a referral to a local audiology service, and a separate referral to a falls service who will work with Funmi to prevent and recover from falls. The social worker checks how confident they are with the plan, and Funmi's brother admits he is worried about the audiology appointment. The social worker asks him what might improve his confidence. He says he will visit ahead to check where the toilet facilities are. The social worker shows them a resource for checking accessibility online which they are both pleased with and will use again. The practice social worker then shows them the local drop-in alcohol intervention service which includes an accessible community garden. Funmi says she will think about it. They agree to follow-up on this conversation at Funmi's formal care-planning appointment which is due in a month.

Pause and reflect

We invite you to reflect on the different approaches of the hospital team that requested the scan, the GP who negotiated an alternative, but directed the focus of discussion, and the practice social worker who simply asked, 'What matters to you, and what would make a difference?' What were the relative impacts on the patient and carer? What were the relative social, environmental and economic costs (triple bottom line)? How do you balance and integrate disease management with patient and carer priorities?

Structural approaches

The House of Care

There is a clear rationale for proactive care for people living with long-term health conditions regardless of multimorbidity. Apart from the obvious impacts of poorly controlled disease on a patient's symptoms and social participation, healthcare needs and costs rise if complications ensue. The socioeconomic rationale of proactive care led several health insurers in the USA to develop a range of models of care for people with long-term conditions such as the 'Kaiser Pyramid' which stratifies patients according to

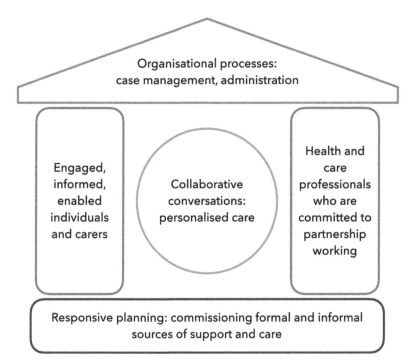

Figure 18.1 The House of Care model includes key organisational processes, collaborative conversations and responsive planning. Adapted from Roberts et al. 2019 (79)

need (56), and the 'Chronic Care Model' which aims to improve outcomes through integrated care (57,58). These models were adapted to the UK context and introduced as the House of Care (59,60) (Figure 18.1).

Organisational processes:
- Case finding and stratification of patients into tiers to identify people who can self-manage or who have risk factors (tier 1), people with health conditions that need regular review (tier 2), and people with multimorbidity or complex needs who require individual case management (tier 3).
- Ensuring healthcare is free at the point of need so that patients and carers are not disincentivised from engaging with proactive and preventive measures.
- Ensuring case management is integrated and organised around people rather than specialisms and managed by a healthcare professional that knows them (usually a generalist with specialist input as needed) to avoid duplication and repetition.

- Separating routine tests, structured education and specialist investigations from care-planning conversations, so that there is time and headspace for forward planning.
- Sharing test results and information with patients and carers in advance of care-planning conversations so that they come prepared and informed and are able get the most out of their appointment.

Collaborative conversations:
- Healthcare professionals that are committed to partnership working and trained with advanced communication skills such as health coaching and shared decision-making.
- Sharing information and sharing decisions, so that no decision is made about a person without involving them, and they have ownership and control when planning next steps.
- Opening up care-planning conversations beyond the biomedical, to invite reflection on what matters to the patient, and what would make a difference to them.
- Assuming people have strengths as well as needs by inviting them to set personal goals that they find important, and to commit to specific actions that they find manageable and achievable, through coaching conversations.

Responsive planning:
- Supporting access to community groups and non-healthcare services through social prescribing (see Chapters 11 and 17) to support well-being and address the determinants of health in addition to pathology.
- Ensuring health and community services are aligned to patients' needs, through responsive commissioning, enabling choice, and patient and public involvement.

The partnership approaches (shared decision-making and care-planning conversations) that are central to this model are supported nationally in the UK through a workforce development programme known as Personalised Care.

Personalised care

Personalised care is considered one of the cornerstones of a sustainable healthcare system (61), and is being operationalised internationally (62,63). Personalised care is not to be confused with personalised medicine which aims to target therapeutics through genetic profiling (64). Rather, it is about engaging people as active partners in their own healthcare and wellbeing. The rationale is strong: patients and carers are arguably healthcare's most under-rated resource. Finding ways to engage people in the decisions that affect them, rather than applying a one-size-fits-all approach, has been shown to improve the quality of those decisions, reduce decision conflict, reduce unwanted interventions and improve adherence to chosen options (65,66). Coaching people who have difficulty managing their long-term health problems has been shown to achieve better outcomes than purely disease-focused case management (67). Giving people with enduring care needs the autonomy to spend their care budgets as they choose, helps them to achieve better quality of life, and leaves patients and carers feeling more confident and empowered (68). Involving people and communities in social interventions, rather than purely medical ones, can improve feelings of control and self-confidence, reduce social isolation and can have positive impacts on health-related behaviours including weight loss, healthier eating and increased physical activity (69).

This chapter introduces the core communicative strategies of health coaching and shared decision-making and discusses how these might be brought together in a personalised care-planning consultation. Chapters 11 and 17 describe how clinical generalists work collaboratively with link workers and other community and social care professionals to address the social determinants of health and wellbeing through community interventions.

Example 18.2: The Personalised Care Institute

The Personalised Care Institute (PCI) was commissioned by NHS England in 2019, to help achieve an ambition to deliver personalised care to 2.5 million people by 2024, a vision that was set out in the NHS Long Term Plan (70). The PCI was tasked with writing a national curriculum for personalised care, and training at least 75,000 health and care professionals by 2024. The personalised care curriculum was written by subject-matter experts and stakeholders including patient and carer representatives in 2019/20. It underpins the PCI's free open access e-learning courses (71) and the courses offered by accredited training providers. Since its launch in 2020, the PCI has steadily gained national attention, and at the time of writing, the PCI was on track to meet its educational targets. Feedback from health and care professionals who have completed the PCI's courses has been extremely positive about the quality of the resources, and the impact it will have upon their practice.

As well as providing training for clinicians and healthcare professionals about personalised care, the Personalised Care Institute accredits training providers to deliver training for new roles that support the implementation of personalised care in practice. These roles include social prescribing link workers, health and wellbeing coaches, and care coordinators. The training for these roles is underpinned by the Personalised Care Curriculum, and the workforce development frameworks for each of the roles (72). Understanding these roles, and learning how to collaborate with them, can be helpful when supporting people who live with multimorbidity.

The PCI curriculum (72) describes six components: shared decision-making, personalised care and support planning, social prescribing and community-based support, supported self-management, enabling choice, and personal health budgets. The target populations for each component are based on their stratified needs, illustrated in Figure 18.2.

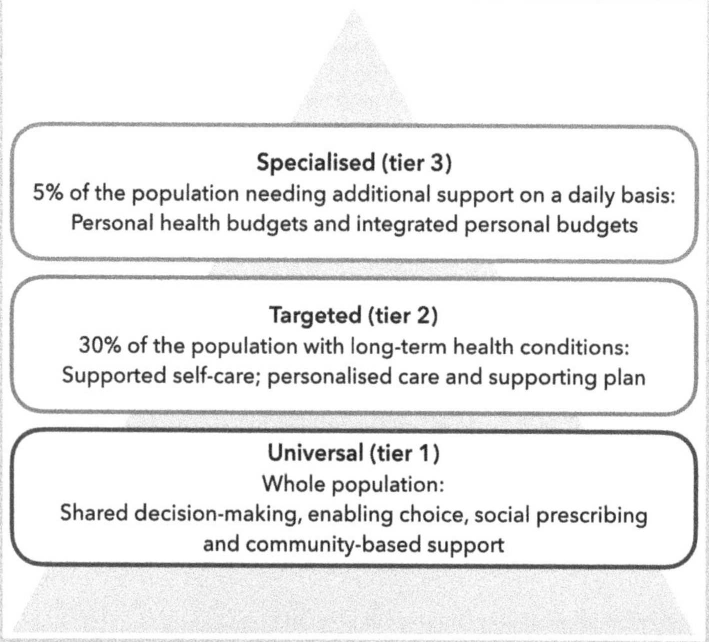

Specialised (tier 3)
5% of the population needing additional support on a daily basis:
Personal health budgets and integrated personal budgets

Targeted (tier 2)
30% of the population with long-term health conditions:
Supported self-care; personalised care and supporting plan

Universal (tier 1)
Whole population:
Shared decision-making, enabling choice, social prescribing and community-based support

Figure 18.2 The interventions and target populations of the personalised care programme. Adapted from NHS England 2019 (62)

Personalised care and support planning

Personalised care planning is not the same as treatment planning, which might focus on treating a specific condition or symptom. Nor is it a notification of what is going to be done to a person. It has been described as a systematic process of 'solution focussed forward planning, which acknowledges the experience and expertise of the patient/carer. It brings together traditional clinical issues with what is most important to the individual, supporting self-management, coordinating complex care and signposting to social prescribing' (73).

Care-planning appointments are part of the regular, proactive care offered to patients with multimorbidity. These appointments are typically longer than acute clinical consultations and are ideally separated from routine tests and structured patient education (such as how to use inhalers/insulin) so that the focus is on a personalised forward plan. It is important that patients and carers come prepared to these appointments with the information they need to make decisions, for example, having been sent recent test results or prompts for areas they might like to discuss.

Personalised care and support planning is underpinned by the organisational processes and responsive commissioning outlined in the House of Care, above. These processes support case finding, preparation before the appointment, and responsive commissioning that supports solutions after the appointment. The appointment itself involves generic communicative strategies such as listening and explaining, and more advanced strategies such as coaching and shared decision-making. Clinicians need to recognise which communicative processes are needed for which situation. In practice, shared decision-making often overlaps with health coaching as any plan involves a balance between risks, burdens, benefits and preferences as well as active forward engagement (74).

Health coaching

It can be tempting as a healthcare professional in a care-planning conversation, to tell people what the matter is with them and what they should do to improve their outcomes, for example, lose weight or take their medicines more regularly. Telling the patient what to do can create an illusion of progress, particularly for the clinician, as the patient now has all the necessary information they need to move forward. The chances are, however, that the patient already knows what they should be doing, and there may be complex reasons why they are not. Health coaching is a different approach which invites individuals to focus on something that is important to them, effectively setting their own agenda, and then to develop their own solutions through a guided process. Coaching can help to build a sense of ownership and is a process that can be repeated by the patient or carer, increasing their confidence in their personal problem-solving abilities.

There are many different models that fall under the broad umbrella term 'coaching', some of which are discussed in Chapters 15 and 17. Models include motivational interviewing (75), conversations inviting change (76), the StACC model (structured agenda-free coaching conversations) (77) and T-GROW (topic, goal, reality check, options, way forward) (78). Some are more directive (for example, focusing on a specific risk factor such as alcohol, or symptom such as pain), some more structured (for example, using defined steps and numerical importance/confidence scales) and some less structured (for example, focusing on personal narrative). However, they share many common features and communicative strategies. A structured, agenda-free approach is outlined in Table 18.2 (adapted from the StACC model (77) and Year of Care (79)).

Table 18.2   A structured agenda-free coaching model

Engaging	Relationship-building, setting expectations, the healthcare professional explaining their role and the purpose of the meeting
Information sharing	Patient and/or carer(s) telling their 'story': how they have been since the last appointment and why; what has been going well and less well. Health or care professional listening with curiosity, sharing relevant information and evidence as needed, discussing any test results and options.
Agreeing on the patient's agenda	The patient or carer deciding on what is most important to them now, or the area(s) they would like to focus on first.
Clarifying +/- importance scale	Confirming their agenda: how important is it to them? Repeat agenda-setting as needed. What would positive change look or feel like? What does the patient or carer think might help?
Goal setting	Turning their agenda into a specific, measurable, achievable goal. How will they know when they have achieved their goal?
Action planning	Exploring different ways of achieving their goal. Deciding on which strategy or strategies to take. Breaking the strategy into manageable steps and agreeing when and how to take the first step(s).

(continued)

Table 18.2   (Cont.)

Problem-solving +/- confidence scale	Exploring their confidence in taking the first step. What might improve their confidence? What if ... questions. What might get in the way of the first step, and what can they do about any barriers?
Follow-up	Recording and sharing the plan. Offering follow-up, with repeat agenda-setting or problem-solving as necessary.

Shared decision-making

Shared decision-making similarly involves a shift in the relationship between healthcare professionals and patients: respecting their autonomy, relationship-building, and curiosity about their values and needs (74). For busy clinicians who are used to a more prescriptive approach, negotiating decisions can initially feel burdensome; however, it also brings practical, ethical and psychological benefits. Patients are more likely to engage if they feel they have ownership of their decisions, and it can reduce 'decision anxiety' for clinicians if they know they are respecting their patients' informed wishes. Shared decision-making, however, is not simply shifting the burden of a decision on to the patient, but is a collaborative act: sharing information and building consensus. If clinicians are genuinely committed to partnership working and individuals are engaged, informed and empowered, then shared decision-making becomes both invited and expected.

At its most basic, shared decision-making about a specific test, treatment or course of action involves a discussion about the benefits, risks and alternatives, including doing nothing, as well as a discussion about the patient or carer's circumstances, values and preferences. Many common clinical decisions are supported by published 'patient decision aids' or 'decision support tools' which might include pictorial representations of risk/benefit ratios. In practice, however, statistics do not always govern how people make decisions or cover the kinds of decisions they need to make which may be multifactorial and highly personalised – for example, whether to move into assisted accommodation or remain at home. Furthermore, decisions are not always discrete events at one point in time, but rather distributed processes that may include other professionals, friends and family, involve autonomous information gathering and be revisited over time (80). Shared decision-making needs to address the power dynamics that are implicit within a practitioner–patient relationship; particularly so for people with multimorbidity who may have had their autonomy eroded through ill health. Elwyn suggests three types of

Table 18.3 The 'Three Talk' model of shared decision-making

Team talk	Indicating choice Providing support Identifying goals	We need to decide together which option … /whether to … Let's work together to make a decision that suits you. What matters to you? Who might you want to discuss this with? What information do you need? [Provide information e.g. patient decision tool]
Option talk	Comparing alternatives Discussing harms and benefits	What did you think of the information? [+/- clarification] What are your concerns about each choice, including doing nothing? What would the benefits of each choice be for you?
Decision talk	Getting to informed preferences Making preference-based decisions	Can you exclude any choices? Which choice are you leaning towards? Are you ready to decide?
Active listening	Attending closely to what is said with curiosity, checking understanding	Tell me more about … What do mean by …
Deliberation	Thinking carefully about options and preferences	Deliberation: often away from the consultation, with friends and family, over time, supported by self-directed information seeking.

talk within shared decision-making: team talk, option talk and decision talk which are underpinned by two processes: active listening and deliberation (Table 18.3 – adapted from Elwyn and colleagues (74)).

Example 18.3: Aran's personalised care-planning appointment

Aran (they/them) is a 20-year-old college student who has anxiety, obesity and recently diagnosed type 2 diabetes. Aran mobilises with a wheelchair following a childhood spinal injury. Aran was recently prescribed an array of tablets but takes them infrequently. Aran lives at home with their mother, but finds this difficult.

Aran received a letter inviting them to a 20-minute personalised care-planning appointment at their GP practice in two weeks' time. Aran's GP practice has various care-planning invitation letter templates for different conditions. The practice sent Aran a letter that was tailored for mobility impairment, mental health and diabetes. The letter included a visual prompt asking Aran to rate how they were coping. Next, it listed a range of topics that might or might not be important: washing, eating and drinking, exercise, pain, falls, mobility, memory, feeling down or stressed, loneliness, relationships and sex, feeling scared, sleep, continence, smoking, alcohol or drugs, taking medicines, preventing future health problems, their care package, support from family and carers, finances.

Aran was invited to list what was going well, what needed to change, what was important to them, and any ideas they had. The letter also included results from a check-up two weeks ago: glycosylated haemoglobin, lipid profile, renal function, body mass index, blood pressure, foot checks, and a prompt for an eye test. The letter explained and graded each test result into high, medium or low risk. There was a space for Aran to write their questions or thoughts against each result. Aran's glycosylated haemoglobin, cholesterol and body mass index were graded as high risk. Aran spent some time going through the letter and looked up cholesterol and glycosylated haemoglobin online. Aran noted that both could lead to serious complications over time, but could be improved by taking medicines more regularly, or by dietary change and exercise, or both. Aran wrote on their letter that losing weight felt important, but impossible and took it to their appointment.

After greeting Aran and ensuring they were comfortable, the practice nurse explained that they would spend about half the appointment discussing how Aran had been since they last met and going through any questions they had, and the rest of the appointment planning ahead. Aran shared the completed prompt letter and said they felt generally OK but were anxious to lose weight as they wanted to avoid taking medicines if possible. After exploring this, the nurse asked if there was anything else. Aran explained that living at home had become difficult since starting college. Aran felt their mother 'fussed' a lot since the spinal injury. After exploring this, the nurse asked what Aran wanted to focus on first. Aran felt that losing weight might solve several issues, so they agreed to start there. Aran explained that losing weight felt impossible as their mobility problem meant they had difficulty exercising. The nurse asked if Aran had any other ideas about how they could lose weight. Aran said eating differently might be easier. The nurse asked Aran to describe a typical day's food and drink. Aran said their mother provided healthy meals, but also offered up to six snacks each day, mostly crisps, snack bars and soft drinks. The nurse asked Aran what an achievable change might be. Aran thought they could cut down to one snack each day and try drinking tea instead of soft drinks. The nurse asked how confident Aran was in achieving this. Aran admitted, not very. Aran didn't want to cause offence by refusing snacks from their mother. The nurse asked what Aran felt would help. After discussing several options, Aran settled on involving their mother in the plan and getting them to count the snacks. Aran and the practice nurse spent a few moments designing a snack diary. The nurse asked Aran if there was anything else that might improve their confidence. Aran said no, they felt confident they could do this. The nurse asked if a follow-up phone call in a couple of weeks would be helpful. Aran agreed. They also agreed to repeat Aran's tests in a few months' time to see if there had been an improvement.

Pause and reflect

We invite you to reflect on the above example. Who was doing most of the work in this appointment? Do you feel Aran had sufficient understanding of the risks and benefits of the different options (medicines, lifestyle changes, or both) for addressing their risk factors? What were the risks and advantages of sharing test results with Aran before the appointment? Would change have happened without this care-planning process? List the factors that led to Aran's dietary change. Compare these factors to the default consultation: telling Aran to take their medicines more regularly and to lose weight. Both aim to attend to biomedical and lifestyle factors, but which approach is more likely to support action or change?

Educational approaches

Chapter 6 articulated some of the challenges that clinical education can produce for generalism. A clinical learner is taught to diagnose, treat and be 'the expert'. Teaching, learning and assessment often focus on systems and conditions, instead of focusing on the unique circumstances of the person. The limitations and constraints of a technical biomedical model when dealing with the epistemological uncertainties of multimorbidity can be associated with significant distress in learners (81). Learning to practise personalised care, however, can be a challenge for health and social care professionals, especially if they are used to being advice-givers or if they do not see personalised approaches being modelled around them.

For learners to 'buy into' personalised care and develop as 'person-centred' clinicians, a realist review suggested three key educational elements are needed (82):

- Priming: information should be given on what person-centredness is, what it means for learners and their patients, and why it is important.
- Meaningful experiences: learners need an active role in the clinical workplace, where they can understand patient narratives over time.
- Opportunities to process experiences: learners need a safe space to reflect, process and challenge their previous assumptions.

The cognitive apprenticeship model of learning (Figure 18.3, adapted from Stalmeijer after Collins and colleagues (83)) outlines the tacit steps in a learner's journey from novice to expert within a community of practice and embodies the steps outlined above.

For personalised care, a cognitive apprenticeship might start with watching these approaches modelled by experts, supplemented with pre-reading or an online course such as the modules provided open access

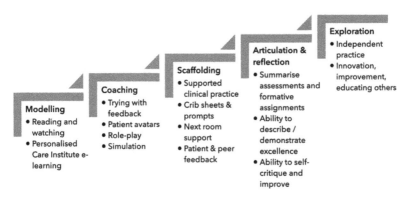

Figure 18.3 A cognitive apprenticeship in personalised care. Adapted from Stalmeijer (83) after Collins and colleagues

by the Personalised Care Institute (71). This could be followed by initial skills development, for example through role play using the Personalised Care Institute's patient avatars, or simulation-based learning opportunities with direct feedback from patient educators and/or advanced practitioners. Once the learner feels able to find the right words, they might progress to clinical practice, scaffolded by crib sheets, patient and peer feedback, or next-room support. Once learners can articulate and reflect on their developing practice, they progress towards independent exploration and mastery learning, finally becoming experts themselves.

Assessment approaches

It is important to assess whether the clinicians of today and tomorrow have the skills, knowledge and confidence to support people who live with multimorbidity. If multimorbidity and personalised care do not feature in a learner's assessment, then learning about them is likely to become marginalised. Chapter 7 articulated the tensions between reductionist assessment methods and the complexities of generalist forms of clinical practice. Internationally, written examinations, including many national licensing examinations, are increasingly based on multiple-choice formats (84). These typically invite the learner to select 'the single best' management option for a given clinical presentation, whereas in multimorbidity there may be differing perspectives on what the most appropriate way forward is. Practical assessments such as OSCEs or PACES promote standardised approaches to clinical skills and tend not to assess more complex practices associated with multimorbidity care such as collaborative working and relationship-based care. There is a need for more complex assessment formats that drive learners and teachers to engage with multimorbidity and personalised care (see Chapters 6 and 7 for further discussion).

Chapter 7 introduces a range of assessment modalities that are potentially more suited to generalist forms of clinical practice. These include structured workplace-based assessments such as case-based discussions (85,86). Workplace-based assessments are not without challenges, including failure to fail, but can be helpful as formative assessments (to promote reflection and growth) or hurdle assignments (to drive learning behaviours by requiring tasks to be completed) (87). The Simulated Consultation Assessment (SCA), recently introduced by the UK's Royal College of General Practitioners, is a form of assessment that is potentially suited to assessing generalist approaches to multimorbidity in pass/fail examinations. The SCA involves 12 short whole consultation simulations over a 9-month period, each marked by a different examiner with opportunities for feedback to promote reflection and growth. Ideally, an authentic assessment would allow a learner to work with all the resources that a generalist would normally use, including patient records, online guidelines, local referral options and other sources of support.

Bridging the gap between education and practice

The House of Care is a whole systems approach and 'clinicians committed to partnership working' is just one pillar. Training alone is unlikely to be enough to change the delivery of care in practice. In addition to attending training, practitioners must also *want* to change *and* have the right structural and cultural opportunities (see Chapter 9). They need to believe that new ways of practising are better than the alternative, and feel encouraged that change will be acceptable to others. It may also be necessary to make physical changes to working environment or changes to their working processes to ensure appointments are long enough, that the right patients are identified and invited for care planning, that patients and carers come prepared for collaborative conversations, that distractions such as form filling and requests for diagnostic tests are minimised, and that there are community referral pathways and resources to support the full spectrum of people's needs.

Conclusion

People who live with chronic ill health or disability have highly individualised strengths and needs. These can fluctuate and vary not only according to a person's health and condition(s), but also in relation to their social, environmental and economic contexts. Multimorbidity is challenging to address through protocolised approaches which are the mainstay of evidence-based medicine. This has arguably led to a mismatch between the needs of people who live with multimorbidity, and the prioritisation of interventions to support them. A breadth of research methodologies are needed to explore the experiences and strategies necessary to meet the needs of people negotiating multimorbidities. One key effective approach is personalised care, which treats people as experts in their own situation, and works with them to address what matters to them. It involves professionals, patients and carers integrating and using a range of available knowledge, and sharing information, power and responsibility. Personalised care is built on core communicative competencies including coaching conversations and shared decision-making and is supported through proactive systems, coordinated teamworking, and engagement with social and community resources as well as healthcare.

Example 18.4: Multimorbidity module, intercalated Primary Care BSc at UCL

This module was established in 2021 and jointly led by the Centre for Ageing Population Studies and the School of Pharmacy at UCL, encouraging interprofessional learning between undergraduate pharmacy and medical students. It runs over a term and explores core debates and challenges, introducing and critically evaluating how health and social care systems support patients with multiple long-term conditions. During weekly interactive workshops, students hear from leading researchers about: ageing and illness, frailty, mental health and loneliness, polypharmacy, social prescribing, health inequalities, drugs and alcohol, and finally complementary medicine. Assessment includes a group presentation and a two-thousand-word essay, based on any aspect of the lectures. Feedback shows the learners value learning with and from others from different clinical courses. This encourages interprofessional learning and builds on previous interprofessional education experienced in earlier pre-clinical years.

For further information: www.ucl.ac.uk/epidemiology-health-care/study/undergraduate/ibsc-primary-care-research-and-clinical-practice/ibsc-primary-care-and-clinical

Further resources

The Personalised Care Curriculum and e-learning resources
- www.personalisedcareinstitute.org.uk/

References

1. Johnston MC, Crilly M, Black C, Prescott GJ, Mercer SW. Defining and measuring multimorbidity: a systematic review of systematic reviews. *Eur J Public Health*. 2019;29(1):182–9.
2. Harrison C, Britt H, Miller G, Henderson J. Examining different measures of multimorbidity, using a large prospective cross-sectional study in Australian general practice. *BMJ Open*. 2014;4(7):e004694.

3. Ho IS-S, Azcoaga-Lorenzo A, Akbari A, Black C, Davies J, Hodgins P et al. Examining variation in the measurement of multimorbidity in research: a systematic review of 566 studies. *The Lancet Public Health*. 2021;6(8):e587–e97.

4. Skou ST, Mair FS, Fortin M, Guthrie B, Nunes BP, Miranda JJ et al. Multimorbidity. *Nature Reviews Disease Primers*. 2022;8(1):48.

5. Tang LH, Thygesen LC, Willadsen TG, Jepsen R, la Cour K, Frølich A et al. The association between clusters of chronic conditions and psychological well-being in younger and older people – a cross-sectional, population-based study from the Lolland-Falster Health Study, Denmark. *J Comorb*. 2020;10:2235042x20981185.

6. Sheridan PE, Mair CA, Quiñones AR. Associations between prevalent multimorbidity combinations and prospective disability and self-rated health among older adults in Europe. *BMC Geriatrics*. 2019;19(1):198.

7. Schousboe JT, Vo TN, Kats AM, Langsetmo L, Diem SJ, Taylor BC et al. Depressive symptoms and total healthcare costs: roles of functional limitations and multimorbidity. *J Am Geriatr Soc*. 2019;67(8):1596–603.

8. Quiñones AR, Allore HG, Botoseneanu A, Newsom JT, Nagel CL, Dorr DA. Tracking multimorbidity changes in diverse racial/ethnic populations over time: issues and considerations. *The Journals of Gerontology: Series A*. 2019;75(2):297–300.

9. Vetrano DL, Roso-Llorach A, Fernández S, Guisado-Clavero M, Violán C, Onder G, et al. Twelve-year clinical trajectories of multimorbidity in a population of older adults. *Nature Communications*. 2020;11(1):3223.

10. van den Akker M, Buntinx F, Roos S, Knottnerus JA. Problems in determining occurrence rates of multimorbidity. *J Clin Epidemiol*. 2001;54(7):675–9.

11. Violan C, Foguet-Boreu Q, Flores-Mateo G, Salisbury C, Blom J, Freitag M et al. Prevalence, determinants and patterns of multimorbidity in primary care: a systematic review of observational studies. *PLoS One*. 2014;9(7):e102149.

12. Barnett K, Mercer SW, Norbury M, Watt G, Wyke S, Guthrie B. Epidemiology of multimorbidity and implications for health care, research, and medical education: a cross-sectional study. *The Lancet*. 2012;380(9836):37–43.

13. Cassell A, Edwards D, Harshfield A, Rhodes K, Brimicombe J, Payne R et al. The epidemiology of multimorbidity in primary care: a retrospective cohort study. *British Journal of General Practice*. 2018:bjgp18X695465.

14. van Blarikom E, Fudge N, Swinglehurst D. The emergence of multimorbidity as a matter of concern: a critical review. *BioSocieties*. 2023;18:614–31.

15. Kingston A, Robinson L, Booth H, Knapp M, Jagger C. Projections of multi-morbidity in the older population in England to 2035: estimates from the Population Ageing and Care Simulation (PACSim) model. *Age and Ageing*. 2018;47(3):374–80.

16. Xu Y, Geldsetzer P, Manne-Goehler J, Theilmann M, Marcus M-E, Zhumadilov Z et al. The socioeconomic gradient of alcohol use: an analysis of nationally representative survey data from 55 low-income and middle-income countries. *The Lancet Global Health*. 2022;10(9):e1268–e80.

17. Ryan A, Wallace E, O'Hara P, Smith SM. Multimorbidity and functional decline in community-dwelling adults: a systematic review. *Health Qual Life Outcomes*. 2015;13:168.

18. Menotti A, Mulder I, Nissinen A, Giampaoli S, Feskens EJ, Kromhout D. Prevalence of morbidity and multimorbidity in elderly male populations and their impact on 10-year all-cause mortality: The FINE study (Finland, Italy, Netherlands, Elderly). *J Clin Epidemiol*. 2001;54(7):680–6.

19. Salisbury C, Johnson L, Purdy S, Valderas JM, Montgomery AA. Epidemiology and impact of multimorbidity in primary care: a retrospective cohort study. *Br J Gen Pract*. 2011;61(582):e12–21.

20. Frølich A, Ghith N, Schiøtz M, Jacobsen R, Stockmarr A. Multimorbidity, healthcare utilization and socioeconomic status: A register-based study in Denmark. *PLoS One*. 2019;14(8):e0214183.

21. Fortin M, Bravo G, Hudon C, Lapointe L, Almirall J, Dubois MF et al. Relationship between multimorbidity and health-related quality of life of patients in primary care. *Qual Life Res*. 2006;15(1):83–91.

22. Walker V, Perret-Guillaume C, Kesse-Guyot E, Agrinier N, Hercberg S, Galan P et al. Effect of multimorbidity on health-related quality of life in adults aged 55 years or older: results from the SU.VI.MAX 2 cohort. *PLoS One*. 2016;11(12):e0169282.

23. Vancampfort D, Koyanagi A, Hallgren M, Probst M, Stubbs B. The relationship between chronic physical conditions, multimorbidity and anxiety in the general population: a global perspective across 42 countries. *General Hospital Psychiatry*. 2017;45:1–6.

24. Melis R, Marengoni A, Angleman S, Fratiglioni L. Incidence and predictors of multimorbidity in the elderly: a population-based longitudinal study. *PLoS One*. 2014;9(7):e103120.

25. Mujica-Mota RE, Roberts M, Abel G, Elliott M, Lyratzopoulos G, Roland M et al. Common patterns of morbidity and multi-morbidity and their impact on health-related quality of life: evidence from a national survey. *Qual Life Res*. 2015;24(4):909–18.

26. Fortin M, Stewart M, Poitras ME, Almirall J, Maddocks H. A systematic review of prevalence studies on multimorbidity: toward a more uniform methodology. *Ann Fam Med*. 2012;10(2):142–51.

27. Armocida B, Monasta L, Sawyer S, Bustreo F, Segafredo G, Castelpietra G et al. Burden of non-communicable diseases among adolescents aged 10–24 years in the EU, 1990–2019: a systematic analysis of the Global Burden of Diseases Study 2019. *The Lancet Child & Adolescent Health*. 2022;6(6):367–83.

28. Mackey LM, Doody C, Werner EL, Fullen B. Self-management skills in chronic disease management: what role does health literacy have? *Med Decis Making*. 2016;36(6):741–59.

29. Sørensen K, Van den Broucke S, Fullam J, Doyle G, Pelikan J, Slonska Z et al. Health literacy and public health: a systematic review and integration of definitions and models. *BMC Public Health*. 2012;12(1):80.

30. Arokiasamy P, Uttamacharya U, Jain K, Biritwum RB, Yawson AE, Wu F et al. The impact of multimorbidity on adult physical and mental health in low- and middle-income countries: what does the study on global ageing and adult health (SAGE) reveal? *BMC Medicine*. 2015;13(1):178.

31. Sinnott C, Mc Hugh S, Browne J, Bradley C. GPs' perspectives on the management of patients with multimorbidity: systematic review and synthesis of qualitative research. *BMJ Open*. 2013;3(9):e003610.

32. Mair FS, May CR. Thinking about the burden of treatment. *BMJ: British Medical Journal*. 2014;349:g6680.

33. Rosbach M, Andersen JS. Patient-experienced burden of treatment in patients with multimorbidity – a systematic review of qualitative data. *PLoS One*. 2017;12(6):e0179916.

34. DuGoff EH, Canudas-Romo V, Buttorff C, Leff B, Anderson GF. Multiple chronic conditions and life expectancy: a life table analysis. *Medical Care*. 2014;52(8):688–94.

35. Rizzuto D, Melis RJF, Angleman S, Qiu C, Marengoni A. Effect of chronic diseases and multimorbidity on survival and functioning in elderly adults. *J Am Geriatr Soc*. 2017;65(5):1056–60.

36. Palladino R, Tayu Lee J, Ashworth M, Triassi M, Millett C. Associations between multimorbidity, healthcare utilisation and health status: evidence from 16 European countries. *Age and Ageing*. 2016;45(3):431–5.

37. Lehnert T, Heider D, Leicht H, Heinrich S, Corrieri S, Luppa M et al. Review: health care utilization and costs of elderly persons with multiple chronic conditions. *Med Care Res Rev*. 2011;68(4):387–420.

38. Bower P, Macdonald W, Harkness E, Gask L, Kendrick T, Valderas JM et al. Multimorbidity, service organization and clinical decision making in primary care: a qualitative study. *Fam Pract*. 2011;28(5):579–87.

39. O'Brien R, Wyke S, Guthrie B, Watt G, Mercer S. An 'endless struggle': a qualitative study of general practitioners' and practice nurses' experiences of managing multimorbidity in socio-economically deprived areas of Scotland. *Chronic Illn*. 2011;7(1):45–59.

40. Hughes LD, McMurdo MET, Guthrie B. Guidelines for people not for diseases: the challenges of applying UK clinical guidelines to people with multimorbidity. *Age and Ageing*. 2012;42(1):62–9.

41. Ridd M, Shaw A, Salisbury C. 'Two sides of the coin' – the value of personal continuity to GPs: a qualitative interview study. *Family Practice*. 2006;23(4):461–8.

42. Boyd CM, Kent DM. Evidence-based medicine and the hard problem of multimorbidity. *Journal of General Internal Medicine*. 2014;29(4):552–3.

43. Academy of Medical Sciences. Multimorbidity: a priority for global health research. Academy of Medical Sciences; 2018.

44. Tinetti ME, Fried T. The end of the disease era. *Am J Med*. 2004;116(3):179–85.

45. Bull C, Callander EJ. Current PROM and PREM use in health system performance measurement: still a way to go. *Patient Experience Journal*. 2022;9(1):12–8.

46. Reeves R. The friends and family test is a foe to the NHS. *Health Serv J*. 2013;7.
47. Elton L. Goodhart's Law and performance indicators in higher education. *Evaluation & Research in Education*. 2004;18(1–2):120–8.
48. Mercer SW, Howie JGR. CQI-2 – a new measure of holistic interpersonal care in primary care consultations. *British Journal of General Practice*. 2006;56(525):262–8.
49. Locock L, Skea Z, Alexander G, Hiscox C, Laidlaw L, Shepherd J. Anonymity, veracity and power in online patient feedback: A quantitative and qualitative analysis of staff responses to patient comments on the 'Care Opinion' platform in Scotland. *Digital Health*. 2020;6:2055207619899520.
50. Ruta DA, Garratt AM, Leng M, Russell IT, MacDonald LM. A new approach to the measurement of quality of life: the Patient-Generated Index. *Medical Care*. 1994;32(11):1109–26.
51. Osborne RH, Elsworth GR, Whitfield K. The Health Education Impact Questionnaire (heiQ): an outcomes and evaluation measure for patient education and self-management interventions for people with chronic conditions. *Patient Education and Counseling*. 2007;66(2):192–201.
52. Moss-Morris R, Weinman J, Petrie K, Horne R, Cameron L, Buick D. The revised illness perception questionnaire (IPQ-R). *Psychology & Health*. 2002;17(1):1–16.
53. Hibbard JH, Mahoney ER, Stockard J, Tusler M. Development and testing of a short form of the patient activation measure. *Health Serv Res*. 2005;40(6 Pt 1):1918–30.
54. Schmittdiel J, Mosen DM, Glasgow RE, Hibbard J, Remmers C, Bellows J. Patient Assessment of Chronic Illness Care (PACIC) and improved patient-centered outcomes for chronic conditions. *J Gen Intern Med*. 2008;23(1):77–80.
55. Leedham-Green K. Personalised Care: What do people with lived experience of multimorbidity want from their health and care professionals? 2023. Unpublished report. Imperial College London on behalf of the Personalised Care Institute.
56. Goodwin J. Long term conditions: how to manage them? *Geriatric Medicine*. 2006;36(1):17–30.
57. Wagner EH, Austin BT, Von Korff M. Organizing care for patients with chronic illness. *Milbank Quarterly*. 1996:511–44.
58. Ham C. The ten characteristics of the high-performing chronic care system. *Health Economics, Policy & Law*. 2010;5(1):71–90.
59. Coulter A, Kramer G, Warren T, Salisbury C. Building the House of Care for people with long-term conditions: the foundation of the House of Care framework. *British Journal of General Practice*. 2016;66(645):e288–e90.
60. Coulter A, Roberts S, Dixon A. Delivering better services for people with long-term conditions. Building the house of care. The King's Fund; 2013.
61. European Steering Group on Sustainable Healthcare. Acting Together: A roadmap for sustainable healthcare. White paper. 2014.
62. NHS England. Universal Personalised Care: Implementing the comprehensive model. 2019.
63. Krist AH, Tong ST, Aycock RA, Longo DR. Engaging Patients in Decision-Making and Behavior Change to Promote Prevention. *Stud Health Technol Inform*. 2017;240:284–302.
64. Ricciardi W, Boccia S. New challenges of public health: bringing the future of personalised healthcare into focus. *European Journal of Public Health*. 2017;27(suppl_4):36–9.
65. Politi MC, Wolin KY, Légaré F. Implementing clinical practice guidelines about health promotion and disease prevention through shared decision making. *Journal of General Internal Medicine*. 2013;28(6):838–44.
66. Boss EF, Mehta N, Nagarajan N, Links A, Benke JR, Berger Z et al. Shared decision making and choice for elective surgical care: a systematic review. *Otolaryngology – Head and Neck Surgery*. 2016;154(3):405–20.
67. Gordon NF, Salmon RD, Wright BS, Faircloth GC, Reid KS, Gordon TL. Clinical effectiveness of lifestyle health coaching: case study of an evidence-based program. *Am J Lifestyle Med*. 2016;11(2):153–66.
68. Jones K, Forder J, Caiels J, Welch E, Glendinning C, Windle K. Personalization in the health care system: do personal health budgets have an impact on outcomes and cost? *Journal of Health Services Research & Policy*. 2013;18(2_suppl):59–67.
69. Moffatt S, Steer M, Lawson S, Penn L, O'Brien N. Link Worker social prescribing to improve health and well-being for people with long-term conditions: qualitative study of service user perceptions. *BMJ Open*. 2017;7(7):e015203.
70. NHS England. The NHS Long Term Plan. 2019. Available from: www.longtermplan.nhs.uk/publication/nhs-long-term-plan/ (accessed 23 March 2024).

71. Personalised Care Institute. Your Learning Options. 2019. Available from: www.personalisedcareinstitute.org.uk/your-learning-options/ (accessed 23 March 2024).
72. Personalised Care Institute. The Personalised Care Curriculum. 2020. Available from: www.personalisedcareinstitute.org.uk/wp-content/uploads/2021/06/The-personalised-care-curriculum.pdf (accessed 20 March 2024).
73. Year of Care Partnerships. Personalised care and support planning, 2023. Available from: www.yearofcare.co.uk/personalised-care-and-support-planning (accessed 23 March 2024).
74. Elwyn G, Dehlendorf C, Epstein RM, Marrin K, White J, Frosch DL. Shared decision making and motivational interviewing: achieving patient-centered care across the spectrum of health care problems. *Annals of Family Medicine*. 2014;12(3):270–5.
75. Miller WR, Rollnick S. *Motivational Interviewing. Preparing People for Change*. The Guilford Press; 2002.
76. Launer J. *Narrative-Based Practice in Health and Social Care: Conversations inviting change*. 2nd edn. Routledge; 2018.
77. Henry K. Structured Agenda-free Coaching Conversation ('StACC') Model. Know Your Own Health; 2022. Available from: https://kyoh.org/StACC-model (accessed 4 January 2023).
78. Downey M. *Effective Coaching: Lessons from the Coaches' Coach*. Texere; 2003.
79. Roberts S, Eaton S, Finch T, Lewis-Barned N, Lhussier M, Oliver L et al. The Year of Care approach: developing a model and delivery programme for care and support planning in long term conditions within general practice. *BMC Family Practice*. 2019;20(1):153.
80. Rapley T. Distributed decision making: the anatomy of decisions-in-action. *Sociology of Health & Illness*. 2008;30(3):429–44.
81. Evans L, Trotter DR. Epistemology and uncertainty in primary care: an exploratory study. *Family Medicine*. 2009;41(5):319–26.
82. Bansal A, Greenley S, Mitchell C, Park S, Shearn K, Reeve J. Optimising planned medical education strategies to develop learners' person-centredness: a realist review. *Medical Education*. 2022;56(5):489–503.
83. Stalmeijer RE. When I say … cognitive apprenticeship. *Medical Education*. 2015;49(4):355–6.
84. Price T, Lynn N, Coombes L, Roberts M, Gale T, de Bere SR et al. The international landscape of medical licensing examinations: a typology derived from a systematic review. *Int J Health Policy Manag*. 2018;7(9):782–90.
85. Norcini JJ, Blank LL, Duffy FD, Fortna GS. The mini-CEX: a method for assessing clinical skills. *Annals of Internal Medicine*. 2003;138(6):476–81.
86. Norcini J, Burch V. Workplace-based assessment as an educational tool: AMEE Guide No. 31. *Medical Teacher*. 2007;29(9–10):855–71.
87. Daelmans HE, Mak-van der Vossen MC, Croiset G, Kusurkar RA. What difficulties do faculty members face when conducting workplace-based assessments in undergraduate clerkships? *Int J Med Educ*. 2016;7:19–24.

Index